The Impact of Artificial Intelligence on Healthcare Industry

Volume 1: Non-Clinical Applications

Editors

Mustafa Berktas, Rector
Department of Medical Microbiology
Izmir Bakircay University, Izmir Türkiye

Abdulkadir Hiziroglu
Management Information Systems Department
Izmir Bakircay University, Izmir Türkiye

Ahmet Emin Erbaycu
Department of Chest Diseases
Izmir Bakircay University, Izmir Türkiye

Orhan Er
Department of Computer Engineering
Izmir Bakircay University, Izmir Türkiye

Sezer Bozkus Kahyaoglu
Department of Accounting and Finance
Izmir Bakircay University
and
Financial Governance Department
University of South Africa, South Africa

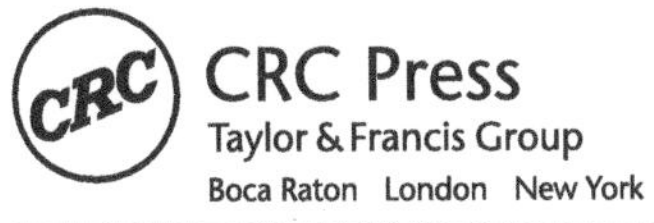

CRC Press
Taylor & Francis Group
Boca Raton   London   New York

CRC Press is an imprint of the
Taylor & Francis Group, an **informa** business

A SCIENCE PUBLISHERS BOOK

First edition published 2025
by CRC Press
2385 NW Executive Center Drive, Suite 320, Boca Raton FL 33431

and by CRC Press
4 Park Square, Milton Park, Abingdon, Oxon, OX14 4RN

CRC Press is an imprint of Taylor & Francis Group, LLC

Library of Congress Cataloging-in-Publication Data (applied for)

ISBN: 978-1-032-77566-1 (hbk)
ISBN: 978-1-032-80097-4 (pbk)
ISBN: 978-1-003-49540-6 (ebk)

DOI: 10.1201/9781003495406

Typeset in Palatino
by Prime Publishing Services

Foreword

The rapid evolution of technology over the past few decades has brought forth numerous advancements, transforming various sectors, and none more profoundly than the healthcare industry. Among these technological innovations, Artificial Intelligence (AI) stands out as a game-changer, holding the potential to revolutionize both clinical and non-clinical facets of healthcare. It is with great pleasure and anticipation that I recommend "The Impact of Artificial Intelligence on Healthcare Industry, Volume 1: Non-Clinical Applications," edited by Sezer Bozkuş Kahyaoğlu et al. This comprehensive volume, the first in a series, investigates the transformative power of AI beyond the clinical environment. It is structured meticulously to provide readers with an in-depth understanding of how AI is reshaping non-clinical applications within healthcare. Comprising twelve insightful chapters, the book covers a broad spectrum of topics, offering a robust framework and diverse perspectives on the subject.

The initial chapters lay the groundwork with a general framework on the impact of AI in the health industry. These sections set the stage by illuminating the foundational principles and overarching trends that underscore the adoption of AI in healthcare. Readers are introduced to the key concepts and the significant role AI plays in enhancing operational efficiency, improving patient care delivery, and optimizing various administrative processes. As the book progresses, it deals with specific non-clinical applications of AI. Here, the authors explore various regional cases, highlighting the global reach and adaptability of AI technologies in different healthcare settings. These chapters provide valuable insights into the unique challenges and opportunities faced by healthcare systems across different regions, offering readers a comparative analysis that enriches their understanding of the global AI landscape.

One of the standout sections of this volume focuses on AI-based health data. The importance of data in driving AI innovations cannot be overstated. The authors discuss the complexities of health data, including its collection, management, and analysis. They investigate health big data modeling and analytics, demonstrating how AI can uncover hidden patterns and insights that can lead to more informed decision-making and policy formulation. In exploring intelligent diagnosis and treatment systems, the book reveals how AI is being harnessed to develop sophisticated algorithms that can assist healthcare professionals in diagnosing diseases more accurately and swiftly. The advent of smart health and AI applications in mobile technologies is another fascinating area covered in this volume. With the proliferation of smartphones and wearable devices, AI-powered mobile health applications are becoming increasingly popular, offering personalized health monitoring and support to individuals. Further, the book addresses AI-supported design of biomedical materials and devices, showcasing the innovative ways in which AI is driving advancements in medical technology. The role of AI in health services management is also examined, highlighting how AI can streamline operations, reduce costs, and enhance the overall efficiency of healthcare delivery.

One of the critical areas discussed is the implementation of AI in the healthcare supply chain. This section outlines the prospects and challenges associated with integrating AI into supply chain management, emphasizing the potential for AI to improve supply chain resilience, accuracy, and responsiveness. Moreover, the book provides a thorough analysis of AI in public health and health policies. The authors discuss how AI can contribute to better public health outcomes through improved surveillance, prevention strategies, and policy-making processes. The concluding chapter ushers readers into the new era of healthcare, marked by the increasing use of AI in quality and accreditation processes. This section underscores the profound impact of AI on healthcare quality assurance and the pursuit of excellence in healthcare standards.

"The Impact of Artificial Intelligence on Healthcare Industry, Volume 1: Non-Clinical Applications" is a timely and essential contribution to the body of knowledge on AI in healthcare. It offers a holistic view of the non-clinical applications of AI, providing valuable insights for healthcare professionals, policymakers, researchers, and anyone interested in the future of healthcare. As we stand on the brink of a new era in healthcare, this volume serves as a guiding light, illuminating the path towards a more efficient, effective, and equitable healthcare system empowered by artificial intelligence.

Sezer Bozkus Kahyaoglu et al. (the editors) and the esteemed contributors have done an exceptional job in compiling this volume.

Their expertise and vision provide a solid foundation for understanding the complexities and potential of AI in transforming healthcare. I am confident that this book will be a valuable resource and inspire further exploration and innovation in the field of AI in healthcare.

Hamid R. Tizhoosh
Professor
Department of Artificial Intelligence and Informatics
Mayo Clinic, Rochester, MN, USA
June 7, 2024

Preface

Mustafa Berktas, Rector
Izmir Bakircay University, Izmir Türkiye
mustafa.berktas@bakircay.edu.tr

Today, the digitalization process is experiencing a new era and undergoing new developments. An important aspect of these developments is the emergence of computer-based machines that work on the basis of human intelligence. This technological progress is characterized by the fact that many tools, from machines containing computers to robots, have gained the ability to perform intelligent activities like humans. Artificial intelligence applications have emerged as a result of these technological innovations and are defined as intelligent tools that have the ability to carry out intelligent activities the way that humans can perform them. In this new stage, scientific and technological structures are changing with artificial intelligence. This technological change leads to the transformation of systems and processes. This change in the basic structure of technology has initiated a new era with the algorithmic integration of artificial intelligence applications.

In the communication age, digitalization has initiated the process of storing and transferring physical information in digital media. This process has contributed to the development of artificial intelligence with techniques such as machine learning and deep learning, which enable the processing, classification and rapid access of information. Artificial intelligence applications stand out as one of the most important developments that will change economic, social and scientific activity processes after the Industrial Revolution.

Artificial intelligence offers a new opening by transferring applications that can mimic human thinking, learning and understanding processes to machines through algorithms and programming languages. This new opening, together with digitalization in the field of healthcare, enables rapid processing of clinical information, which facilitates the evaluation processes of doctors, experts and decision-makers and accelerates the decision-making process.

Considering the knowledge gained in the past, it is clear that healthcare sector is the area where artificial intelligence will be used and the data to be processed can be made useful in the fastest way. Artificial intelligence will positively affect the training process of doctors and specialists, especially decision-makers, and lead to significant changes in health sciences education plans.

Artificial intelligence seeks the cooperation of different disciplines and fields of science by providing basic knowledge on the use of artificial intelligence toolsand their integration with the knowledge required by each speciality. Therefore, it is necessary to establish a common language in the various fields of science and to organize education and training structures in accordance with these new developments.

The knowledge production process in the field of health and medicine is based on clinical experiences and decisions. The process of transforming these decisions into digital information and transferring them to artificial intelligence–based technical tools highlights a new field in medical science. In the new era, this field will take its place in a "non-clinical" health science discipline. From this point of view, the first volume of this work is designed to cover the non-clinical field and is presented to the readers as a resource. In the second volume of the work, artificial intelligence applications in clinical sciences and experiences from clinics will be presented.

I would like to take this opportunity to sincerely thank the authors of all the chapters, editors and valuable faculty members who contributed to the volume for their support. I wish this work to take its place as a basic resource for practitioners and researchers and to be useful to all our colleagues by contributing to the literature.

Contents

Abbreviations List

2FA	two-factor authentication
6LoWPAN	IPv6 over Low-Power Wireless Personal Area Networks
ADC	analog-to-digital converter component
AI	artificial intelligence
ALV	artificial lung ventilation
ANN	Artificial Neural Network
ARIMA	autoregressive integrated moving average
AUC	Area Under the ROC curve
BGP	Binary Gabor Pattern
BMI	body mass index
BPNN	Back Propagation Neural Network
BRIEF	Binary Robust Independent Elementary Features
BSIF	Binarized Statistical Image Features
CART	Classification and Regression Tree
CBAM	convolutional block attention module
CCPA	California Consumer Privacy Act
CCTA	coronary computed tomography angiography
CENTRIST	CENsus Transform hISTogram
CNN	Convolutional Neural Networks
COPPA	Children's Online Privacy Protection Act
CRM	Customer Relationship Management
CT	Computed Tomography
DT	Decision Trees
DWT	Discrete Wavelet Transform
ECG	electrocardiogram
ECPA	Electronic Communications Privacy Act
EEG	electroencephalography

EHRs	electronic health records
EU	European Union
FD	Fractal Dimension
FD-LBP	Frequency Decoded Local Binary Patterns
FFNN	Feed Forward Neural Network
GANs	generative adversarial networks
GDPR	General Data Protection Regulation
GLCM	Gray Level Co-Occurrence Matrix
GLDZM	Gray-Level Distance-Zone
GLRLM	Gray-Level Run-Length
GLSZM	Gray-Level Size-Zone
GPS	Global Positioning System
HA	Hybrid architectures
HIPAA	Health Insurance Portability and Accountability Act
HMIS	Health Management Information System
HRV	heart rate variability
HSC	healthcare supply chain
IoMT	Internet of Medical Things
IoT	Internet of Things
KNN	K-Nearest Neighbor
LBP	Local Binary Patterns
LGPD	General Data Protection Law
LMICs	low- and middle-income countries
LPQ	Local Phase Quantization
LR	Logistic Regression
LSTM	Long Short-Term Memory
LUS	Lung Ultrasound
MEMS	Micro Electromechanical System
ML	machine learning
MLP	Multi-Layer Perceptron
MLSD	Ministry of Labour and Social Development
MOHSP	Ministry of Health and Social Protection
MRI	magnetic resonance imaging
mRMR	minimum Redundancy and Maximum Relevance algorithm
MSER	Maximally Stable Extremal Regions
MV	missing value
NASA	National Aeronautics and Space Administration
NB	Naïve Bayes
NGLDM	Neighboring Gray-Level Dependence Matrix
NGTDM	Neighborhood Gray-Tone Difference
NIMSR	National Resource Management Information System
NLP	Natural Language Processing
NTC	negative temperature coefficient

PCA	principal component analysis
PDPA	Personal Data Protection Act
PHOG	Pyramid Histogram of Oriented Gradients
PII	personally identifiable information
PPG	Photoplethysmography
QLR-BP	Quaternionic Local Ranking Binary Pattern
RF	Random Forest
RFE	Recursive Feature Elimination
RFID	Radio Frequency Identification
RNN	recurrent neural network
sAE	stacked AutoEncoder
SDGs	Sustainable Development Goals
SEIR	susceptible, exposed, infectious, then susceptible
SF	Social Fund
SFLA	Shuffled Frog Leaping Algorithm
SFTA	Segmentation-based Fractal Texture Analysis
SIR	Susceptible, Infectious, or Recovered
SMOTE	Synthetic Minority Oversampling Technique
SRS	State Registration Service
SSA	Salp Swarm Optimization Algorithm
SSFM	Single-Stage Feature Enhancement Module
SSL	Semi-supervised Learning
STL	Seasonal-Trend decomposition method
STS	State Tax Service
SURF	Speeded Up Robust Features
SVM	Support Vector Machine
TSA	Training Signal Annealing
UIOBL	University of Iowa Orthopedic Biomechanics Laboratory
URDSZ	Unified Repository (Storage) of Data and Health Services of the Kyrgyz Republic
VAEs	Variational autoencoders
WHO	World Health Organization
XGBoost	Linear eXtreme Gradient Boosting–Linear
XGBoost–Tree	eXtreme Gradient Boosting–Tree

Chapter 1

The Impact of Artificial Intelligence on the Health Industry: General Framework on Non-clinical Applications

Mustafa Berktas[1], Ahmet Emin Erbaycu[2], Kadir Hiziroglu[3], Orhan Er[4] and Sezer Bozkus Kahyaoglu[*,5]

[1]Izmir Bakircay University, Department of Medical Microbiology, Rector, ORCID: 0000-0002-4413-0435; Email: mustafa.berktas@bakircay.edu.tr

[2]Izmir Bakircay University, Department of Chest Diseases, ORCID: 0000-0001-6618-6774; Email: ahmet.erbaycu@bakircay.edu.tr

[3]Izmir Bakircay University, Department of Management Information Systems, ORCID: 0000-0003-4582-3732; Email: kadir.hiziroglu@bakircay.edu.tr

[4]Izmir Bakircay University, Department of Computer Engineering, ORCID: 0000-0002-4732-9490; Email: orhan.er@bakircay.edu.tr

[5]Izmir Bakircay University, Department of Accounting and Finance, University of South Africa, Financial Governance Department, ORCID: 0000-0003-2865-3399; Email: sezer.bozkus@bakircay.edu.tr

INTRODUCTION

Artificial intelligence (AI), or machine intelligence in the literature, has rapidly penetrated every aspect of our lives. With regard to machine

*For Correspondence: Sezer Bozkus Kahyaoglu (sezer.bozkus@bakircay.edu.tr)

intelligence, we can say that it is a field of computer science in which a machine is programmed with an intelligent approach to perform the tasks that a human normally performs in various fields (Tsang et al. 2020). Machine intelligence is essentially based on the use of AI techniques for computers and machines to understand, analyze, and learn every stage and structure of relevant data through algorithms specifically designed for the need (Sasubilli et al. 2020). The most important reason for the rapid progress of AI and its widespread use in various fields in all aspects of our lives is the recognition that research, application, and development activities go beyond computer science and require a systematic approach to interdisciplinary work (Herath and Mittal 2022, Kılıç and Bozkuş Kahyaoğlu 2024). Accordingly, AI project teams are intertwined with researchers working on data sciences such as statistics and mathematics, as well as researchers with experience in different fields such as sociology, psychology, philosophy, and linguistics (Ali et al. 2022). Medicine occupies a special place among scientific fields. Due to its complex structure, the difficulty and cost of obtaining data on patient health and the effects of treatment methods makes the need for AI even more critical and a priority. In this context, this study attempts to make a contribution based on non-clinical applications within the framework of basic needs in the health sector.

Considering the general structure and functioning of the healthcare sector, the diversity of data, complexity of business processes and high operational risks are the salient features. Due to these characteristics, the healthcare sector has the capacity to generate more complex and big data than other sectors (Wu et al. 2016, McKinsey 2023). AI is proving to be the most important remedy in this regard. The scope of AI in the healthcare sector is very broad, including hardware, software, and services (Market Research Futures 2024). This is also evident in recent studies on the size of the healthcare market.

As the world's population continues to grow and age, the need to expand the scope of healthcare services and deliver them quickly is expected to increase. Therefore, there is a need for innovative AI solutions to increase the effectiveness and efficiency of healthcare without increasing costs. Recently, technological developments in the healthcare sector have reached a stage where AI can perform tasks that healthcare professionals sometimes cannot, with the speed, simplicity, reliability, and meticulousness that AI can provide at a lower cost (Sqalli and Al-Thani 2019, Zhou et al. 2021, Zhou 2020). Key applications based on AI technologies include big data, machine learning applications, and robots that are used to detect and measure the operational risks of the services provided in the healthcare sector (Hossen and Karmoker 2020, Dharani and Krishnan 2021, Duan et al. 2011).

It is a fact that big data is generated by healthcare professionals, such as "electronic health records (EHRs)", "medical imaging data", and various healthcare data from many monitoring devices, including health tracking devices and apps (Antoniou et al. 2018, Liu et al. 2020, Xie et al. 2020, McKinsey 2023). Big data and developments in the health sector are very extensive. In light of this, we have divided our study into two volumes. The first volume presents developments based on non-clinical applications of AI. Our main aim in this work is to discuss all aspects of the impact of AI on non-clinical healthcare applications and to identify current developments based on the literature. The main topics discussed here are global and regional issues with a systematic approach as shown in Figure 1.1, starting from big data under the domain of the health sector, through health data analytics, health policy, health management, and health supply chain to smart devices and treatment technologies.

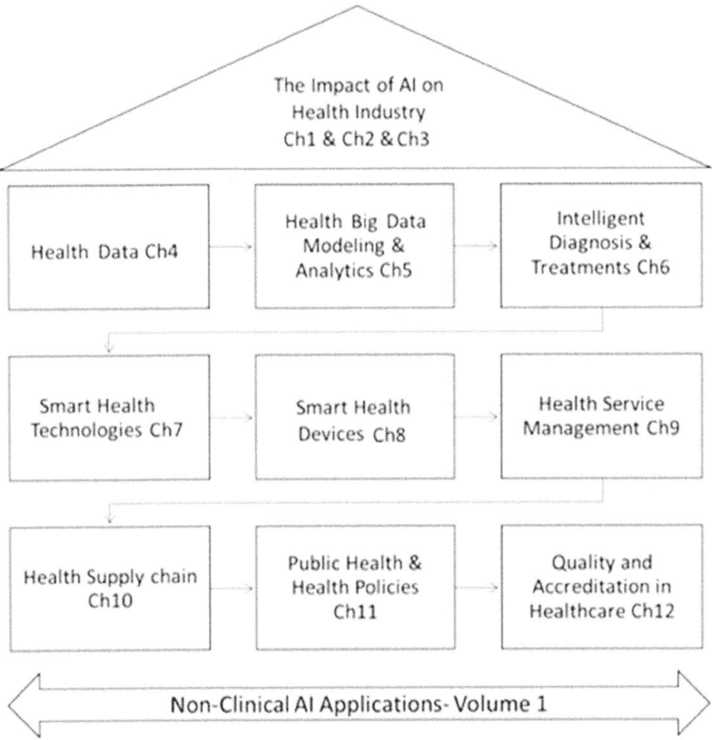

Figure 1.1   The scope of work.
Source: Prepared by the authors.

The health sector has a structure that follows and implements innovations most closely, and in this respect, we hope to contribute to the health professionals who provide this, to adapt to the digital working environment based on algorithms with AI techniques and machine learning, as well as medical domain knowledge. Based on the predictions that healthcare robots will dominate the sector in the future, policy recommendations are presented to improve the working environment of the sector within the framework of the information explained in each of the following chapters. It also demonstrates the challenges, and the managerial and policy development needs to address them to demonstrate the "big picture".

NON-CLINICAL APPLICATIONS OF AI IN THE HEALTH INDUSTRY: THE BIG PICTURE

This study, which discusses non-clinical health sector applications based on AI, aims to reveal the subject in all its aspects, present a vision to health professionals within the framework of future expectations, and make recommendations to policymakers. The organization of the book is given in Figure 1.1. We can summarize the content of the chapters as follows to establish the vision for the big picture.

Chapter 1 is prepared as a general perspective and introduction to the book. General information about the scope of the first volume and the themes of all chapters are mentioned. Our aim here is to present the flow of value-added information clearly within the framework of the fields and topics of interest to the reader and to reveal the connections between the chapters to show the big picture for health professionals and researchers in this field.

In Chapter 2, it is explained where and how AI is used in non-clinical applications, by taking advantage of the capabilities of metaheuristic approaches as one of the innovative application areas of AI. Here, Chapter 2 aims to contribute to the literature by analyzing how meta-scientific approaches are used in predictive analysis, health monitoring, and health management as the most important contribution areas in the healthcare industry. In this context, frequently used algorithms and optimization techniques are presented such as genetic algorithms and bat algorithms. Application areas and value-added aspects of these algorithms and techniques are discussed.

Chapter 3 presents the general view of the health sector in Central Asia and the Turkish world and the studies on AI applications. General trends in the Central Asia region are explained, and the difficulties encountered and the gains made in the digital transformation process in connection with the smart healthcare system development needs and expectations are discussed through country examples. Recommendations for policymakers are presented, especially by revealing the need for change in AI-based strategies, policies, and legislation in the health sector.

In Chapter 4, comprehensive content has been prepared to draw attention to the importance of health data. The generation of synthetic data has been extensively studied to enable the widespread use of AI in the healthcare sector. AI applications are accepted as an important tool for use in various business processes and treatments in the healthcare sector. The uses and sources of health data, which have great potential to improve treatment outcomes and influence public health policy, are very diverse. For example, it plays a critical role in areas such as clinical decision-making, public health surveillance, medical research and innovation, resource allocation, and health policy implementations. Health data plays a key role in the fast development and widespread use of AI applications. Examples of areas where AI contributes to healthcare include improving patient outcomes, identifying disease trends, and developing new treatments. AI algorithms are developed rapidly all over the world in areas such as disease diagnosis, personalized treatment planning, drug discovery, and medical research. However, there are also risks caused by this situation. The points that need to be taken into consideration in the health data production process are emphasized upon and the things that need to be done in terms of data security are explained. This chapter also provides recommendations for the careful management of AI, within the framework of the risks that may arise during its use in healthcare, to protect patient privacy and ensure ethical use.

Chapter 5 contains information on analytics and modeling of big data in conjunction with the previous chapter. The main purpose of this chapter is to comprehensively explain the requirements to effectively benefit from big data in the health industry. Here, the authors explain the importance of a robust health data modeling framework and present the key elements of the process in this context. The health data modeling framework includes data preprocessing steps such as cleansing, integration, and transformation to ensure data quality and usability. Additionally, the framework is designed to support theoretical studies on the implementation and analytics of data mining, treatment management, and recommendation systems to improve medical diagnosis and treatment. When evaluated from this perspective, big data modeling and analytics in healthcare reveal the potential to revolutionize the healthcare industry by improving the decision-making process, patient outcomes, and the overall quality of healthcare services. However, while presenting this potential, the authors provide balanced information and indicate that the challenges must be overcome. Accordingly, it is revealed that the full potential of big data in healthcare should be realized in improving healthcare delivery and patient care by applying effective data modeling frameworks.

Chapter 6 provides comprehensive information about smart diagnostic and treatment systems in the healthcare sector. Regarding this issue, the authors examine the results obtained by data visualization of viruses based on smart systems and machine learning and deep learning algorithms during the pandemic period that has recently affected the whole world. The necessity and strategic importance of early diagnosis and treatment of the Covid-19 virus, which poses fatal risks all over the world, based on smart systems during the pandemic period, is discussed. In this respect, the smart treatment and diagnostic devices developed for the diagnosis and treatment of viruses during the pandemic are explained based on intelligent modeling approaches and current literature. The smart systems, smart tools, and techniques used to ensure consistent diagnosis and rapid treatment of the Covid-19 virus have been researched by the authors and presented based on the literature as a whole.

In Chapter 7, comprehensive information is provided about smart health services, which have significant potential in the health sector and are expected to become widespread in the future. Smart health and applications of AI in mobile technologies are the main topics of this chapter. In general, the provision of smart health services is based on the use of data obtained by analyzing daily human activities for smart health monitoring. Thus, by performing smart health monitoring, it is possible to diagnose the diseases of the relevant people early and fight them on time. At the same time, it is possible to bring patients and physicians together on a single platform through this system. Smart healthcare services collect information about the patient or the patient's environment. Smartwatches, heart belts, and activity wristbands are examples of wearable devices that collect data. As part of a smart healthcare system, numerous sensors are also used to collect information about the patient's environment. The data collected by all these sensors can be sent to a cloud via the patient's mobile devices. Here, it can be analyzed using AI algorithms on a platform that creates health big data. The most important contribution in this way is that it enables early intervention to the patient through rapid and consistent analysis of the health data in question. This section gives an overview of the sensors used in smart health applications and explains how they work. It also focuses on communication technologies used by mobile smart health applications.

Chapter 8 explains the basic definition and concept of biomedical engineering, the subject covered, and provides an approach to contribute to the correct positioning of this field by defining its interaction with other engineering fields for the health sector. The position of biomedical engineering requires an interdisciplinary perspective at the intersection of engineering, biology, and medical sciences. In this chapter, the definition and study areas of biomedical engineering, biomechanics, biomaterials, biomedical devices, and medical imaging systems, and the integration of AI into biomedical material and device design are examined. It includes scientific activities carried out as part of a systematic field of research aimed at the development of processes, devices, and procedures used in the diagnosis and treatment of medical conditions, aiming to provide efficient and effective healthcare services. Therefore, the overall structure of this field relies on collaboration between engineers, scientists, and medical professionals to overcome complex challenges in the health sector. This chapter provides insights into the diverse applications of biomedical engineering and the role of interdisciplinary approaches in improving health outcomes. Biomaterials, an important component of biomedical engineering, are materials designed to be used in contact with biological systems. They find applications in a variety of medical fields, including implants, diagnostic devices, and tissue engineering. Biomaterials play an important role in the advancement of medical technology. When evaluated from this perspective, its importance can be understood better, and it can be stated that it is not a coincidence that biomedical engineering has a significant presence in the global market. This chapter aims to be a comprehensive resource for researchers, professionals, and students interested in the field, encouraging further advances in biomedical engineering and related disciplines to add value to the relevant literature and public health. In this context, according to the authors, it is possible to improve the scope and quality of services offered in the healthcare sector through AI applications while also enabling cost control.

Chapter 9 focuses on the opportunities and challenges of using AI-applied healthcare technology and explores the latest developments in AI-based applications and their impact on the healthcare industry. In this chapter, AI medical techniques in the literature are reviewed with comprehensive research methods and the findings are presented for discussion. An overview of the various AI applications currently in use or under development is provided. This study aims to contribute to the development of AI-based studies in healthcare management by providing a multi-level overview of the current literature. It is observed that various types of diseases and epidemics are emerging day by day, triggered by the pandemic period. When evaluated from this perspective, there has recently been a great demand for the use of smart health information technologies in the prediction and treatment of diseases, rehabilitation of diseases, clinical decision-making, and management of health services. AI applications are accepted as a strategic technique to meet this demand. AI is used in various fields, including medicine, to analyze large amounts of medical data, including whole genome sequencing, clinical images, and various types of medical records of patients. For example, numerous AI applications are used in the healthcare industry, including online appointment scheduling, healthcare management and discovery of new drugs for patients' treatments, online records in hospitals, digitization of medical information, calls, and notifications for follow-up appointments. Another reason for this is the need for smart healthcare service delivery as a result of the insufficient number of employees in the healthcare sector and the increase in operational workload. Given this scenario, according to the authors, AI applications can play an important role in providing a wider range and higher standard of healthcare services at an affordable expense.

Chapter 10 focuses on the healthcare supply chain (HSC) as an integral part of the healthcare industry. This chapter aims to examine the current uses and future potential of AI in the healthcare supply chain, the challenges involved, and considerations for successful implementation within the framework of developing HSC. As is well known, all over the world, healthcare services is among the sectors that grows rapidly and demands efficient intelligent services and products to meet the increasing needs of patients. In this context, to support the growth trend, healthcare providers need a reliable supply chain to ensure the timely availability of necessary medical supplies. However, the HSC has a complex structure that is affected by international developments. Everyone has experienced an example of this during the Covid-19 pandemic. It is apparent that hospitals around the world do not always operate effectively, as seen during the Covid-19 pandemic, wherein hospitals faced shortages of essential items such as vaccines, ventilators, masks, and personal protective equipment. In this respect, supply chain approaches based on AI applications are offered as a permanent solution to this situation. AI applications have the potential to improve stages of the supply chain process, allowing medical professionals to eliminate operational inefficiencies and provide rapid patient care. AI-enabled smart systems can provide critical information such as vital medical supply requirements that help clinicians make better decisions by taking into account factors such as patient conditions, demographic information, and location. The important point here is that before AI can be used appropriately to increase the efficiency of the healthcare supply chain, several obstacles must be overcome. In this context, the authors reveal the effects of lack of data, high implementation costs, and lack of experience on the part of healthcare personnel. This chapter will present studies on the application of AI in the healthcare supply chain to fill a knowledge gap and explore the numerous potential issues this entails.

Chapter 11 discusses the implications of using AI in the field of public health and the basic needs that arise from it. As a generally accepted approach, the widespread use of AI in the health sector has created significant changes in the field of health in general and public health in particular. The point that the authors want to emphasize here is that while AI in health stands out in fields such as radiology, pathology, and dermatology, public health applications do not receive enough attention. The main reason for this is that public health is less prominent because the results of public health practices are realized in the longer term than therapeutic health services. However, it is critical that public health interventions cover large segments of society and that health problems can be detected and tackled before they become devastating. For this reason, the widespread use of AI applications in public health emerges as a fundamental necessity for carrying out improvements in this field. Although AI technologies are not as prominent as other areas of health or are not prioritized in the literature, they have application areas that contribute positively to public health. It is possible to define areas of contribution directly and indirectly. Direct contributions include surveillance systems, epidemic management, early diagnosis of diseases, monitoring of disease risk factors, and vaccine studies. The indirect contributions are in areas such as facilitating the collection and processing of health records, enabling non-medical records to identify health risks and diseases in society, accurate and rapid diagnosis of diseases, and increasing academic studies. According to the authors, it is easier to benefit from patient-oriented AI applications to improve public health, especially with the widespread use of smartphones. Given the lack of resources and the large burden of disease in developing countries, it is possible for these countries to benefit from appropriate public health initiatives. AI has some proven successes in public health, but more evidence is needed to protect and support its role in public health. In this context, this chapter aims to contribute by trying to fill this gap in the literature.

Chapter 12 covers quality and accreditation practices to ensure assurance and sustainability of service standards in the healthcare sector. Technological changes that are accelerating day by day in the field of health services and affecting the whole world necessitate the reorganization of accreditation programs to adapt to the pace of the age. According to the information obtained as a result of the authors' research and compilation of literature, health-related issues will be prominent in the coming years. It is stated that five main trends will be evident: sustainable health systems, genomic revolution, technological developments, global demographic dynamics, and new care models based on knowledge-driven approaches (Cebeci and Hızıroğlu 2016). Reflecting on these health-themed trends related to accreditation, standards, and policies, it appears that digitalization, AI, and telemedicine applications will gain importance in creating new standards and methodologies.

The accreditation methodology will require organizing in a way that focuses on individuality, such as healthy behavior and healthy decision-making, and evaluates the entire system rather than being specific to the institution. Similarly, in terms of sustainability, it will tend to transform accreditation standards into a more flexible structure that will facilitate adaptation to changes. Based on this, the chapter discusses how AI can be used in the accreditation practices of the health sector, its advantages, and issues awaiting solutions. Thus, policy recommendations are presented according to the requirements in the quality and accreditation process in the health sector.

CONCLUDING REMARKS AND FUTURE EXPECTATIONS

Digitalization and innovation-based developments in the health sector are expected to continue unabated. While this situation is seen as positive, it also requires some preparation and early diagnosis of potential risks. It is important to note that while technological developments and innovations are constantly shaping the healthcare sector, healthcare professionals need to adapt their technical and digital skills at the same pace. In the current situation, the healthcare industry is experiencing difficulties. At the same time, it is necessary to determine the grey areas of AI applications that may lead to ethical violations and algorithmic discrimination, and to take precautions to ensure the security of health data management (Kılıç and Bozkuş Kahyaoğlu 2024). At this point, it would be appropriate to closely monitor quality, accreditation and compliance with legal regulations as basic indicators of corporate risk management in the healthcare industry. Based on this, it is important for all researchers to contribute to uncovering the impact of AI applications in the healthcare sector based on knowledge-driven models and to pay attention to ethical compliance in the development of new-generation AI algorithms (Hızıroğlu et al. 2022).

The application of AI in medicine is based on important technological developments in the computer and electronic-based tools and smart devices of clinics, which are the application part of the medical field. However, the preparation and processing of information that will facilitate the use of these tools and accelerate the processes of diagnosis and treatment is a new era for AI in the healthcare industry. From this point of view, the importance of AI in the creation of tools for the classification of information that will be generated in current clinical processes and its use in diagnosis and treatment also requires a change in medical education (McKinsey 2023). Therefore, to understand and easily apply AI and knowledge-generation processes used in health, and to draw inferences from the available information, i.e. health big data, the need for new learning programs that provide a deep understanding of knowledge and use of AI languages for medical education comes to the fore. Medical science is at the forefront of the process of compiling value-added information from clinical practice and drawing conclusions from it. However, it can serve as an application area for interdisciplinary fields from image processing to biochemistry, and from biochemistry to the application of physical sciences to medicine.

Depending on the integration of this interdisciplinary knowledge in diagnosis and treatment and its potential to assist doctors' decision-making procedure in clinical processes, the need for healthcare personnel to have the necessary on-the-job training and education to handle the information produced by the clinic to assist this process will bring about new development in specialty training. How should the knowledge of basic mathematics and statistics domain knowledge required for the knowledge-generation processes of AI be imparted to gain expertise in the field is also an issue that needs to be discussed. Existing advances have led to a tendency to apply the basic AI knowledge to all branches of science. It seems that a trend will emerge wherein there will be distinction between the clinical and the non-clinical in the healthcare industry (Noorbakhsh-Sabet et al. 2019, Park et al. 2022).

There is a great need for interdisciplinary work and collaboration with other industries to efficiently manage all the health-related issues discussed here and to achieve successful outcomes through early diagnosis of risks. It would be appropriate to make strategic decisions and generate smart healthcare and public policies with a global AI perspective, considering the vital role of the healthcare industry in ensuring the sustainability of social welfare all over the world. This study aims to contribute to the emerging needs from this perspective.

REFERENCES

Ali, O., Murray, P., Muhammed, S., Dwivedi, Y.K. and Rashiti, S. 2022. Evaluating organizational level IT innovation adoption factors among global firms. Journal of Innovation & Knowledge. 7(3): 100213.

Antoniou, Z.C., Panayides, A.S., Pantzaris, M., Constantinides, A.G., Pattichis, C.S. and Pattichis, M.S. 2018. Real-time adaptation to time-varying constraints for medical video communications. IEEE Journal of Biomedical and Health Informatics. 22(4): 1177–1188.

Cebeci, H.I. and Hızıroğlu, A. 2016. Review of business intelligence and intelligent systems in healthcare domain. *In:* Celebi, N. (ed.). Intelligent Techniques for Data Analysis in Diverse Settings, 192–206. IGI Global.

Dharani, N. and Krishnan, G. 2021. ANN based COVID-19 prediction and symptoms relevance survey and analysis. The 5th International Conference on Computing Methodologies and Communication. 1805–1808.

Duan, L., Street, W.N. and Xu, E. 2011. Health-care information systems: data mining methods in the creation of a clinical recommender system. Enterprise Information Systems. 5: 169–181.

Herath, H.M.K.K.M.B. and Mittal, M. 2022. Adoption of artificial intelligence in smart cities: A comprehensive review. International Journal of Information Management Data Insights. 2(1): 100076.

Hızıroğlu, A., Pişirgen, A., Özcan, M. and İlter, H.K. 2022. Artificial intelligence in healthcare industry: A transformation from model-driven to knowledge-driven DSS. Artificial Intelligence Theory and Applications. 2(1): 41–58.

Hossen, M.S. and Karmoker, D. 2020. Predicting the probability of Covid-19 recovered in South Asian countries based on healthy diet pattern using a machine learning approach. The 2nd International Conference on Sustainable Technologies for Industry 4.0. 1–6.

Kılıç, M. and Bozkuş Kahyaoğlu, S. 2024. The interaction of artificial intelligence and legal regulations: social and economic perspectives. pp. 3–13. *In:* Kılıç, M. and Kahyaoğlu, S.B. (eds). Algorithmic Discrimination and Ethical Perspective of Artificial Intelligence. Accounting, Finance, Sustainability, Governance & Fraud: Theory and Application. Springer, Singapore.

Liu, J., Ma, J., Li, J., Huang, M., Sadiq, N. and Ai, Y. 2020. Robust watermarking algorithm for medical volume data in internet of medical things. IEEE Access. 8: 93939–93966.

Market Research Futures. 2024. Artificial intelligence market research report, https://www.marketresearchfuture.com/thank-you-sample?report_id=5681 (accessed on 24 January 2024).

McKinsey. 2023. Healthcare practice—tackling healthcare's biggest burdens with generative AI, https://www.mckinsey.com/industries/healthcare/our-insights/tackling-healthcares-biggest-burdens-with-generative-ai (accessed on 24 January 2024).

Noorbakhsh-Sabet, N. Zand, R. Zhang, Y. and Abedi, V. 2019. Artificial intelligence transforms the future of health care. The American Journal of Medicine. 132(7): 795–801.

Park, S., Bekemeier, B., Flaxman, A. and Schultz, M. 2022. Impact of data visualization on decision-making and its implications for public health practice: a systematic literature review. Informatics for Health and Social Care. 47(2): 175–193.

Sasubilli, S.M., Kumar, A. and Dutt, V. 2020. Machine learning implementation on medical domain to identify disease insights using TMS. The International Conference on Advances in Computing and Communication Engineering. 1–4.

Sqalli, M.T. and Al-Thani, D. 2019. AI-supported health coaching model for patients with chronic diseases. The 16th International Symposium on Wireless Communication Systems. 452–456.

Tsang, K.C.H., Pinnock, H., Wilson, A.M. and Ahmar Shah, S. 2020. Application of machine learning to support self-management of asthma with mHealth. The 42nd Annual International Conference of the IEEE Engineering in Medicine & Biology Society (EMBC). 5673–5677.

Wu, J., Li, H., Cheng, S. and Lin, Z. 2016. The promising future of healthcare services: when big data analytics meets wearable technology. Information & Management. 53(8): 1020–1033.

Xie, X., Zang, Z. and Ponzoa, J.M. 2020. The information impact of network media, the psychological reaction to the COVID-19 pandemic and online knowledge acquisition: evidence from Chinese college students. Journal of Innovation & Knowledge. 5(4): 297–305.

Zhou, L. 2020. A rapid, accurate and machine-agnostic segmentation and quantification method for CT-based COVID-19 diagnosis. IEEE Transactions on Medical Imaging. 39(8): 2638–2652.

Zhou, R., Zhang, X., Wang, X., Yang, G., Guizani, N. and Du, X. 2021. Efficient and traceable patient health data search system for hospital management in smart cities. IEEE Internet of Things Journal, 8(8): 6425–6436.

Chapter 2

Non-clinical Applications of Artificial Intelligence

Hilal Arslan[1,*], Betul Aygun[2] and Orhan Er[3]

[1]Department of Software Engineering,
Ankara Yıldırım Beyazıt University, Ankara, Türkiye
ORCID: 0000-0002-6449-6952; Email: hilalarslan@aybu.edu.tr

[2]Softtech Software Technologies Research Development Inc.,
Ankara, Türkiye
ORCID: 0000-0001-9610-9235; Email: Betul.Aygun@softtech.com.tr

[3]Department of Computer Engineering,
Izmir Bakırcay University, Izmir Türkiye
ORCID: 0000-0002-4732-9490; Email: orhan.er@bakircay.edu.tr

INTRODUCTION

From clinical decision-making and diagnosis to health service management and patient engagement, applications of artificial intelligence (AI) can be found in a wide range of sectors of the healthcare industry. Medical images like X-rays and CT scans can be analyzed with AI to help diagnose diseases and conditions. This can assist with working on the precision and speed of the diagnosis. AI can be also used to analyze big data to find new drug candidates and figure out how well they will work. This can assist with speeding up the medication revelation process and the offering of new medicines for sale to the public. Furthermore, AI can be utilized to investigate electronic health

---

*For Correspondence: Hilal Arslan (hilalarslan@aybu.edu.tr)

records to improve customized treatment plans. This may assist in advancing the outcomes of treatment and lowering the likelihood of side effects. Moreover, healthcare providers can receive real-time guidance and recommendations from AI during patient care. The probability of making medical mistakes can be reduced and the accuracy and consistency of clinical decision-making can be enhanced by this. Finally, healthcare organizations can use AI to improve service delivery and optimize operations. Costs can be cut, productivity can be increased, and patient satisfaction can rise as a result.

AI-based techniques hold great promise to pave the way to determine applications that may be divided into clinical and non-clinical applications. When developing and implementing AI solutions for healthcare, it is essential to take into account the differences between these two areas of application. First, while non-clinical applications of AI primarily focus on enhancing healthcare organizations' administrative and operational functions, clinical applications of AI primarily improve clinical decision-making, diagnosis, and treatment. Second, non-clinical applications of AI rely primarily on organizational data, such as billing and supply chain data, while clinical applications of AI rely primarily on patient-specific data, such as medical images and electronic health records. Third, while non-clinical applications of AI may be subject to certain regulatory requirements, such as those related to data privacy and security, clinical applications of AI are subject to a different set of regulations, such as those set by the food and drug administration, to ensure patient safety and efficacy. Finally, while non-clinical applications of AI may have an indirect impact on patient outcomes, such as increasing organizational efficiency and decreasing costs, clinical applications of AI have a direct impact on patient outcomes, such as diagnosis accuracy and treatment efficacy.

In this chapter, we investigate AI-based methodologies in the health industry and we review non-clinical applications of AI. In the next section, we review metaheuristic methods used in medicine. The third section discusses AI methods used in non-clinical applications that are predictive analytics, health monitoring, and health management. The last section presents the discussions and conclusions.

METAHEURISTIC METHODS USED IN MEDICINE

An overview of the AI methods is given in Figure 2.1. In this chapter, we focus on natural computing (metaheuristic) methods rather than the traditional approaches. Next, we briefly explain natural computing methods used in medicine.

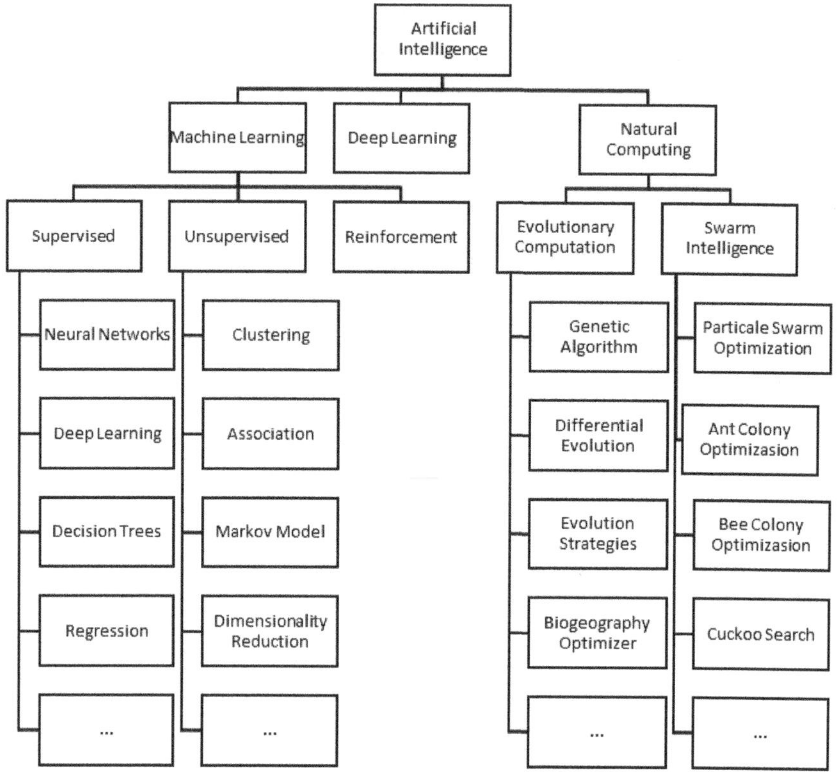

Figure 2.1   Overview of the artificial intelligence methods.

Spider monkey optimization (Bansal et al. 2014) is a metaheuristic algorithm inspired by spider monkey social behaviour and foraging technique. This algorithm is used to address complicated optimization issues. As the first step of the algorithm, in the population initialization, a colony of spider monkeys is created to represent probable solutions.

Each spider monkey represents a potential solution. The second step is position updating. Each spider monkey's position is updated depending on its current location and the locations of other monkeys in the population. This update is achieved by utilizing mathematical equations that imitate spider monkey social activity. The third step is fitness evaluation. The objective function of the optimization problem to each spider monkey's location is applied to determine its fitness. The objective function defines the quality of a certain solution. The fourth step is selection. To construct the next generation, the spider monkeys with the highest fitness scores are chosen. This phase guarantees that better solutions are more likely to be picked for replication. The next step is reproduction. Crossover and mutation procedures are applied to the selected spider monkeys to produce novel solutions. Another step is the replacement. Some of the old population with freshly produced children is replaced. Finally, these steps are repeated until a satisfactory solution is obtained.

The shuffled frog leaping algorithm (SFLA) (Zhen el al. 2009) is a nature-inspired optimization technique based on a frog's leaping action. It combines local search, global search, and information sharing among frogs to effectively explore and exploit the solution space. The algorithm seeks to discover the optimum or near-optimal solution to a given optimization problem by emulating frog behaviour. The first main step of the algorithm is the initialization step. In this, a frog population is created and each frog represents a potential solution to the optimization issue. The population is separated into subgroups. The second step is local search. To enhance the individual frog's solutions, a local search is performed and this stage permits the frogs to explore their local search space for better options. Next, the fitness function of each frog is evaluated to determine the quality of the solution. Thereafter, the frogs are sorted according to their fitness levels. The rating defines the likelihood that a frog will be chosen for the global search step. In the global search step, the best-ranked frogs from each subgroup are chosen to build a global frog pool. The next step is shuffling. To make novel frog pairings, the global frog pool is shuffled. This stage mimics frog leaping behaviour in which they communicate information to other frogs in order to explore other portions of the search space. After this, local improvement is applied to enhance solutions. This stage enables the prospective solutions to be fine-tuned. Finally, replacement strategy is applied and this process is continued until the termination criterion is met.

Cuckoo search (Yang and Deb 2013) is a metaheuristic method and mimics the behaviour of cuckoo birds. The method searches for the optimal or near-optimal solution to a given optimization problem by mimicking the reproductive behaviour of cuckoos. The main steps of the algorithm are described here. In the initialization step, a cuckoo nest population is created with each nest representing a potential solution to the optimization problem. The nests are often formed randomly in the search space. The second step is the survey flight step. In this step, each cuckoo performs a Levy flight, a random step that follows a very tail-heavy distribution. This step helps the cuckoos explore the search space more effectively and potentially find better solutions. After the fitness functions are evaluated, the host selection step is performed. In this step, the best nests are selected from the population based on their fitness values. These nests reflect the best solutions found so far. In cuckoo egg-laying step, each cuckoo bird lays an egg, denoting a probable solution. Based on particular parameters, such as fitness or random selection, the cuckoo replaces the nest of a randomly selected host.

Next, the cuckoo population abandons certain nests, generally based on likelihood. Within the search field, abandoned nests are replaced by newly produced nests. The algorithm is repeated until termination criteria are met.

Bat algorithm (Gandomi et al. 2012) is inspired by bat echolocation activity. It is employed in the solution of difficult optimization issues. In the initialization step, a bat colony is created and each bat represents a potential solution. The bats are placed at random throughout the search space. Each bat navigates and explores the search space using echolocation. They use ultrasonic pulses to detect the distance and quality of surrounding solutions by listening to echoes. The next step is updating the frequency and loudness. In this step, the frequency and loudness of each bat are improved. The frequency defines how quickly the bat searches the search space whereas the loudness defines the strength of the transmitted pulses. After this, each bat's frequency and volume are updated based on the knowledge retrieved from echolocation. Next, the fitness of each bat's solution is evaluated to define the quality of the solution. A bat may occasionally conduct a global search by randomly seeking a new solution outside of its current local area. This stage encourages global investigation of the search space. After the global search, the local search is performed for fine-tuning and exploration of the search space. These steps are repeated until the optimum solution is achieved.

Grey wolf optimization (Mirjalili et al. 2014) mimics the social structure and hunting behaviour of grey wolves. In the initialization step, a grey wolf population is scattered at random around the search area. After the fitness function of each wolf is evaluated, alpha, beta, and delta wolves are determined with respect to their fitness values. The best solution is represented by alpha wolf so far, and the second and third best solutions are represented by beta and delta wolves, respectively. Next, each wolf's position is updated with respect to its current position as well as the positions of the alpha, beta, and delta wolves. The alpha wolf wields the most power, followed by the beta and delta wolves. To obtain feasible solutions, wolves which are outside the search space limits are repositioned. Finally, these steps are repeated until the desired solution is obtained.

Whale optimization algorithm (Mirjalili and Lewis 2016) mimics the social behaviour of humpback whales. The steps of the algorithm are similar to the algorithms described above. After initialization and fitness evaluation steps, the best whale called the leader is determined among the current population. Next, each whale's position is updated with respect to its current position as well as the leader position. To improve the solution, some whales might exhibit encircling behaviour wherein the whales circle around the leader. Hence, the local performance of the whales is improved. The next step is bubble net feeding. Some whales may use a bubble net to catch and concentrate prey. This behaviour is reproduced in the context of the algorithm by applying random disturbances to the locations of the whales.

Dragonfly algorithm (Meraihi et al. 2020) mimics collective behaviour of dragonflies and knowledge passing among them. After initialization and evaluation of the fitness function, there is leader selection similar to the whale optimization algorithm. Based on their fitness levels, the best dragonflies in the population, known as leaders, are identified. The number of leaders can be predetermined or chosen dynamically. Next, each dragonfly updates its position with respect to the fitness function as well as the positions of leaders. Dragonflies engage in prey capture behaviour by shifting their places to areas with greater fitness values.

NON-CLINICAL APPLICATIONS OF AI

In this section, we review AI methods focusing on natural computing methods used in non-clinical applications, which are predictive analytics, health monitoring, and health management.

Predictive Analytics

There is a remarkable increase in the number of people who have some type of disease as an aftermath of various kinds of pandemics. Hence, the data in the health sector has increased remarkably and it is vital to analyze the big data accurately as well as efficiently. A number of statistical, probabilistic, and optimization methods are used by AI techniques to learn from the past and find meaningful patterns in huge, unstructured, and complicated datasets. In the literature, state-of-the-art AI techniques have been proposed to analyze massive data and predict patient outcomes. Hence, people who may be at risk of developing a particular illness have been identified before the illness gets worse. For example, Figure 2.2 presents steps for detecting Covid-19 disease from X-ray images using AI techniques.

Recently, several metaheuristic techniques have been proposed for disease diagnosis. Spider monkey optimization was used for predicting confirmed and negative cases of Covid-19 and also deaths due to the disease (Chander et al. 2020). This technique achieved less mean square error and had a better performance than other techniques. Furthermore, spider monkey optimization was used for diabetes classification and the method achieved higher accuracy (Cheruku et al. 2017). SFLA was used for detecting brain illness and Alzheimer's disease and the method presented satisfactory fusion results (Huang et al. 2019). SFLA

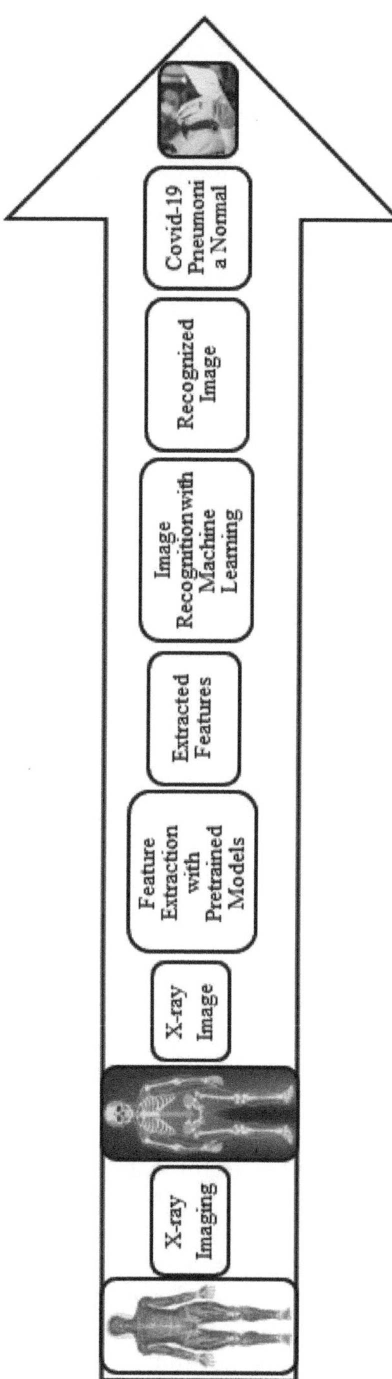

Figure 2.2   Steps for Covid-19 diagnosis using AI techniques.

was also used with convolutional neural networks (CNN) for detecting retinal disease (Ding et al. 2020). Their method achieved 96.7% accuracy. Furthermore, SFLA was used with tabu search for segmentation of MRI images to determine brain tumour (Sirisha and Haritha 2021). Cuckoo search optimization was used for diagnosing heart disease and diabetes with an accuracy of 91% (Gadekallu and Khare 2017). Bat algorithm was used for prediction of heart disease (Reddy and Khare 2016), and diabetes mellitus (Soliman and ElHamd 2015). Ant lion optimization was used for diagnosing chronic kidney diseases (Shankar et al. 2018), influenza (Hu et al. 2019), and Alzheimer's disease (Chitradevi et al. 2020). Grey wolf optimization was used for determining lung disease (Gupta et al. 2019), brain tumour (Geetha and Gomathi 2020), diabetes (Shankar and Manikandan 2020), and coronary artery disease (Shankar and Manikandan 2020). Moth flame optimization was used for identifying Alzheimer's disease (Sayed et al. 2016), pulmonary emphysema (Isaac et al. 2020), brain tumour, and somatization (Luo et al. 2019). Whale optimization algorithm was used for the classification of chronic liver (Rajathi and Jiji 2019), Covid-19 (Elghamrawy and Hassanien 2020), and lung tumour (Zamani and Nadimi-Shahraki 2016). Dragonfly algorithm was used for detecting skin diseases (Melbin and Raj 2019), classification of MRI images of brain (Bharanidharan and Rajaguru 2019), infant cry (Hariharan et al. 2018), and cancer diagnosis (Medjahed et al. 2017).

Health Monitoring

Patient monitoring can be achieved through AI by using sensors or some other devices shown in Figure 2.3. Thus, doctors can determine potential problems before a disease becomes worse. In case of ageing population, early detection in health monitoring through home control is increasing due to the advancement and development of technology. The rapid ageing of the global population has a considerable impact on the rise in expectations of healthy life. By gathering and analyzing health data, the services of health monitoring can help the patient by addressing a variety of complicated health concerns on a broad scale. Health monitoring is an on-going clinical trial process that makes sure that health is tracked in accordance with the established protocols and standard operating procedures.

In the literature, several state-of-the-art techniques have been discussed for monitoring human activities in the health sector. A systematic review on ambient supported living was presented by Qureshi et al. (2021) in order to understand how ambient supported living encourages and supports patients with heart disease in self-management in order to lower associated mortality and morbidity. They

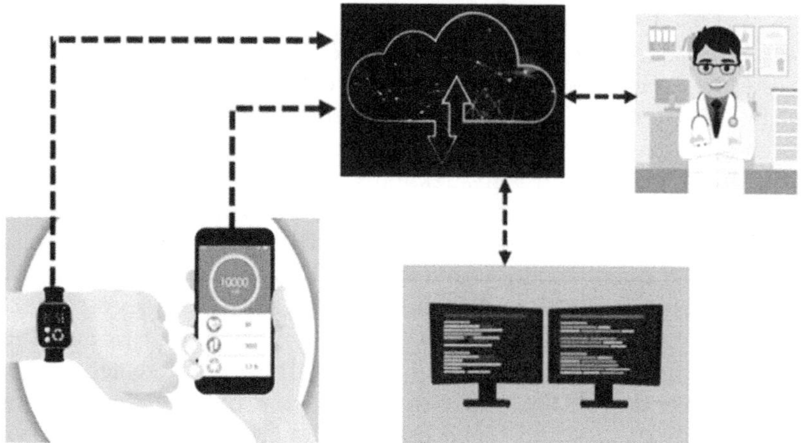

Figure 2.3   Remote patient monitoring.

divided their study into four major categories, including self-monitoring, wearable technology, clinical management systems, and deep learning–based methods for diagnosing heart disease. A complete analysis of the integrated research focused on machine health monitoring was published by Zhao et al. (2019). In another study, through the use of physiological and natural signs, Debauche et al. (2020) presented a cloud-based health monitoring framework for fog Internet of Things (IoT) to provide pertinent information regarding daily living activities. Their method gave healthcare professionals the ability to monitor a patient's well-being and made modifications for elderly or lone patients. The strategy in their paper also offered an assessment of clinical practice and turnaround times. The clinical experts might clearly evaluate the details throughout this examination, which made it easier for them to naturally accept any inconsistencies that were found.

Health Management

By giving patients individualized advice for eating habits, exercise, and other lifestyle aspects, AI can assist them in managing their health. Thus, patients' general quality of life can be enhanced and their health-related decisions made better. Recently, several AI-based health management studies have been introduced. Khan and Yairi (2018) published a review about deep learning methods for health management. Their experimental results presented that AI demonstrated remarkable benefits for fault diagnosis.

Some of the AI techniques applied to health monitoring system are shown in Figure 2.4. The goal of health management is to collect suitable data from multiple sensor sources and perform the appropriate processing, such as detecting important features and fault diagnosis.

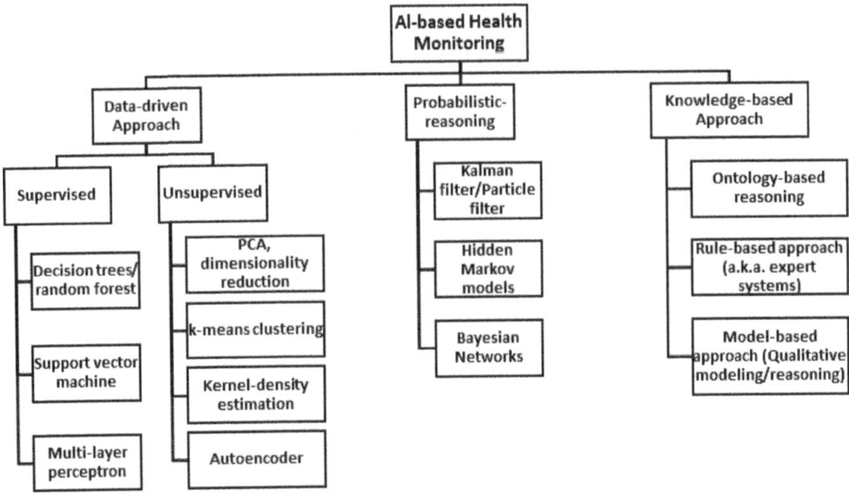

Figure 2.4　AI-based methods for health management (adapted from Khan and Yairi [2018]).

Next, we investigate supervised and unsupervised learning techniques for health management. First, we discuss supervised methods. Ash et al. (1993), Rao et al. (2015), Spina et al. (2002), and Bajwa and Kulkarni (2000) applied decision tree methods for achieving health system management. Thus, making decision using breaches is easy. Yan (2006) and Yang et al. (2008) used random forests for health system management. When compared to decision trees, random forest had a better performance and provided fast and accurate decisions. The Naive Bayes method was implemented by Kumar et al. (2014) and Ng et al. (2014) for health system management using less data. Support vector machines were used by Fuertes et al. (2016), Salem et al. (2014), and Li et al. (2011). Their methods were efficient for large data and provided higher accuracy. The disadvantages of their methods were that they required large amounts of memory and depended on the kernel selection with parameters. Multilayer perceptron was used by Marsland (2013) for health management. Their methods required less number of parameters but were prone to overfitting. Second, we discuss unsupervised methods. The k-means clustering method was performed by Soualhi et al. (2013). This method required short training time. Lei et al. (2013) and He et al. (2012) performed adaptive resonance theory for health management and their method had the ability to model non-linear clusters in a short time. Self-organizing maps were used by Tibaduiza et al. (2012) to achieve health management. The advantages of this method are that it has robust training times and data are mapped easily. However, determining input weights is difficult in this method. Finally, hidden Markov models were used by Zhou et al. (2016) for health management.

CONCLUSION AND DISCUSSION

There are major benefits and drawbacks of using AI techniques in non-clinical and clinical applications of medicine, and these offer suggestions for future research areas. AI methods can be used to analyze large data, medical records as well as lab results. Furthermore, AI methods can extract meaningful information by analyzing medical images to help with accurate and timely diagnoses. Thanks to AI methods, we can determine potential health risks before systems manifest. Thus, early precautions can be taken. Moreover, systems including AI reduce the burden on professionals in the field of medicine by automating repetitive tasks like medical documentation. With the advent of deep learning methods, we can accurately analyze medical images and detect anomalies. On the other hand, there are some drawbacks too of AI methods. The usage of AI methods reduces patient–doctor interactions. Data privacy is another issue. These methods require large amounts of personal data and concerns about privacy and ethical considerations may be raised. Moreover, some AI models provide black-box results that are difficult to interpret.

In this chapter, we touched upon non-clinical applications of AI by exploiting the capabilities of metaheuristic approaches. We analyzed how these approaches have been used in predictive analysis, health monitoring, and health management.

REFERENCES

Ash, D., Gold, G., Seiver, A. and Hayes-Roth, B. 1993. Guaranteeing real-time response with limited resources. Artificial Intelligence in Medicine. 5(1): 49–66.

Bajwa, A.R. and Kulkarni, D. 2000. Engine data analysis using decision trees. The 36th Joint Propulsion Conference, American Institute of Aeronautics and Astronautics.

Bansal, J.C., Sharma, H., Jadon, S.S. and Clerc, M. 2014. Spider monkey optimization algorithm for numerical optimization. Memetic Computing. 6(1): 31–47.

Bharanidharan, N. and Rajaguru, H. 2019. Dementia MRI classification using hybrid dragonfly based support vector machine. 2019 IEEE R10 Humanitarian Technology Conference (R10-HTC). (47129): 45–48.

Chander, S., Padmanabha, V. and Mani, J. 2020. Jaya spider monkey optimization-driven deep convolutional LSTM for the prediction of Covid'19. Bio-Algorithms and Med-Systems. 16(4): 20200030. https://doi.org/10.1515/bams-2020-0030.

Cheruku, R., Edla, D.R. and Kuppili, V. 2017. SM-RuleMiner: spider monkey based rule miner using novel fitness function for diabetes classification. Computers in Biology and Medicine. 81: 79–92.

Chitradevi, D., Prabha, S. and Prabhu, A.D. 2020. Diagnosis of Alzheimer disease in MR brain images using optimization techniques. Neural Computing and Applications. 33(1): 223–237.

Debauche, O., Mahmoudi, S., Mahmoudi, S.A., Manneback, P., Bindelle, J. and Lebeau, F. 2020. Edge computing and artificial intelligence for real-time poultry monitoring. Procedia Computer Science. 175: 534–541.

Ding, W., Sun, Y., Ren, L., Ju, H., Feng, Z. and Li, M. 2020. Multiple lesions detection of fundus images based on convolution neural network algorithm with improved SFLA. IEEE Access. 8: 97618–97631.

Elghamrawy, S. and Hassanien, A.E. 2020. Diagnosis and prediction model for Covid-19 patient's response to treatment based on convolutional neural networks and whale optimization algorithm using CT images. medRxiv. Retrieved from http://dx.doi.org/10.1101/2020.04.16.20063990.

Fuertes, S., Picart, G., Tourneret, J.-Y., Chaari, L., Ferrari, A. and Richard, C. 2016. Improving spacecraft health monitoring with automatic anomaly detection techniques. SpaceOps 2016 Conference. Presented at the SpaceOps 2016 Conference, Daejeon, Korea. doi:10.2514/6.2016-2430.

Gadekallu, T.R. and Khare, N. 2017. Cuckoo search optimized reduction and fuzzy logic classifier for heart disease and diabetes prediction. International Journal of Fuzzy System Applications, 6(2): 25–42.

Gandomi, A.H., Yang, X.-S., Alavi, A.H. and Talatahari, S. 2012. Bat algorithm for constrained optimization tasks. Neural Computing and Applications: 22(6): 1239–1255.

Geetha, A. and Gomathi, N. 2020. A robust grey wolf based deep learning for brain tumour detection in MR images. Biomedical Engineering/Biomedizinische Technik. 65(2): 191–207.

Gupta, N., Gupta, D., Khanna, A., Rebouças Filho, P.P. and de Albuquerque, V.H.C. 2019. Evolutionary algorithms for automatic lung disease detection. Measurement. 140: 590–608.

Hariharan, M., Sindhu, R., Vijean, V., Yazid, H., Nadarajaw, T., Yaacob, S., et al. 2018. Improved binary dragonfly optimization algorithm and wavelet packet based non-linear features for infant cry classification. Computer Methods and Programs in Biomedicine. 155, 39–51.

He, H., Caudell, T.P., Menicucci, D.F. and Mammoli, A.A. 2012. Application of adaptive resonance theory neural networks to monitor solar hot water systems and detect existing or developing faults. Solar Energy. 86(9): 2318–2333.

Hu, H., Li, Y., Bai, Y., Zhang, J. and Liu, M. 2019. The improved antlion optimizer and artificial neural network for Chinese influenza prediction. Complexity. 2019, 1–12.

Huang, C., Tian, G., Lan, Y., Peng, Y., Ng, E.Y.K., Hao, Y., et al. 2019. A new pulse coupled neural network (PCNN) for brain medical image fusion empowered by shuffled frog leaping algorithm. Frontiers in Neuroscience. Vol. 13. Frontiers Media SA. https://doi.org/10.3389/fnins.2019.00210.

Isaac, A., Nehemiah, H.K., Isaac, A. and Kannan, A. 2020. Computer-aided diagnosis system for diagnosis of pulmonary emphysema using bio-inspired algorithms. Computers in Biology and Medicine. 124: 103940.

Khan, S. and Yairi, T. 2018. A review on the application of deep learning in system health management. Mechanical Systems and Signal Processing. 107: 241–265.

Kumar, H., Kumar, T. R., Amarnath, M. and Sugumaran, V. 2014. Fault diagnosis of bearings through vibration signal using Bayes classifiers. International Journal of Computer Aided Engineering and Technology. 6(1): 14–28.

Lei, Y., Han, D., Lin, J. and He, Z. 2013. Planetary gearbox fault diagnosis using an adaptive stochastic resonance method. Mechanical Systems and Signal Processing. 38(1): 113–124.

Li, K., Zhang, Y.L. and Li, Z.X. 2011. Application research of Kalman filter and SVM applied to condition monitoring and fault diagnosis. Applied Mechanics and Materials. 121–126: 268–272.

Luo, J., Chen, H., Hu, Z., Huang, H., Wang, P., Wang, X., et al. 2019. A new kernel extreme learning machine framework for somatization disorder diagnosis. IEEE Access. 7: 45512–45525.

Marsland, S. 2013. Novelty detection in learning systems. Neural Computing Surveys. 3(2): 157–195.

Medjahed, S.A., Saadi, T.A., Benyettou, A. and Ouali, M. 2017. Kernel-based learning and feature selection analysis for cancer diagnosis. Applied Soft Computing. 51: 39–48.

Melbin, K. and Raj, Y.V. 2019. An enhanced model for skin disease detection using dragonfly optimization based deep neural network. Third International Conference on I-SMAC (IoT in Social, Mobile, Analytics and Cloud) (I-SMAC). 346–351.

Meraihi, Y., Ramdane-Cherif, A., Acheli, D. and Mahseur, M. 2020. Dragonfly algorithm: a comprehensive review and applications. Neural Computing and Applications. 32(21): 16625–16646.

Mirjalili, S., Mirjalili, S.M. and Lewis, A. 2014. Grey wolf optimizer. Advances in Engineering Software. 69: 46–61.

Mirjalili, S. and Lewis, A. 2016. The whale optimization algorithm. Advances in Engineering Software. 95: 51–67.

Ng, S.S., Xing, Y. and Tsui, K.L. 2014. A Naive Bayes model for robust remaining useful life prediction of lithium-ion battery. Applied Energy. 118: 114–123.

Qureshi, M.A., Qureshi, K.N., Jeon, G. and Piccialli, F. 2021. Deep learning-based ambient assisted living for self-management of cardiovascular conditions. Neural Computing and Applications. 34(13): 10449–10467.

Rajathi, G.I. and Jiji, G.W. 2019. Chronic liver disease classification using hybrid whale optimization with simulated annealing and ensemble classifier. Symmetry. 11(1): 33.

Rao, P.S., Mohan, S. and Chindam, V. 2015. AI based on-board diagnostic and prognostic health management system. Annual Conference of the Prognostics and Health Management Society. 73–102.

Reddy, G.T. and Khare, N. 2016. An efficient system for heart disease prediction using hybrid OFBAT with rule-based fuzzy logic model. Journal of Circuits, Systems and Computers. 26(4): 1750061.

Salem, O., Guerassimov, A., Mehaoua, A., Marcus, A. and Furht, B. 2014. Anomaly detection in medical wireless sensor networks using SVM and linear regression models. International Journal of E-Health and Medical Communications. 5(1): 20–45.

Sayed, G.I., Hassanien, A.E., Nassef, T.M. and Pan, J.-S. 2016. Alzheimer's disease diagnosis based on moth flame optimization. pp. 298–305. *In:* Pan, J.-S., Lin, J.W., Wang, C.H. and Jiang, X. (eds). Genetic and Evolutionary Computing. ICGEC 2016. Advances in Intelligent Systems and Computing, Vol. 536. Springer, Cham.

Shankar, G.S. and Manikandan, K. 2020. Remote diagnosis of diabetics patient through speech engine and fuzzy based machine learning algorithm. International Journal of Speech Technology. 23(4): 789–798.

Shankar, K., Manickam, P., Devika, G. and Ilayaraja, M. 2018. Optimal feature selection for chronic kidney disease classification using deep learning classifier. IEEE International Conference on Computational Intelligence and Computing Research (ICCIC). 1–5.

Sirisha, P. and Haritha, D. 2021. Hybrid shuffled frog leaping algorithm with probability dispersal method for tumor detection in 3D MRI braintumor images. IOP Conference Series: Materials Science and Engineering. 1074(1): 012001.

Spina, P.R., Torella, G. and Venturini, M. 2002. The use of expert systems for gas turbine diagnostics and maintenance. Proceedings of the ASME Turbo Expo 2002: Power for Land, Sea, and Air. Volume 2: Turbo Expo 2002, Parts A and B. Amsterdam, The Netherlands. June 3–6, 2002. pp. 127–134. ASME. https://doi.org/10.1115/GT2002-30033.

Soliman, O.S. and ElHamd, E.A. 2015. A chaotic levy flights bat algorithm for diagnosing diabetes mellitus. International Journal of Computer Applications. 111(1): 36–42.

Soualhi, A., Clerc, G. and Razik, H. 2013. Detection and diagnosis of faults in induction motor using an improved artificial ant clustering technique. IEEE Transactions on Industrial Electronics. 60(9): 4053–4062.

Tibaduiza, D.A., Mujica, L.E. and Rodellar, J. 2012. Damage classification in structural health monitoring using principal component analysis and self-organizing maps: damage classification in SHM using PCA and SOM. Structural Control and Health Monitoring. 20(10): 1303–1316.

Yan, W. 2006. Application of random forest to aircraft engine fault diagnosis. The Proceedings of the Multiconference on "Computational Engineering in Systems Applications". 468–475.

Yang, B.-S., Di, X. and Han, T. 2008. Random forests classifier for machine fault diagnosis. Journal of Mechanical Science and Technology. 22(9): 1716–1725.

Yang, X.-S. and Deb, S. 2013. Cuckoo search: recent advances and applications. Neural Computing and Applications. 24(1): 169–174.

Zamani, H. and Nadimi-Shahraki, M.H. 2016. Feature selection based on whale optimization algorithm for diseases diagnosis. International Journal of Computer Science and Information Security. 14(9): 1243–1247.

Zhao, R., Yan, R., Chen, Z., Mao, K., Wang, P. and Gao, R.X. 2019. Deep learning and its applications to machine health monitoring. Mechanical Systems and Signal Processing. 115: 213–237.

Zhen, Z., Wang, D. and Liu, Y. 2009. Improved shuffled frog leaping algorithm for continuous optimization problem. 2009 IEEE Congress on Evolutionary Computation, Trondheim, Norway. 2992–2995. doi: 10.1109/ CEC.2009.4983320.

Zhou, H., Chen, J., Dong, G., Wang, H. and Yuan, H. 2016. Bearing fault recognition method based on neighbourhood component analysis and coupled hidden Markov model. Mechanical Systems and Signal Processing. 66–67: 568–581.

Chapter 3

Non-clinical Applications of Artificial Intelligence in Health Sector: Regional Cases

Ainura Turdalieva*,[1] and Razia Abdieva[2]

[1]Department of Economics, Kyrgyz-Turkish Manas University,
ORCID: 0000-0001-5545-5561; Email: aynura.turdaliyeva@manas.edu.kg

[2]Department of Economics, Kyrgyz-Turkish Manas University,
ORCID: 0000-0002-9438-1558; Email: razia.abdieva@manas.edu.kg

INTRODUCTION

The healthcare sector around the world is embracing artificial intelligence (AI). As it develops, AI has the potential to improve every aspect of organizations, and it is crucial to improving the effectiveness and accessibility of healthcare services. The use of innovative technologies and reliable, up-to-date data can ensure high quality healthcare services.

The Central Asian countries started giving priority to digitalization and development of information and communications technology (ICT) for the modernization of national economies and society in the early 2000s. At present, all Central Asian countries are running national digitalization programs; these programs are called "Digital Strategy" in three out of five countries: "Digital Kazakhstan 2018–2022", "Digital

*For Correspondence: Ainura Turdalieva (aynura.turdaliyeva@manas.edu.kg)

Kyrgyzstan 2019–2023", and "Digital Uzbekistan—2030". Tajikistan and Turkmenistan have prioritized their digital transformation programs as part of a broader national development program and/or digital economy. The examples for these are the "Concept of the Digital Economy in the Republic of Tajikistan", arising from the "National Development Strategy of the Republic of Tajikistan for the Period up to 2030", and the digitalization of Turkmenistan based on the "Concept of Development of the Digital Economy in Turkmenistan for 2019–2025" (Hakimov 2023).

In this chapter, the application of AI in healthcare in select Central Asian countries—Kazakhstan, Uzbekistan, Kyrgyzstan, and Tajikistan—has been analyzed. The discussion is based on official documents such as National Strategy, the National Strategy for the Development of the Health Sector, and Roadmap for the implementation of the digital transformation concept.

AI IN KAZAKHSTAN'S HEALTHCARE

Kazakhstan developed its own digital health action plan based on the state-approved "Digital Kazakhstan" program adopted on December 12, 2017, wherein the government announced the use of AI in the health care sector.

The initiative asserts digitalization of healthcare thereby minimizing the number of medical errors and enhancing the quality and speed of service, as well as the quality of managerial decision-making (Digital Kazakhstan 2017: 21). Digitalization of healthcare involves both further informatization of the industry with the introduction of an interoperability platform and the development of mobile healthcare, as well as the introduction of breakthrough technologies of augmented reality, machine learning and AI in the processes of teaching students, diagnosing and managing treatment plans (Digital Kazakhstan 2017: 21).

The targets of the program include building the healthcare integration platform which implies the possibility of flexible interaction of medical systems with each other and with external systems, the possibility of creating an ecosystem of applications for end users that are integrated with wearable devices, mobile applications created by commercial companies, as well as the introduction of an electronic health passport for every citizen of the country (Digital Kazakhstan 2017: 21).

By creating regional medical information systems, the collected data will be used for medical statistics, analytics and appropriate decision-making using big data technology. This will make it possible to transition to paperless healthcare, optimize and improve the efficiency of the assistance provided, and ensure the continuity of the assistance provided between different levels and medical organizations. Secure access to key medical information will be provided for all participants in the care process, including the patient himself. Through personalized notifications and alerts, including through mobile technologies, the involvement of the population in the process of protecting their own health and the formation of a healthy lifestyle will be ensured.

Acting as a central hub of medical information, electronic health passports will provide timely and reliable information to patients and medical workers, as well as health care authorities and insurance providers (Digital Kazakhstan 2017: 53–54).

Another framework for digitalization health care is the Concept for the Development of Health Care in the Republic of Kazakhstan until 2026, which includes the main approaches to the development of the healthcare system.

The process of implementation of the strategy and program is marked by both achievements and problems. To enable access to medical information systems, all healthcare organizations at the level of cities and district centers are provided with 100% access to the Internet; at the level below district centers and in remote rural areas, access to the Internet is 86.7% (Concept for the Development of Health Care 2022: 32).

On an ongoing basis, healthcare facilities have been equipped with an IT infrastructure with an Internet connection, data is being transferred to the Smart Data Ukimet analytical platform, and measures have been planned and launched to integrate Medical Information System (MIS) with the Ehealth core (Concept for the Development of Health Care 2022: 32).

There are about 20 mobile applications in the Kazakhstan segment of digital mobile solutions in the field of healthcare, with the help of which the people can evaluate the work of medical organizations, provide their feedback, and choose a clinic according to criteria and reviews (Concept for the Development of Health Care 2022: 32).

However, the existing databases (47 information systems) are fragmented and not integrated into a single information space, and there is no single industry operator, which complicates the interaction of different levels and healthcare services, does not ensure the continuity of information, and limits the ability analysis.

There are several problems related to infrastructure development and digitalization of healthcare system such as insufficient availability of digital services in medical organizations in remote rural areas; lack of a single industry operator in the field of e-health; more than 47 disparate information systems (monolithic outdated Information System (IS) architecture) (Concept for the Development of Health Care 2022: 33).

Development of a single digital health space (eHealth) will ensure the consolidation of medical information received from different sources around a particular patient through the integration of information systems in the field of healthcare and improve the quality of public services in electronic format. In order to ensure an integrated approach to the implementation of the platform model throughout Kazakhstan, a single operator for digitalization in the field of healthcare will be identified.

The eHealth architecture will contribute to the full and comprehensive formation of national electronic health passport of citizens, which will improve the quality and accessibility of medical care focused on the needs of citizens, as well as contribute to the implementation of continuous monitoring of the health of patients and seamless provision of medical services.

Duplication of functions in different information systems, untimely updating of data, and fragmentation of information systems will be excluded (Concept for the Development of Health Care 2022: 57).

National electronic health passports and electronic passports of medical institutions will be issued, and comprehensive measures will be implemented to automate the formation of demand for drugs and medical devices: the launch of a unified classifier of medicines and medical devices, the introduction of labeling and control of the movement and balance of medicines, reengineering and digital transformation of business processes from drug registration to diagnostic processes.

As part of the projects to develop technologies for augmented and virtual reality (AV/VR), AI in healthcare, along with the introduction of software, it will be planned to purchase equipment for medical organizations that is compatible with digital systems for processing, storing and transmitting medical images (Concept for the Development of Health Care 2022: 57).

However, there are still many large areas of the healthcare system that are not covered by digitalization and do not use modern opportunities to increase efficiency.

Despite all the advantages of digital health, the problem of patients' and medical staff's low levels of digital literacy needs to be resolved. Physicians, nurses, and young employees are trained by public health authorities and developers to improve their digital skills.

The main issues with digitalizing healthcare today are the shortage of highly skilled specialists, inadequate IT infrastructure in clinics, overabundance of MIS providers (over 30), and the numerous integrations with Ministry of Healthcare (MoH) services that are experiencing performance issues. The situation is made worse by the absence of a unified health information environment (Arslanova 2021).

National medical facilities are already entirely equipped with computer and Internet technologies in urban and district centers. However, health services in inaccessible rural locations face difficulties in this regard. The IT infrastructure of medical facilities in inaccessible regions will be upgraded as part of a significant public–private partnership (PPP) initiative to connect these communities to the Internet (Arslanova 2021).

One of the areas of Kazakhstan healthcare that needs more development is AI. Personalized medicine will become a reality as digital medicine and AI become more widely used.

In Kazakhstan, the process of digitalization and the use of AI in medicine takes place according to internal dynamics. Also, this process is not fully implemented due to the existing problems such as insufficient availability of digital services in medical organizations in remote rural areas because of the low availability of the Internet; existing databases are fragmented and not integrated into a single information space; there is no single industry operator, which complicates the interaction between different levels and health services.

AI IN HEALTHCARE OF UZBEKISTAN

The "Digital Uzbekistan—2030" strategy launched the digitalization, active development, and widespread adoption of information technologies in healthcare in Uzbekistan.

In accordance with the strategy "Digital Uzbekistan—2030" and in order to create favorable conditions for the accelerated introduction of AI technologies and their wide application in the country, to ensure the availability and high quality of digital data, training of qualified personnel was approved through digital transformation programs at the regional and sectoral levels (Decree of the President of the Republic of Uzbekistan 2021).

As part of the digital transformation of regions and industries in 2020–2022, it was planned to increase access to the Internet, lay fiber-optic lines and develop mobile communication networks, introduce information systems, electronic services and other software products in the economic development of regions, organize training in the basics of programming, introduce information systems and software products to automate management processes, and improve digital literacy and skills (Resolution of the President of the Republic of Uzbekistan, February 17, 2021).

There has been defined a list of pilot projects that will be carried out in 2020–2022, involving residents of the technical park of software products in healthcare: the application of AI technologies to the detection of pneumonia based on human lung computed tomography analysis and early stage breast cancer based on mammography analysis (Sarymsakova 2021).

A program of measures to study and implement AI in 2021–2022 has been approved in accordance with the guidelines of the "Digital

Uzbekistan—2030" strategy. This program includes framing a strategy for the development of AI, forming a regulatory framework, building a domestic ecosystem of innovation in the field, and gaining access to information technologies.

The Decree of the President of the Republic of Uzbekistan on "Additional Measures to Digitize the Healthcare System" (Yangi Uzbekiston 2023) provides the creation of a digital healthcare platform, the implementation of a database complex for medical and preventive institutions at all levels, and the development of software.

Uzbekistan and KfW Bank inked grant and loan agreements to fund the project "Support for Reforms on Digitalization of Healthcare" over a period of 12 years. An action plan for the digitalization of the healthcare system in 2023–2025 was approved, and it proposes the implementation of the electronic prescription system (reimbursement); development of the "electronic sanatorium" platform that makes it possible to purchase a ticket for the sanatorium and monitor the waitlist and availability; putting into place the cancer-register information system to keep an electronic list of cancer patients; creation of the "passport of health of mother and child" electronic system; the establishment of a single platform through which individuals can acquire brochures and certifications of temporary incapacity; and technical and economic project metrics for "support for reforms in the digitalization of health care" (Decree of the President of the Republic of Uzbekistan, "On Additional Measures for Digitalization of the Healthcare System", dated May 1, 2023 (Yangi Uzbekiston 2023)).

In accordance with the resolution "On Measures for the Effective Organization of Digitalization in the Healthcare Sector" (Azizov 2021), it has been planned to create a limited liability company "IT-Med" under the Ministry of Health on the basis of the state unitary enterprise, "Center for the Development of Information and Communication Technologies".

It will design information solutions for hospitals, clinics, and other medical organizations. It is also entrusted with the tasks of optimizing, rationalizing, standardizing, and automating processes in the healthcare system and organizations, developing technical and economic parameters and concepts, implementing policies and standards for information technology and communications in the field of medicine and pharmaceuticals, implementing and maintaining a single complex of information systems "eHealth", as well as ensuring their integration with other information systems (Azizov 2021).

The application of AI in healthcare has been initiated by the Ministry of Health of Uzbekistan. Thus, together with partners, it is working on a project to provide a platform for processing radiological medical images using AI in all healthcare entities, and is also upgrading equipment, telecommunications infrastructure, and software (Zdrav 2021).

Uzbekistan intends to use AI to develop capability to recognize a stroke in the first four hours, according to the National Chamber of Innovative Healthcare (National Chamber of Innovative Healthcare, 2023), together with partners from Kazakhstan, there are plans to launch a pilot project to provide medical services in the field of diagnosing ischemic and hemorrhagic strokes based on an automated system (SPUTNIK Uzbekistan 2023).

Uzbekistan started developing a turbine artificial lung ventilation (ALV) equipment controlled by AI. The concept of the research was presented during the First Educational Forum for Anesthesiologists and Resuscitators in Nukus (Ministry of Higher Education, Science and Innovations of the Republic of Uzbekistan 2023). Therefore, in Uzbekistan, the usage of AI is not yet common; there are cases of pilot initiatives.

APPLICATION OF AI IN THE HEALTH SECTOR OF KYRGYZSTAN

In 2018, the National Strategy for 2018–2040 was developed in Kyrgyzstan. The strategy pays particular attention to digitalization and information technology. This indicates that the widespread introduction of information technology in production and management should become a development policy priority. Digitization of the economy and widespread use of innovative and advanced technologies drive growth competitiveness of the country, and welfare and security of the population (Ministry of Economy and Commerce of the Kyrgyz Republic 2018).

Strengthening primary healthcare is one of the objectives of social development. Online consultations, telemedicine, etc., will be developed at the primary healthcare level. As a result, full coverage of the population with access to quality primary health care is expected to be achieved.

Currently, the Ministry is also developing an appropriate regulatory legal act to lay down the procedure for organizing and providing medical care using telemedicine in order to create a favorable climate for the development of telemedicine in the Kyrgyz Republic (UNICEF 2022).

In the context of the fight against infectious diseases, mention must be made of the necessity to review the system of data collection and analysis for the main infectious diseases (including the most dangerous and socially important ones) using modern ICT, disaggregated by sex, age, socio-economic indicators, etc.

The "Roadmap for the Implementation of the Digital Transformation Concept 'Digital Kyrgyzstan 2019–2023'" aims to create the Central

System of the Unified Repository (Storage) of Data and Health Services of the Kyrgyz Republic (URDSZ) by 20 September 2021, to develop a unified format for the "electronic medical record of the patient" by 20 March 2020, and to develop a regulation on the information system "electronic medical record of the patient" and implement it in healthcare organizations after integrating it with the single repository (storage) of health data and services by 20 December 2021 (The Government of the Kyrgyz Republic, 2019).

The roadmap also seeks to implement digital services for patients that capture electronic appointment with a doctor, referral/redirection to healthcare organizations, and online interaction with patients; implement the National Database of Medicines and Medical Devices; implement the information system "emergency (ambulance) medical care"; implement the integrated information system "radiology (PACS)"; create and implement the integrated information system "laboratory"; develop a catalog of electronic clinical protocols; introduce an online platform for tracking the quality of medical care; and develop telemedicine technologies and distance education during 2020 and 2022 (The Government of the Kyrgyz Republic, 2019).

In the period up to 2023, the cities of Bishkek, Osh, and Karakol will have a completely modernized ambulance system. The key measures will be the introduction of an automated control system with the use of modern innovative technologies, logistics, the revision of legislation, increase in the capacity of the system's employees and their motivation, and the improvement of the standard of assistance. As a result, the service time for the population is expected to be reduced to 20 minutes and the pre-hospital mortality rate to 70% of the total.

It is necessary to create an information system for healthcare that is capable of providing uniform and centralized data processing, information security, access to information systems in real time using efficient software products and integration with other information systems such as State Registration Service (SRS), State Tax Service (STS), Social Fund (SF), and Ministry of Labor and Social Development (MLSD). First of all, it is necessary to integrate the databases used in the payment systems for medical services at all levels of care in order to create a patient-oriented system of organization and financing of medical care. There will also be revised procedures and approaches to funding high technologies.

As part of the implementation of the Presidential Enactment 2021, "On Urgent Measures to Develop the Healthcare Sector and Improve the Quality of Life and Health of the Population in the Kyrgyz Republic", the digital transformation plan "Digital Kyrgyzstan 2019–2023" and the development program to 2030 "Healthy People—Prospering Land", the Ministry of Health of the Kyrgyz Republic has developed a number of digital infrastructure products to increase the availability of medical care and improve its efficiency.

Bakyt Dzhangaziyev, Deputy Minister of Health for Digital Development of the Kyrgyz Republic, indicated that the Ministry of Health of the Kyrgyz Republic has defined the digitalization of healthcare as one of its priority areas. To this end, the Ministry has identified a target model for the development of digital health, as well as tasks for 2022, in which the individual is at the center. Also, in 2023, the Ministry will move from developments aimed at solving problems related to automation of activities within the healthcare system to digital solutions that will be felt by the population—this is by obtaining various certificates, online registration to polyclinics, and online interaction with business (Djaparova 2022).

Digital Health Profile, the ILab laboratory information system, the National Resource Management Information System (NIMSR), the IEmdoo immunization information system, and others are the first in a series of national digital products that will form a unified digital ecosystem for the healthcare system. Digitalization of healthcare leads to increase in accountability, accessibility, and effectiveness. Therefore, the automation of activities within the health system for digital solutions is now necessary (KABAR 2022).

Digitization has been actively pursued in Kyrgyzstan in recent years. It can be seen in many fields such as electronic document circulation, education, and economy. But one of the most important is medicine. The importance of healthcare reform was fully recognized during the pandemic, especially in the first year (KABAR 2022).

APPLICATION OF AI IN THE HEALTH SECTOR OF TAJIKISTAN

In Tajikistan, the Public Health Strategy for the period up to 2030 defines the process of reforms in the healthcare system and provides ways for further development of the public health sector. The strategy contributes to the integration of the international obligations of the Republic of Tajikistan in relation to the Sustainable Development Goals (SDGs). The aim of the strategy is to accelerate progress towards universal coverage of the population of the Republic of Tajikistan with affordable, quality healthcare by strengthening the strategic management system, achieving sustainable financing and human resources, and developing modern technologies.

In this reform, special attention was given to the establishment of the Health Management Information System (HMIS) which will be used by the Ministry of Health and Social Protection of the Population in making informed decisions in all critical areas of management, setting reporting standards and real-time information exchange, and ensuring a high level of security and confidentiality of patient information. In addition, the HMIS can improve the administration, implementation, and monitoring of expenditures and establish fruitful partnerships with stakeholders. The HMIS informs the decision-making process at every level of the system to support the rational purchase of public health services.

In spite of the efforts by the government towards digitalization of the health sector, there are still a number of issues in the development of management information systems and digital health such as lack of appropriate legislation to ensure the effective implementation of HMIS, e-health, digital health and telemedicine (World Health Organization 2020). Some of the other issues are as follows:

- **Fragmentation of health information systems:** In recent years, with the support of the Government of the Republic of Tajikistan and the European Union (EU), a Unified Health Management Information System has been created, operating on the basis of DHIS2 (Unified Health Management Information System), which allows, in accordance with the adopted national indicators, to generate online information about the health status of the population and activities of healthcare institutions. In addition, separate healthcare structures have chaotically developed their information systems piecemeal, which has led to the fragmentation of health information systems, the dispersal and weakening of responsibility, and the competing interests of various actors from different sectors. The quality of some data production is not in line with the approved standards. One of the most pressing issues in health information technology is analyzing and adopting national health data standards.

- **Excessive data and reporting requirements:** Health workers, especially at the primary healthcare level, are overwhelmed by excessive demands for data and reporting. Another problem is that the little information that is produced is not actually used for decision-making.

- **Inadequate funding:** Establishing a national network of institutions to implement HMIS requires careful estimation/forecasting of all costs, which should be properly budgeted and funded to ensure smooth implementation.

- **Underdeveloped information technology and communication infrastructure and administrative capacity:** The information technology and communication infrastructure is underdeveloped, underfunded, and unevenly distributed.

The main goal is to improve the management information system and expand the digitalization and telemedicine systems of health and social protection, which consists of the following tasks (World Health Organization 2020):

- streamline the regulatory framework to support the development of the HMIS and digital and telemedicine healthcare;
- strengthen the digital infrastructure of the Ministry of Health and Social Protection;
- strengthen the administrative and human resources capacity of the Ministry of Health and Social Protection to use digital platforms and provide telemedicine and digital medical services to the population;
- develop a National Investment Plan to support the development of HMIS, digital medicine, and telemedicine services.

In Tajikistan, the active process of digitalization started in 2018. The Ministry of Health and Social Protection of the Population of the Republic of Tajikistan has developed a roadmap for the implementation of an action plan to improve the health management information system for the period from 2018 to 2020 (Rizoev 2019). The Unified Health Management Information System has been developed with the support of the Government of the Republic of Tajikistan and in cooperation with the EU. Tajikistan has begun the transition to paperless medical records and has been actively implementing mobile applications in recent years (Dialog 2019).

CONCLUSION AND RECOMMENDATIONS

Digitalization of the health sector in Central Asia has rapidly increased during the last few years. The pioneer was Kazakhstan, where digitalization process started in 2017, and since 2019 it has been consulting with Tajikistan for the digitalization of the health sector. The Covid-19 pandemic accelerated the digitalization process in this sector.

In Kazakhstan, the process of digitalization and the use of AI in healthcare are driven by internal dynamics. The lack of a single industry operator complicates interactions between various levels and health services; this process is not fully implemented as a result of other issues too, such as the limited availability of digital services in medical organizations in remote rural areas due to the reduced Internet access.

In Uzbekistan, the digitalization of healthcare and the introduction of AI requires improving the infrastructure that will expand access to the Internet, developing mobile communication networks, introducing information systems and software products to automate management processes, and improving digital literacy and skills.

Some steps that have begun to be taken in this region are use of digital instruments such as telemedicine; creating a unified format for the "electronic medical record of the patient", digital services for patients that capture electronic appointment with a doctor, referral/redirection to healthcare organizations, and online interaction with patients; implementation of the National Database of Medicines and Medical Devices; implementation of the information system "emergency (ambulance) medical care"; implementation of the integrated information system "radiology (PACS)"; creation and implementation of the integrated information system "laboratory"; formation of a catalog of electronic clinical protocols; the introduction of an online platform for tracking the quality of medical care; and the development of telemedicine technologies and distance education.

At the same time, effective digitalization demands appropriate institutional, legal, and infrastructural conditions. In spite of the efforts by governments in digitalization of health sector, there are still a number of issues in the development of management information systems and digital health such as lack of appropriate legislation to ensure the effective implementation of HMIS, e-health, digital health, and telemedicine. The majority of the countries are facing difficulties in building the Internet infrastructure and finding the required employees with the necessary experience. One of the most pressing issues in health information technology is analyzing and adopting national health data standards. The information technology and communication infrastructure is underdeveloped, underfunded, and unevenly distributed. These countries are at the initial stage of digitalization and a lot of issues must be addressed in order to improve this process and increase the efficiency of the health sector. The possibilities for applying AI in healthcare will greatly expand when these issues are resolved, and the quality of healthcare services will improve as a result.

REFERENCES

Arslanova, N. 2021. PROFIT Healthcare Day 2021: digital life—digital health (цифровой жизни—цифровое здоровье) (in Russian). Accessed at https://profit.kz/news/61992/PROFIT-Healthcare-Day-2021-cifrovoj-zhizni-cifrovoe-zdorove/ (on May 23, 2023).

Azizov, Abdulla. 2021. Digitalization in healthcare: transparent, high quality, reliable (Цифровизация в здравоохранении: прозрачно, качественно, надежно) (in Russian). Accessed at https://ssv.uz/ru/news/tsifrovizatsija-v-zdravoo-hranenii-prozrachno-kachestvenno-nadezhno- (on May 20, 2023).

Concept for the development of health care in the Republic of Kazakhstan until 2026. 2022. Resolution of the Government of the Republic of Kazakhstan,

November 24, No. 945 (in Russian). Accessed at https://adilet.zan.kz/rus/docs/P2200000945 (on May 23, 2023).

Decree of the President of the Republic of Uzbekistan. 2021. On approval of the strategy "Digital Uzbekistan—2030" and measures for its effective implementation (in Russian). Accessed at https://lex.uz/docs/5031048?ON DATE2=30.11.2021&action=compare (on May 23, 2023).

Dialog. 2019. Healthcare in Tajikistan goes digital (in Russian). Accessed at https://www.dialog.tj/news/zdravookhranenie-v-tadzhikistane-perekhodit-v-tsifrovoj-format (on May 18, 2023).

Digital Kazakhstan state program. 2017. Decree of the Government of the Republic of Kazakhstan, dated December 12, No. 827 (in Russian). Accessed at https://adilet.zan.kz/rus/docs/P1700000827 (May 22, 2023).

Hakimov, F. 2023. National strategies for digitalization of Central Asian states: challenges and opportunities (Национальные Стратегии Цифровизации Государств Центральной Азии: Вызовы и Возможности) (in Russian). Accessed at https://cabar.asia/wp-content/uploads/2022/10/Policy-Brief_Digitalization_ru_1910.pdf (on May 25, 2023).

KABAR (Kyrgyz National News Agency). 2022. What digital projects have been implemented in the field of healthcare in Kyrgyzstan (in Russian). Accessed at https://kabar.kg/news/kakie-tcifrovye-proekty-realizovany-v-oblasti-zdravookhraneniia-v-kyrgyzstane/ (on May 20, 2023).

Ministry of Economy and Commerce of the Kyrgyz Republic. 2018. National development strategy of The Kyrgyz Republic for 2018–2040 (Национальная Стратегия Развития Кыргызской Республики на 2018-2040 годы) (in Russian). Accessed at https://mineconom.gov.kg/storage/directs/documents/209/15421950795bec078718fff.pdf (on May 5, 2023).

Ministry of Higher Education, Science and Innovations of the Republic of Uzbekistan. 2023. Uzbekistan develops the first turbine ventilator controlled by artificial intelligence (В Узбекистане разрабатывают первый турбинный аппарат ИВЛ под управлением искусственного интеллекта) (in Russian). Accessed at https://aktualno.uz/ru/news/9332 (on May 22, 2023).

National Chamber of Innovative Healthcare. 2023. Accessed at https://uz.sputniknews.ru/20210115/V-Uzbekistane-zapustyat-kazakhstanskiy-proekt-po-bystroy-diagnostike-insulta-15796474.html (on May 22, 2023).

Presidential Decree of February 8, 2021 UP No. 23. On urgent measures to develop the healthcare sector and improve the quality of life and health of the population in the Kyrgyz Republic, https://cbd.minjust.gov.kg/430379/edition/1040960/ru, Retrieved at: 15.07.2023

Resolution of the President of the Republic of Uzbekistan. 2021. On measures to create conditions for the accelerated implementation of artificial intelligence technologies (in Russian), dated February 17. Accessed at https://president.uz/ru/lists/view/4195 (on May 23, 2023).

Rizoev, M. 2019. http://www.polit-asia.kz/kazahstan-pomozhet-v-czifroizaczii-zdravoohraneniya-tadjhijistana/ (accessed on May 17, 2023).

Sarymsakova, Julia. 2021. Artificial intelligence: a legal platform for development (Искусственный интеллект: правовая платформа для развития) (in Russian).

Accessed at https://yuz.uz/ru/news/iskusstvenny-intellekt-pravovaya-platforma-dlya-razvitiya (on May 20, 2023).

SPUTNIK Uzbekistan. 2023. accessed at https://uz.sputniknews.ru/20210115/V-Uzbekistane-zapustyat-kazakhstanskiyproekt-po-bystroy-diagnostike-insulta-15796474.html (on May 22, 2023).

The Government of the Kyrgyz Republic. 2019. Order of the Government of the Kyrgyz Republic dated February 15, 2019 No. 20 On approval of the "Road Map" for the implementation of the Concept of digital transformation "Digital Kyrgyzstan 2019-2023", https://cbd.minjust.gov.kg/216896/edition/1118030/ru

UNICEF. 2022. UNICEF: Telemedicine is being introduced in Kyrgyzstan as part of the digitalization of the healthcare system (Кыргызстане внедряется телемедицина в рамках цифровизации системы здравоохранения) (in Russian). Accessed at https://www.unicef.org/kyrgyzstan/ru/%D0%9F%D1%80%D0%B5%D1%81%D1%81-%D1%80%D0%B5%D0%BB%D0%B8%D0%B7%D1%8B/%D0%B2-%D0%BA%D1%8B%D1%80%D0%B3%D1%8B%D0%B7%D1%81%D1%82%D0%B0%D0%BD%D0%B5-%D0%B2%D0%BD%D0%B5%D0%B4%D1%80%D1%8F%D0%B5%D1%82%D1%81%D1%8F-%D1%82%D0%B5%D0%BB%D0%B5%D0%BC%D0%B5%D0%B4%D0%B8%D1%86%D0%B8%D0%BD%D0%B0-%D0%B2-%D1%80%D0%B0-%D0%BC%D0%BA%D0%B0%D1%85-%D1%86%D0%B8%D1%84%D1%80%D0%BE%D0%B2%D0%B8%D0%B7%D0%B0%D1%86%D0%B8%D0%B8-%D1%81%D0%B8%D1%81%D1%82%D0%B5%D0%BC%D1%8B-%D0%B7-%D0%B4%D1%80%D0%B0%D0%B2%D0%BE%D0%BE%D1%85%D1%80%D0%B0%D0%BD%D0%B5%D0%BD%D0%B8%D1%8F (on May 15, 2023).

World Health Organization. 2020. Health-related SDG targets in Tajikistan: implementation of policies and measures to achieve the SDG health-related targets. Copenhagen: WHO Regional Office for Europe; https://cdn.who.int/media/docs/librariesprovider2/default-document-library/health-related-sdg-targets-in-tajikistan-eng.pdf?sfvrsn=58de0867_4&download=true Retrieved at: 17.07.2023.

Yangi Uzbekiston. 2023. 50.5 million euros will be allocated for the digitalization of healthcare in Uzbekistan (На цифровизацию здравоохранения Узбекистана направят 50,5 млн евро) (in Russian). Accessed at https://yuz.uz/ru/news/na-tsifrovizatsiyu-zdravooxraneniya-uzbekistana-napravyat-505-mln-evro (on May 20, 2023).

Zdrav. 2021. The Celsus AI system for processing radiological images will be implemented in the medical centers of Uzbekistan (ИИ-систему обработки радиологических изображений «Цельс» внедрят в медцентрах Узбекистана) (in Russian). Accessed at https://zdrav.expert/a/636433 (on May 22, 2023).

Chapter 4

Artificial Intelligence–based Health Data

Kamil Akarsu*[,1], Ourania Areta Hiziroglu[2] and Orhan Er[3]

[1]Computer Engineering Department, Izmir Bakircay University, Izmir Türkiye
ORCID: 0000-0001-7715-2801; Email: kamilakarsu94@gmail.com
[2]Management Information Systems Department,
Izmir Bakircay University, Izmir Türkiye
ORCID: 0000-0001-8607-6089; Email: ourania.areta@bakircay.edu.tr
[3]Computer Engineering Department, Izmir Bakircay University, Izmir Türkiye
ORCID: 0000-0002-4732-9490; Email: orhan.er@bakircay.edu.tr

INTRODUCTION

Importance of Health Data

Data regarding people's health and medical services is referred to as health data. It can originate from many different places, including hospitals, clinics, labs, and health insurance providers (Zhang et al. 2023); see Figure 4.1.

The capacity of health data to enhance health outcomes and influence public health policy is what makes it so significant. The following are some applications of health data:

- **Clinical decision-making:** Healthcare professionals use health data to guide clinical decisions. Important details concerning

---

*For Correspondence: Kamil Akarsu (kamilakarsu94@gmail.com)

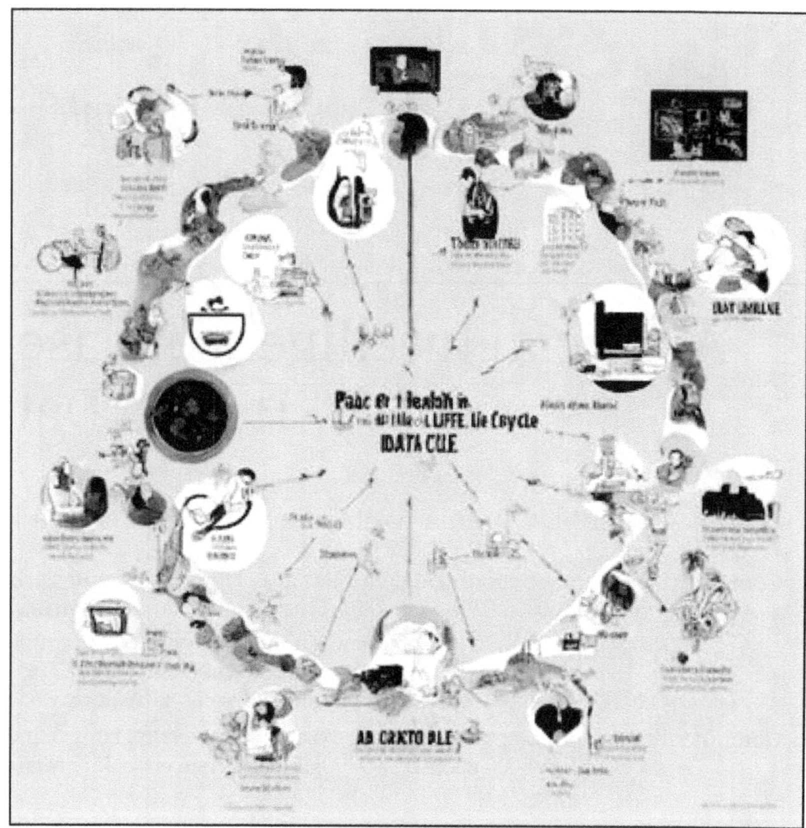

Figure 4.1 Place of health data in the life cycle.
Source: Prepared by the authors.

medical history, present symptoms, and previous therapies can be found in patient health records. To create individualized treatment programs and enhance patient results, this data can be employed.

- **Public health surveillance:** Health information is also used to keep tabs on epidemics and disease outbreaks. This knowledge aids public health professionals in identifying possible population hazards and taking the necessary precautions to stop the spread of infectious illnesses.

- **Medical research and innovation:** Health information is used to create novel cures and treatments. Researchers can identify risk factors for specific diseases and create more effective interventions by examining patterns and trends in health data.

- **Resource distribution:** Health information can also be utilized to more efficiently distribute healthcare resources. Policymakers can direct resources where they are most needed by knowing which populations are more susceptible to specific ailments.

- **Health policy:** Decisions on national, state, and local health policies are based on health data. This data is essential for creating policies that increase access to care, advance health equity, and lower the cost of healthcare.

In conclusion, health data is an essential part of contemporary healthcare systems. It helps public health officials track epidemics and disease outbreaks, lets healthcare professionals make knowledgeable clinical decisions, and influences medical research and innovation. Health data is crucial for resource allocation and health policy decisions as well, which will ultimately lead to better individual and population health outcomes (Shen et al. 2019).

Data Privacy and Security

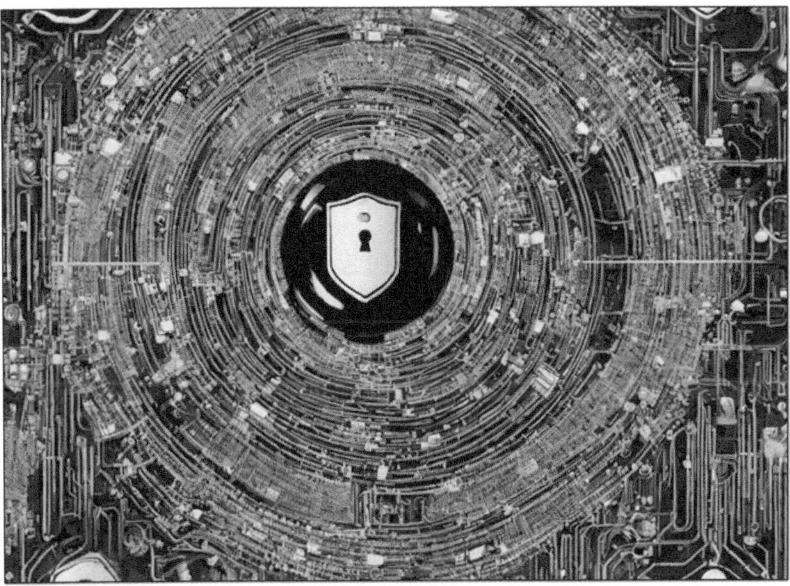

Figure 4.2   Data privacy and security.
Source: Prepared by the authors.

Privacy and security are critical components of any modern system in today's digital world (Gong and Schroeder 2022), see Figure 4.2. Sensitive data must be protected from unwanted access, theft, or misuse more than ever as the volume of data generated and gathered grows exponentially.

The ability of people or organizations to manage who has access to their personal data is referred to as data privacy. Sensitive information like financial data, medical records, or online activity can fall under this category. Many international laws and rules, such the California Consumer Privacy Act (CCPA) and the General Data Protection Regulation (GDPR) of the European Union, defend the right to privacy.

There are several reasons why privacy is vital. It aids in defending people against financial fraud, identity theft, and other types of cybercrime. Additionally, it gives users control over their personal data, empowering them to decide how their data is shared and used.

Data security is the term used to describe the steps taken to guard against unauthorized access, theft, or misuse of data. This can involve both technical and physical security measures such as encryption, firewalls, and access controls, as well as locks, cameras, and alarms (Gupta et al. 2023).

Because it aids in preventing data breaches, cyberattacks, and other security concerns, data security is crucial. Additionally, it helps minimize the risk of data loss or theft by ensuring that critical information is available only to authorized individuals.

There are several best practices that individuals and organizations can follow to ensure data privacy and security:

- **Strong passwords:** For all accounts, including online banking, email, and social media, use strong passwords. An effective password should include at least eight characters and include capital and lowercase letters, numbers, and symbols.

- **Two-factor authentication:** Whenever possible, enable two-factor authentication (2FA). By requiring a second form of authentication in addition to a password, such as a code texted to a mobile device, 2FA adds an extra layer of security.

- Use encryption to safeguard sensitive data both in transit and at rest. Data is encrypted so that only authorized users with the proper decryption key may decode and read it.

- **Regular updates:** Always use the most recent security patches and upgrades to keep all software and firmware current. Cybercriminals may be able to use weaknesses in outdated software.

- **Train employees:** Train employees on privacy and security best practices, including how to spot phishing emails, create strong passwords, and handle sensitive information.

- **Data backups:** Regularly create backup copies of vital data to fend off theft or loss. Backups should be kept in a safe area with only authorized employees being able to access them.

Data security and privacy are essential elements of any contemporary digital system. It is more crucial than ever to guard against unauthorized access, theft, or misuse of sensitive information. Individuals and businesses can contribute to ensuring data privacy and security by adhering to best practices, such as choosing strong passwords, enabling 2FA, and staying current.

Artificial Intelligence and Health Data

Health data and artificial intelligence (AI) are linked and closely related. In order to enhance patient outcomes, recognize illness trends, and create new treatments, AI systems in the healthcare industry rely heavily on health data as a training set. They can generate predictions using the data to develop insights, spot patterns, and enhance patient outcomes. In other words, for AI systems to be useful and effective in the healthcare sector, they need access to health data (Ortega-Calvo et al. 2023).

Every day, the healthcare sector produces enormous volumes of data, including patient-generated data from wearables and other devices, genomic data, electronic health records (EHRs), and medical pictures. AI systems can analyze this data and find patterns, links, and insights that human analysts would not instantly notice (Bag et al. 2023).

To discover disease or abnormalities that human radiologists might overlook, for instance, AI algorithms can be trained on enormous databases of medical pictures. Additionally, they can examine patient information to find risk factors for certain illnesses or ailments and suggest treatments or preventative actions.

The application of AI in medication development is another example. With massive molecular datasets, AI algorithms can be trained to find prospective medication candidates and forecast their efficacy and safety. This could hasten the discovery of new drugs and the release of new treatments

Health data and AI work harmoniously together. Health data is required for AI systems to be useful in the healthcare sector, and AI is required for health data to reach its full potential for enhancing patient outcomes and advancing medical research.

DATA ANONYMIZATION

Anonymization is a data processing technique that removes or alters identifying information, resulting in anonymous data that cannot be associated with any individual. Data anonymization is performed on user data to prevent the disclosure of identity information and sensitive data of data owners present in shared large datasets, to protect their privacy, and to prevent all kinds of attacks that can be made on data owners, as shown in Figure 4.3.

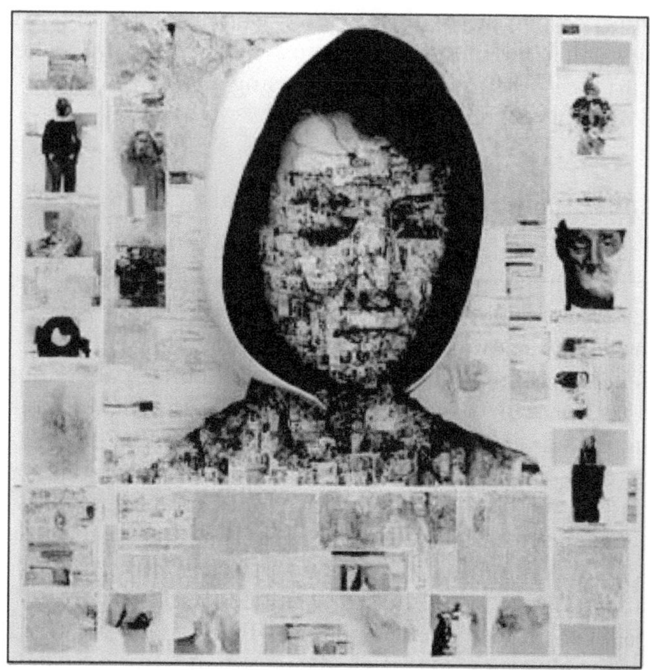

Figure 4.3. Example of data anonymization.
Source: Prepared by the authors.

By analyzing anonymized data, secure and valuable products and features can be created. At the same time, many organizations can securely share anonymized data externally, allowing others to benefit without compromising user privacy.

The anonymization process protects data without changing its type or format. The primary goal of this process is to make data shareable. However, the detection of individual identities through various applications such as computational techniques and background context methods in shared data is a significant problem.

Deliberate actions that result in a breach of anonymity are referred to as "anonymity attacks". In this context, the risk of undoing anonymized personal data through various interventions and returning the anonymized data to an identifiable and distinctive state for real individuals should be investigated and addressed accordingly.

Data Anonymization Techniques

Anonymization is the transformation process on semi-identifying attributes by privacy models to prevent the disclosure of data containing identity and sensitive information. These operations make it difficult to expose the identity information and sensitive data of the data owners present in shared large datasets, while preserving the type and form of the data.

Performing anonymization with an acceptable level of data loss is important in terms of the benefit obtained from big data. An increase in data losses can reduce data quality, leading to a decrease or even complete elimination of the benefit obtained from shared big data.

Different definitions have been made for the concept of anonymization, such as modifying or removing the structure and form of sensitive data while preserving it and hiding privacy-sensitive data.

The primary purpose of the anonymization process is to make the data shareable for various value-added purposes. Big data applications involving data sharing can also bring along privacy violations. Although big data may seem complex, the identity of the data owner or sensitive data can be exposed through various privacy-focused attacks.

There are various anonymization techniques and solutions aimed at protecting data privacy. Fundamentally, these techniques provide protection against record linkage, attribute linkage, table linkage, and probabilistic attacks.

Some commonly used techniques for anonymizing data include:

Data Masking: This is the method of hiding data with modified values. Encryption, tokenization, blurring, shuffling, and invalidation are some of the most used methods in data masking. In data masking, the data format is not changed, only the values are altered; however, this change should be done in such a way that it cannot be detected and reversed. For example, a character value can be replaced with a symbol like "*" or "x". Data masking makes reverse engineering or detection impossible. Any properly implemented method is sufficient for the security of personal data in institutions. Data masking can be done in five different ways:

- Static data masking
- Dynamic data masking
- On-the-fly data masking
- Deterministic data masking
- Statistical data masking

Pseudonymization: This is a data management and identification method that replaces specific identifiers with fake identifiers or pseudonyms, such as changing the identifier "Levent KARTAL" to "Mert DEMİR". Pseudonymization allows the altered data to be used for training, development, testing, and analytics while maintaining statistical accuracy and data integrity, and it protects data privacy. In this process, the sensitive data referred to as a pseudonym is replaced with a fake string. The obtained string is used in a way that will always be the same for the same input. This is done with a hidden key, and only those who know this key can obtain the original data. To enhance data security, this secret key should also be changed periodically.

Generalization: This is the method of intentionally removing some data to make it less identifiable. For example, it is important not to remove the street name when removing the building number from an address. The goal here is to eliminate some identifiers while maintaining the measure of data accuracy. Also, with this method, the values in some fields are replaced with a broader category. For example, generalization can be done by changing the value in the height field to "$\geq$170 cm" or "180 cm $\geq$ height $\geq$160 cm". This change is permanent in sensitive data and is an irreversible process.

Data Swapping: Also known as shuffling and permutation, this is a technique used to rearrange dataset attribute values in a way that will not correspond to the original records. For example, data containing identifier values such as birth date (columns) may have more impact on anonymization than membership type values.

Data Perturbation: This is the method of slightly altering the original dataset by applying techniques that round numbers and add random noise. The value range should be proportional to the distortion. A small base lead to weak anonymization, while a large base can reduce the benefit of the dataset. For example, you can use a base of 5 to round values like age or house number, which is proportional to the original value. You can multiply a building number by 15, and the value can retain its reliability. However, using higher bases like 15 can make age values appear fake.

Synthetic Data: This is the method of using algorithmically generated information with no connection to real events. Synthetic data is used to create artificial datasets instead of modifying or using the original dataset as it is, which could put privacy and security at risk. The process involves creating statistical models based on patterns found in the original dataset. Standard deviations, medians, linear regression, or other statistical techniques can be used to create synthetic data (Kilic et al. 2023).

SYNTHETIC DATA GENERATION

Synthetic Data Concept and Purpose

In the idea of synthetic data, data that has been intentionally made to resemble real-world data is produced, but it is exempt from personally identifiable information (PII). A secure and privacy-preserving substitute for real-world data, which may be sensitive and contain PII that needs to be secured, is what synthetic data is meant to do (Alqudah et al. 2023).

Statistical algorithms and machine learning models are used to create synthetic data, which is created by learning patterns and relationships from existing data and then creating new data based on those patterns. Although statistically similar to real data, the produced data does not include any PII.

There are several advantages to using synthetic data (Murtaza et al. 2023a). It can be used, for instance, to expand currently available datasets or produce whole new datasets that can be used to train machine learning models without jeopardizing the privacy of real-world data. Additionally, without compromising patient privacy, it can be used to create datasets for research and development as well as to test the effectiveness of algorithms and software programs in a controlled setting.

Organizations are increasingly turning to synthetic data as a solution to secure sensitive information while still allowing for useful research. The privacy of personal data is especially crucial in sectors like healthcare and banking.

The idea of synthetic data is an excellent tool for data science and analytics because it offers a safe and private alternative to real-world data while still enabling accurate and successful analysis (Pathare et al. 2023).

Synthetic Data Generation Methods

The process of generating synthetic data can vary depending on the method used, but generally involves the following steps (Zhou and Chiam 2023):

- **Define the data requirements:** The first step is to define the data requirements, such as data types, format, and size. This step is important to ensure that the synthetic data meets the needs of the application.

- **Collect and pre-process the source data:** The next step is to collect the source data, which may be in the form of raw data, a dataset, or a database. The source data may need to be pre-processed to remove sensitive information or outliers that could affect the quality of the synthetic data.

- **Select a method for generating synthetic data:** The next step is to select a synthetic data generation method that is appropriate for the data requirements and application. The choice of method will depend on factors such as data types, complexity, and privacy requirements.

- **Train the synthetic data generation model:** If the chosen method requires a model to be trained, the next step is to train the model using the source data. This step may involve selecting appropriate parameters or hyperparameters and tuning the model to achieve the desired performance.

- **Generate the synthetic data:** Once the model has been trained, the next step is to generate the synthetic data. This may involve sampling from a distribution defined by the model, simulating a real system, or using a machine learning model to generate new data.

- **Evaluate the quality of the synthetic data:** The final step is to evaluate the quality of the synthetic data to ensure that it meets the data requirements and is suitable for the application. This may involve comparing the statistical properties of the synthetic data with the source data, evaluating the performance of machine learning models trained on the synthetic data, or other methods.

Overall, generating synthetic data can be a challenging operation that calls for careful consideration of each application's needs and the data's requirements. Synthetic data that is suitable for a variety of applications can be created by following a method in a way that preserves people's and organizations' privacy.

Parametric Modeling

A technique for creating synthetic data using statistical models that have been trained on real data is known as parametric modeling. The synthetic data is created using a set of parameters in parametric modeling that specify the statistical characteristics of the data (Hernandez et al. 2022).

The process of parametric modeling involves first fitting a statistical model to the existing data. This model can be a simple distribution model, such as a Gaussian or Poisson distribution, or a more complex model, such as a multivariate regression model or a neural network.

By selecting samples from the model's stated distribution, the model can be used to generate new synthetic data once it has been trained. The model's parameters, such as the mean and variance of a Gaussian distribution, can be changed to affect the features of the synthetic data.

Parametric modeling has several advantages over other methods of generating synthetic data. First, it enables a great deal of control over the properties of the generated data, making it appropriate for tasks like testing machine learning models or creating training datasets. Second, compared to other techniques like simulation-based techniques or generative adversarial networks (GANs), it may be more computationally efficient. Last, but not least, parametric modeling can be used to create fake data for a variety of data types, including continuous, discrete, and categorical data.

An effective method to generate synthetic data that may be applied in many different contexts is parametric modeling. Synthetic data can support research and development in fields like healthcare, finance, and the social sciences while safeguarding the privacy of people and organizations by offering a safe and privacy-preserving substitute to real-world data.

Generative Adversarial Networks (GANs)

Synthetic health data can also be produced using GANs. Health information that is artificially manufactured rather than gathered from actual patients is referred to as synthetic health data (Qiu et al. 2023). GANs can be used to generate synthetic health data by training a generator network to produce data samples that resemble real health data, while simultaneously training a discriminator network to discriminate between the real health data and the synthetic data produced by the generator.

The generator network can be trained on a variety of health data types, such as EHRs, medical images, and physiological signals. The generator can produce synthetic health data samples that resemble the real data, while the discriminator evaluates these samples and attempts to distinguish between real and synthetic data (Yilmaz and Korn 2022). Through this adversarial training process, the generator learns to produce synthetic health data that is increasingly similar to the real health data.

The GAN-generated synthetic health data can be helpful in a variety of contexts. For instance, it can be used to supplement genuine health data while maintaining privacy when training machine learning models. The privacy of actual patients can be maintained while allowing the machine learning model to gain knowledge from a larger and more varied set of data by employing synthetic health data. In order to imitate uncommon or complex medical problems that are challenging to record in real-world data, synthetic health data can also be used. This can aid in the better understanding of these disorders and the creation of more efficient remedies by researchers and physicians. However, before being used in clinical applications, synthetic data must be validated and vetted to guarantee its correctness and dependability.

Variational Autoencoders (VAEs)

Variational autoencoders (VAEs) can also be used to generate synthetic health data (Fei et al. 2023). Health information that is artificially created rather than obtained from actual patients is referred to as synthetic health data. By training a VAE to map genuine health data samples onto a lower-dimensional latent space and then creating fresh synthetic health data samples by sampling from the learned latent space distribution, VAEs can be used to create synthetic health data.

Real health data samples are transformed by the VAE's encoder network into a representation in a lower-dimensional latent space, which is subsequently transformed back into the original data space by the decoder network. While regularizing the learned latent space distribution to adhere to a prior distribution, often a standard normal distribution, the VAE learns to minimize the difference between the input data and the reconstructed data. Then, new synthetic health data samples that closely mirror the genuine data can be created by sampling this regularized latent space distribution.

There are several uses for the synthetic health data that VAE generates. For instance, it can be used to augment real health data while maintaining privacy when training machine learning models. The privacy of real patients can be preserved while allowing the machine learning model to gain knowledge from a larger and more varied set of data by employing synthetic health data. Additionally, rare or complex medical diseases that are challenging to capture in real-world data can be simulated using synthetic health data (Caciularu and Goldberger 2023). This may help in the better understanding of these disorders and the creation of more efficient solutions by researchers and medical professionals. However, before being used in clinical applications, synthetic health data must be validated and checked to guarantee its correctness and dependability.

Synthetic Data Applications and Usage Areas

Synthetic data has many applications and uses (as shown in Figure 4.4) in various industries, including healthcare (Yale et al. 2020). Synthetic data is artificially generated data that mimics the statistical properties of real-world data but does not contain PII.

Here are some examples of synthetic data applications and uses:

- **Privacy-preserving machine learning:** Synthetic data can be used to train machine learning models while protecting the privacy of individuals. By using synthetic data instead of real data, organizations can reduce the risk of data breaches and ensure compliance with privacy regulations such as GDPR and the Health Insurance Portability and Accountability Act (HIPAA).

- **Data augmentation:** Synthetic data can be used to increase the size and diversity of datasets used to train machine learning models. This can improve the accuracy and generalization of machine learning models, especially when real data is limited or expensive to obtain.

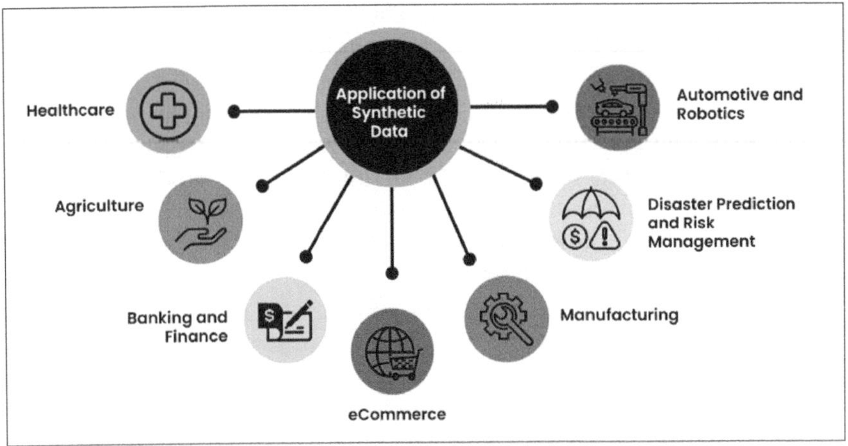

Figure 4.4 Examples of synthetic data applications and uses.
Source: Saherwardi (2023).

- **Simulation and testing:** Synthetic data can be used to simulate rare or complex events that are difficult to observe in real data. This can be useful for testing and evaluating machine learning models in a controlled environment.

- **Fraud detection:** Synthetic data can be used to create realistic fraud scenarios for testing and training fraud detection algorithms.

- **Health data generation:** Synthetic data can be used in healthcare to generate health data patterns for research and development purposes. This can include the generation of synthetic EHRs, medical images, and physiological signals.

Synthetic data can be very helpful in the healthcare industry for generating innovative medical treatments and training machine learning models while maintaining patient privacy. Researchers and doctors can create more precise and efficient medical therapies while lowering the chance of disclosing patients' private health information by employing synthetic data. However, before being used in clinical applications, synthetic health data must be validated and vetted to guarantee its correctness and dependability.

Benefits and Challenges of Synthetic Data Generation

Synthetic data generation has many potential advantages, including privacy protection, cost-effectiveness, diversity, and scalability (Murtaza et al. 2023a). But it also has serious problems with validity, prejudice, and context, among other things. The effectiveness of creating synthetic data depends on careful planning, choosing the right methodologies, and validation, just like with other data-related work.

Its benefits are (Rajotte et al. 2022):

- **Privacy protection:** Synthetic data generation enables organizations to protect sensitive personal information while still providing realistic data for analysis and modeling. This is particularly important in industries such as healthcare, finance, and telecommunications where privacy regulations are strict and data breaches can be costly.

- **Cost-effective:** Synthetic data generation can be a cost-effective alternative to collecting and storing large amounts of real-world data. This is especially true when data is difficult or expensive to obtain.

- **Diversity:** Synthetic data generation can provide a wider range of data than is typically available in real-world datasets. This can lead to more robust and accurate models.

- **Scalability:** Synthetic data generation can produce large amounts of data quickly, making it easier to train and test machine learning models.

Its challenges are (Carvajal-Patiño and Ramos-Pollán 2022):

- **Quality:** Synthetic data must be of sufficient quality to be useful for modeling and analysis. This requires careful selection of modeling techniques and validation methods to ensure that the data is realistic and representative of real-world data.

- **Validation:** Synthetic data generation requires validation to ensure that the data is accurate and useful for the intended application. This can be challenging, especially if the real-world data is complex or poorly understood.

- **Bias:** Synthetic data generation can introduce bias if the models used to generate the data are biased. Careful selection of models and validation methods can help mitigate this risk.

- **Limited context:** Synthetic data may not capture the same context or complexity as real-world data. This may limit the usefulness of synthetic data for certain applications.

AI AND HEALTH DATA

Application of AI Algorithms to Health Data

Algorithms based on AI are being utilized more often in the healthcare sector to analyze patient data, enhance patient outcomes, and streamline healthcare delivery (O'Connor amd Booth 2022). AI methods like machine learning and deep learning may analyze vast volumes of data and find patterns, links, and insights that people would not instantly see.

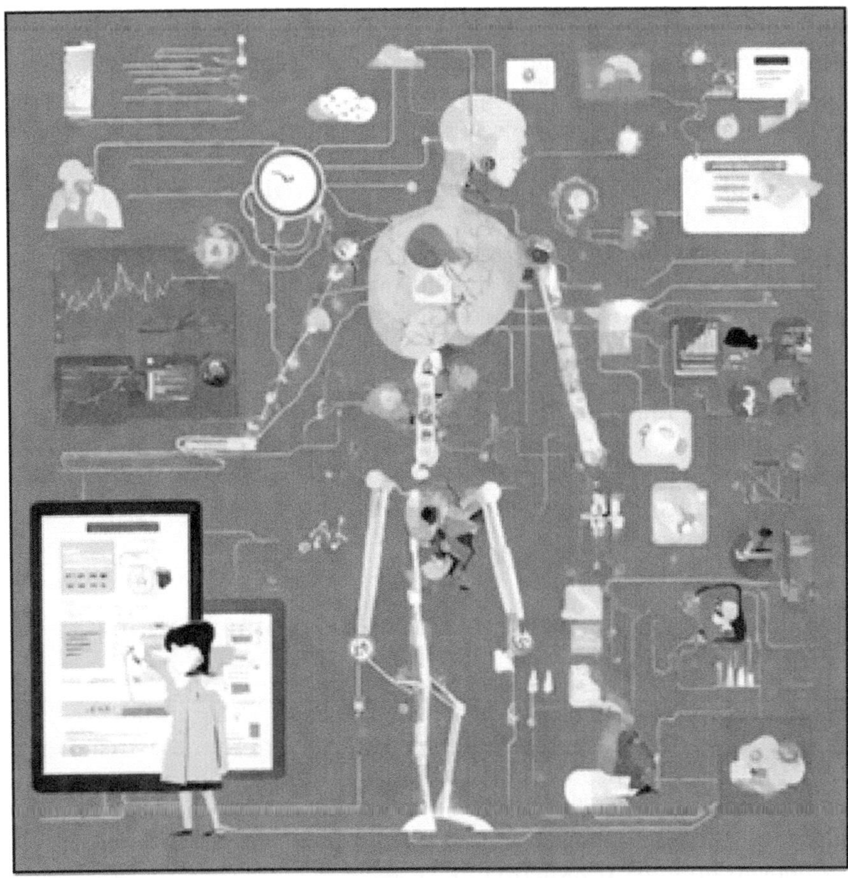

Figure 4.5   Artificial intelligence and health data.
Source: Prepared by the authors.

The diagnosis and prognosis of diseases is one area in which AI algorithms are being used. Machine learning algorithms can assist healthcare professionals in the diagnosis and prediction of diseases by analyzing medical pictures, lab test results, and patient health information. Early discovery and treatment may result from this, improving patient outcomes (Marino et al. 2023).

Additionally, individualized treatment regimens are being developed for patients using AI algorithms. AI can assist medical professionals in developing a treatment plan that is suited to each patient's specific requirements by analyzing a patient's medical history, genetics, and lifestyle factors. This can increase the efficacy of the medication and lower the possibility of side effects.

AI is employed in medication discovery in addition to diagnosis and treatment. AI algorithms can forecast the effectiveness and safety of future pharmaceuticals by analyzing enormous datasets of molecular structures, which expedites the drug discovery process.

Medical research is another area of healthcare where AI is being applied. AI can assist researchers in finding potential correlations and trends by analyzing vast amounts of medical data that would be challenging for humans to notice. This may result in fresh perceptions and medical breakthroughs.

Finally, AI-powered virtual assistants are being created to support patients, keep track of their health, and remind users to take their medications. As a result, patients may be more engaged and likely to follow treatment programs.

Healthcare could be transformed by AI, but there are also ethical issues that need to be resolved. It is crucial to guarantee the confidentiality and privacy of patient data as well as the impartiality and lack of discrimination of AI algorithms. AI is an attractive field of medical research because it has the potential to enhance healthcare outcomes and save costs.

Disease Diagnosis and Treatment Recommendations with AI

Healthcare professionals are increasingly using AI algorithms to help in disease diagnosis and the prescription of appropriate treatments. Large volumes of health data, such as lab test results, patient health records, and medical photographs, can be analyzed by machine learning algorithms to find patterns and associations that may not be immediately evident to humans (Kakileti et al. 2020).

AI algorithms can assist healthcare professionals in diagnosing diseases more quickly and accurately. For instance, machine learning algorithms can analyze medical photos and spot disease symptoms that may be difficult for people to see. This could result in earlier disease detection and treatment, which would benefit patients.

AI can also be used to personalize a patient's course of therapy. For instance, based on a patient's genetic profile, AI algorithms can determine which treatments are most likely to be beneficial for them.

AI algorithms can also assist medical professionals in monitoring a patient's condition and recommending treatments (Dragoni et al. 2023). AI, for instance, can analyze patient health data to spot potential health hazards and notify healthcare professionals about them. This can assist medical professionals in making better treatment decisions and enhancing patient outcomes.

While AI algorithms can be quite accurate in identifying diseases and recommending treatments, it is crucial to remember that they should not take the place of human expertise and judgment. The final diagnosis and recommended course of treatment must still be determined by the healthcare provider, notwithstanding the use of AI algorithms to aid in decision-making. When applying AI algorithms in healthcare, it is also important to keep ethical issues like bias and patient privacy in mind.

Personalized Medicine and AI

In the field of personalized medicine, where medical care is tailored to each patient's unique traits, AI algorithms are being employed more frequently. AI algorithms can assist healthcare professionals in developing individualized treatment plans by analyzing vast volumes of health data, including medical records, genetic information, and lifestyle factors (Khan et al. 2020).

The detection of biomarkers is one application of AI in personalized medicine. Medical professionals can create treatment plans that are specifically suited to the needs of a patient by finding the biomarkers that are particular to that patient. Biomarkers are quantifiable indications of a disease or health condition.

Drug discovery is another area of personalized medicine where AI is being employed. Large databases of molecular structures can be analyzed by AI systems to forecast the effectiveness and safety of future medications (Al-Medfa et al. 2023). Healthcare professionals can increase treatment efficacy and lower the risk of adverse events by developing customized pharmacological treatments based on each patient's unique genetic composition and other features.

AI can also be used to spot potential drug interactions and side effects that could be harmful. AI algorithms can assist healthcare professionals in determining which medications are most likely to be beneficial for a given patient while reducing the possibility of unfavorable drug interactions by analyzing a patient's health data and medication history.

Overall, by developing more efficient and focused treatments, the application of AI in personalized medicine offers the potential to enhance patient outcomes and lower healthcare costs. It is crucial to remember that there are ethical issues, such as bias and patient privacy, that must be taken into account when employing AI in healthcare. Additionally, while AI algorithms can aid healthcare professionals in making more informed decisions, they should not take the place of human judgment and expertise.

REGULATION AND ETHICAL ISSUES

Data Privacy and Security Legislation

In the digital age, where personal data is increasingly being gathered and shared online, privacy and security legislation are crucial issues (Caidi and Ross 2005). Here are some important things to think about:

- Personal information is normally gathered, held, and used in accordance with privacy rules. Names, addresses, phone numbers, email addresses, and social security numbers are among the data included in this.

- The protection of personal information from unauthorized access, use, or disclosure is often governed by data security legislation. This entails actions like data backup, access limits, and encryption.

- The GDPR, which took effect in 2018, is one of the most important pieces of data privacy law in the EU. The GDPR includes stiff penalties for non-compliance and specifies the manner in which personal data must be gathered, stored, and used in the European Union.

- The HIPAA, which outlines criteria for safeguarding the privacy and security of personal health information, is arguably the most significant piece of data security legislation in the US.

- The Children's Online Privacy Protection Act (COPPA), the Electronic Communications Privacy Act (ECPA), and the California Consumer Privacy Act (CCPA) are other significant privacy and security regulations in the US.

- The Privacy Shield pact between the US and the European Union, the Personal Data Protection Act (PDPA) in Singapore, and the General Data Protection Law (LGPD) in Brazil are a few other significant international privacy and security regulations.

- It is crucial to remember that security and privacy laws are always changing as new dangers and technologies appear. In the digital world, securing personal data requires being updated on laws and best practices.

In general, enacting privacy and security laws is essential to safeguarding personal data in the digital age. Particularly when it comes to storing patient health information securely and in accordance with applicable rules and regulations, healthcare providers must take appropriate action.

Ethical Use and Sharing Principles of Synthetic Data

Synthetic data can be utilized to safeguard people's privacy and facilitate more effective analysis, but it is crucial to keep ethical usage and sharing guidelines in mind while working with this kind of data (Bohua et al. 2023).

Making ensuring that synthetic data does not contain any information that could be exploited to identify specific people is a fundamental ethical requirement. To do this, PII including names, addresses, and social security numbers must be deleted or obscured.

Another moral tenet is transparency. Researchers who use synthetic data must be upfront about how it was created and any data constraints. Utilize synthetic data only for research; do not use it for anything else. The synthetic data should not be used for commercial or other reasons, nor should researchers try to re-identify specific persons using it.

Researchers should make sure that access to shared synthetic data is confined to authorized people or organizations and that recipients agree to use the data strictly for study. To make sure that synthetic data adequately reflects real-world data, researchers also need to make sure that it is appropriately tested and reviewed. This includes contrasting the outcomes of analyses using artificial and actual data.

Finally, researchers should think about how their work may affect society and take precautions to lessen any unfavorable repercussions. This entails being open and honest about their processes and findings, as well as considering how their work might influence certain people or groups.

For academics and organizations dealing with this type of data, the ethical usage and sharing of synthetic data is a crucial topic. Researchers can contribute to ensuring the appropriate and open use of synthetic data by adhering to ethical guidelines and best practices.

Different Approaches for Applications in the Private and Public Sectors

Data that is artificially generated but not sourced from actual individuals can mirror real-world data. In the corporate and public sectors of healthcare, synthetic data can be applied in a variety of ways (Goodair and Reeves 2022). Here are some methods for applying fictitious health data in these fields.

Application in the Private Sector

For a variety of purposes in the private sector, such as drug development, medical device testing, and healthcare analytics, synthetic health data is used. The ability of businesses to work with data without jeopardizing individual privacy rights or running the danger of data breaches is one of the main advantages of employing synthetic health data in the private sector.

For instance, without compromising patient privacy, pharmaceutical corporations can create and test new medications using fake health data. Medical device firms can also replicate the effects of their devices on patients using synthetic health data without endangering actual patients.

The development of AI algorithms for the healthcare industry is another private sector use for synthetic health data. Machine learning models can be trained with synthetic health data, enabling businesses to enhance the precision and efficiency of their AI systems. This is especially helpful in fields like medical image analysis, where synthetic health data may be utilized to train AI models to precisely recognize and diagnose medical disorders.

Application in the Public Sector

Synthetic health data can also be applied in the public sector for a variety of purposes, such as epidemiological research, the creation of health policies, and public health initiatives (Dyda et al. 2021). Utilizing synthetic health data in the public sector has several advantages, one of which is that it enables academics to perform studies and analyses without endangering patient privacy or running the risk of data breaches.

For instance, synthetic health data can be used to model the spread of contagious diseases and create countermeasures to epidemics. Additionally, it can be used to analyze population health trends and create public health improvement programs.

The creation of clinical decision support systems is another public sector use for synthetic health data. These algorithms can be trained to generate accurate diagnoses and treatment suggestions using synthetic health data without endangering actual patients.

Though there are numerous potential advantages to using synthetic health data, it is essential to take ethical issues into account. A crucial factor is making sure that artificial health data does not include any information that might be used to identify specific people. Researchers should be open and honest about the limits of the data they use when employing synthetic health data. Additionally, it is recommended that artificial health data be utilized for research and not for other purposes.

Researchers should make sure that access to shared synthetic health data is confined to authorized parties and that these parties agree to use the data strictly for study when they provide it. To make sure that synthetic health data accurately represents real-world data, researchers also need to ensure that it is appropriately tested and assessed.

This includes contrasting the outcomes of analyses performed using artificial and actual health data.

Overall, there are numerous possible uses for synthetic health data in both the public and private sectors. Researchers and organizations can contribute to ensuring that synthetic health data is utilized in a responsible and transparent manner by adhering to ethical principles and best practices.

FUTURE PERSPECTIVES

AI-based Health Data Analysis and Management

In recent years, the use of AI in healthcare has become increasingly common (Grainger 2007). AI algorithms can analyze large amounts of health data to identify patterns and relationships that would be difficult or impossible for humans to detect. This can lead to more accurate diagnoses, personalized treatment plans, and improved patient outcomes.

One of the most important applications of AI in healthcare is the analysis of medical images. AI algorithms can be trained to analyze medical images, such as X-rays and magnetic resonance imaging (MRI), to identify potential areas of concern. This can help radiologists and other healthcare professionals make more accurate and timely diagnoses, leading to earlier treatment and better patient outcomes.

Another application of AI in healthcare is the analysis of EHRs. The EHRs contain a wealth of information about a patient's health, including medical history, diagnoses, medications, and lab test results (Huang et al. 2023). AI algorithms can analyze this data to identify patterns and relationships that can be used to improve patient care. For example, AI algorithms can help identify patients who are at high risk of developing a particular condition, allowing healthcare providers to intervene early and potentially prevent the condition from developing.

AI can also be used to improve the management of healthcare resources. By analyzing data on patient demand and resource availability, AI algorithms can help healthcare providers optimize resource allocation and scheduling, reducing waiting times, and improving the efficiency of healthcare delivery (Onno et al. 2023).

However, the use of AI in healthcare also raises important ethical and privacy concerns. The sensitive nature of health data means that it must be handled with care to protect patient privacy and ensure ethical use. The development of robust data security and privacy policies is therefore critical to the responsible use of AI in healthcare. AI has enormous potential to improve healthcare delivery and patient outcomes, but its use must be guided by careful ethical considerations and a commitment to protecting patient privacy and ensuring responsible use of health data.

The future of Anonymization and Synthetic Data Generation Techniques

As health data becomes more widely available and valuable for research and innovation, there is a growing need for techniques that can ensure the privacy and security of sensitive health information. Anonymization and synthetic data generation are two techniques that can help protect the privacy of health data while still allowing for analysis and research (Kossen et al. 2021).

In the future, the use of these techniques is likely to increase as more data becomes available and privacy concerns become more prominent (Pathare et al. 2023). However, there are likely to be challenges and opportunities as these techniques develop and mature.

One challenge that is likely to arise is the need to balance privacy and utility. While anonymization and synthetic data generation can help protect privacy, they can also reduce the utility of the data for research and analysis. As a result, there may be a need for new techniques that can better balance these competing concerns.

Another challenge is the need for better tools and techniques to evaluate the effectiveness of anonymization and synthetic data generation techniques. As these techniques become more sophisticated and complex, it may be difficult to determine how well they work and whether they actually protect privacy.

On the other hand, there are likely to be opportunities for new and innovative applications of these techniques in healthcare. For example, synthetic data generation could be used to create large datasets for research purposes or to generate simulated data for testing and validation of healthcare applications.

In addition, advances in machine learning and AI are likely to play an important role in the future of anonymization and synthetic data generation. For example, AI algorithms could be used to improve the accuracy and quality of synthetic data generation or to identify potential weaknesses in anonymization techniques.

The future of anonymization and the synthetic generation of health data is likely to be shaped by a combination of challenges and opportunities. As health data continues to play a critical role in research and innovation, it will be important to continue to develop and refine these techniques to ensure that they can meet the evolving needs of patients, researchers, and health professionals (Murtaza et al. 2023b).

New Technologies and Applications

One promising technology is differential privacy, a technique that adds noise to data to protect privacy while still allowing meaningful analysis. Differential privacy has already been applied to health data and has been shown to be effective in protecting privacy while still allowing useful analysis (Rashidi et al. 2022).

Another emerging technology is homomorphic encryption, which allows data to be analyzed without ever being decrypted. This technique could be used to allow the analysis of sensitive healthcare data while keeping the data completely private.

In addition, there are several new applications of synthetic data generation in healthcare. For example, synthetic data could be used to simulate the effects of different treatments or interventions or to generate large datasets for research purposes. Synthetic data could also be used to create realistic patient avatars that could be used to train healthcare professionals or test medical devices and software.

Machine learning and AI are also playing an increasingly important role in anonymization and synthetic data generation (Pollack et al. 2019). AI algorithms have the capacity to enhance the precision and quality of generating synthetic data or to detect potential flaws in anonymization methods.

Many new technologies and applications are emerging in the fields of anonymization and synthetic data generation techniques for health data. As health data becomes more widely available and valuable for research and innovation, it will be important to continue to develop and refine these techniques to ensure that patient privacy is protected while still allowing for meaningful analysis and innovation in healthcare.

RESULT AND CONCLUSION

This chapter has comprehensively examined the importance of health data, the use of AI with health data, and the generation of synthetic data. Health data, which has great potential for improving health outcomes and influencing public health policy, plays a critical role in areas such as clinical decision-making, public health surveillance, medical research and innovation, resource allocation, and health policy.

AI and health data are closely linked to improve patient outcomes, identify disease trends, and develop new treatments. AI algorithms are used in areas such as disease diagnosis and prognosis, personalized treatment planning, drug discovery, and medical research. However, the use of AI in healthcare must be carefully managed to protect patient privacy and ensure ethical use.

Data anonymization and synthetic data generation are important tools to ensure privacy and security. However, effective use of these techniques carries the risk of re-identification and discrimination of anonymized personal data, and this risk needs to be properly addressed.

Finally, the future of health data and AI is constantly evolving with the emergence of new technologies and applications. This offers the opportunity to further develop anonymization and synthetic data generation techniques in the future, and to further expand the potential of health data and AI. However, it is essential that these developments are managed within the framework of ethical principles and the protection of patient privacy.

In conclusion, the exponential growth of health data, combined with advances in AI, presents significant opportunities to transform healthcare delivery, improve patient outcomes, and accelerate medical research. AI techniques, including machine learning and deep learning, can analyze large volumes of health data and uncover patterns and insights that can lead to more accurate diagnoses, personalized treatment plans, and early disease intervention.

At the same time, the creation of synthetic data serves as an innovative approach to maintaining privacy and security in healthcare, allowing researchers and healthcare providers to use data without compromising patient confidentiality.

Despite these challenges, the future is promising. As technology continues to evolve, the potential of health data and AI can be harnessed even further. However, it is paramount that these advances are managed within the framework of ethical principles, data protection regulations, and a deep commitment to patient privacy. As we move forward, a balanced approach that harnesses the potential of these technologies while ensuring the ethical and responsible use of health data will be essential.

REFERENCES

Al-Medfa, M.K., Al-Ansari, A.M.S., Darwish, A.H., Qreeballa, T.A. and Jahrami, H. 2023. Physicians' attitudes and knowledge toward artificial intelligence in medicine: benefits and drawbacks. Heliyon. 9(4): e14744.

Alqudah, R., Al-Mousa, A.A., Hashyeh, Y.A. and Alzaibaq, O.Z. 2023. A systemic comparison between using augmented data and synthetic data as means of enhancing wafermap defect classification. Computers in Industry. 145: 103809.

Bag, S., Dhamija, P., Kumar Singh, R., Sabbir Rahman, M. and Raja Sreedharan, V. 2023. Big data analytics and artificial intelligence technologies based collaborative platform empowering absorptive capacity in health care supply chain: an empirical study. Journal of Business Research. 154: 113315.

Bohua, L., Yuexin, W., Yakun, O., Kunlan, Z., Huan, L. and Ruipeng, L. 2023. Ethical framework on risk governance of synthetic biology. Journal of Biosafety and Biosecurity. 5(2): 45–56.

Caciularu, A. and Goldberger, J. 2023. An entangled mixture of variational autoencoders approach to deep clustering. Neurocomputing. 529: 182–189.

Caidi, N. and Ross, A. 2005. Information rights and national security. Government Information Quarterly. 22(4): 663–684.

Carvajal-Patiño, D. and Ramos-Pollán, R. 2022. Synthetic data generation with deep generative models to enhance predictive tasks in trading strategies. Research in International Business and Finance. 62: 101747.

Dragoni, M., Eccher, C., Ferro, A., Bailoni, T., Maimone, R., Zorzi, A., et al. 2023. Supporting patients and clinicians during the breast cancer care path with AI: the Arianna solution. Artificial Intelligence in Medicine. 138: 102514.

Dyda, A., Purcell, M., Curtis, S., Field, E., Pillai, P., Ricardo, K., et al. 2021. Differential privacy for public health data: an innovative tool to optimize information sharing while protecting data confidentiality. Patterns. 2(12): 100366.

Fei, R., Wan, Y., Hu, B., Li, A. and Li, Q. 2023. A novel network core structure extraction algorithm utilized variational autoencoder for community detection. Expert Systems with Applications. 222: 119775.

Gong, Y. and Schroeder, A. 2022. A systematic literature review of data privacy and security research on smart tourism. Tourism Management Perspectives. 44: 101019.

Goodair, B. and Reeves, A. 2022. Outsourcing health-care services to the private sector and treatable mortality rates in England, 2013–20: an observational study of NHS privatisation. Articles Lancet Public Health. 7: 638–684.

Grainger, D.W. 2007. Peer review as professional responsibility: a quality control system only as good as the participants. Biomaterial. 28(34): 5199–5203.

Gupta, B.B., Gaurav, A. and Panigrahi, K. 2023. Analysis of security and privacy issues of information management of big data in B2B based healthcare systems. Journal of Business Research. 162: 113859.

Hernandez, M., Epelde, G., Alberdi, A., Cilla, R. and Rankin, D. 2022. Synthetic data generation for tabular health records: a systematic review. Neurocomputing. 493: 28–45.

Huang, X., Yang, F., Zheng, J., Feng, C. and Zhang, L. 2023. Personalized human resource management via HR analytics and artificial intelligence: theory and implications. Asia Pacific Management Review. 28(4): 598–610.

Kakileti, S.T., Madhu, H.J., Manjunath, G., Wee, L., Dekker, A. and Sampangi, S. 2020. Personalized risk prediction for breast cancer pre-screening using artificial intelligence and thermal radiomics. Artificial Intelligence in Medicine, 105, 101854.

Khan, O., Badhiwal. J.H., Grasso, G. and Fehlings, M.G. 2020. Use of machine learning and artificial intelligence to drive personalized medicine approaches for spine care. World Neurosurgery. 140: 512–518.

Kilic, F., Korkmaz, M., Er, O. and Altin, C. 2023. A CNN-based novel approach for classification of sacral hiatus with GAN-powered tabular data set.

Elektronika Ir Elektrotechnika, 29(2): 44–53. https://doi.org/10.5755/J02. EIE.33852

Kossen, T., Subramaniam, P., Madai, V.I., Hennemuth, A., Hildebrand, K., Hilbert, A., et al. 2021. Synthesizing anonymized and labeled TOF-MRA patches for brain vessel segmentation using generative adversarial networks. Computers in Biology and Medicine. 131: 104254.

Marino, D., Carlizzi, D.N. and Falcomatà, V. 2023. Artificial intelligence as a disruption technology to build the Harmonic Health Industry. Procedia Computer Science. 217: 1354–1359.

Murtaza, H., Ahmed, M., Farooq Khan, N., Murtaza, G., Zafar, S. and Bano, A. 2023a. Synthetic data generation: state of the art in health care domain. Computer Science Review. 48: 100546.

Murtaza, H., Ahmed, M., Farooq Khan, N., Murtaza, G., Zafar, S. and Bano, A. 2023b. Synthetic data generation: state of the art in health care domain. Computer Science Review. 48: 100546.

O'Connor, S. and Booth, R.G. 2022. Algorithmic bias in health care: opportunities for nurses to improve equality in the age of artificial intelligence. Outlook and Perspectives. 70(6): P780–782.

Onno, J., Khan, A., Daftary, A. and David, P.-M. 2023. Artificial intelligence-based computer aided detection (AI-CAD) in the fight against tuberculosis: effects of moving health technologies in global health. Social Science and Medicine. 327: 115949.

Ortega-Calvo, A.S., Morcillo-Jimenez, R., Fernandez-Basso, C., Gutiérrez-Batista, K., Vila, M.-A. and Martin-Bautista, M.J. 2023. AIMDP: an artificial intelligence modern data platform. Use case for Spanish national health service data silo. Future Generation Computer Systems. 143: 248–264.

Pathare, A., Mangrulkar, R., Suvarna, K., Parekh, A., Thakur, G. and Gawade, A. 2023. Comparison of tabular synthetic data generation techniques using propensity and cluster log metric. International Journal of Information Management Data Insights. 3: 100177.

Pollack, A.H., Simon, T.D., Snyder, J. and Pratt, W. 2019. Creating synthetic patient data to support the design and evaluation of novel health information technology. Journal of Biomedical Informatics. 95: 103201.

Qiu, X., Wang, S. and Chen, K. 2023. A conditional generative adversarial network-based synthetic data augmentation technique for battery state-of-charge estimation. Applied Soft Computing. 142: 110281.

Rajotte, J.-F., Bergen, R., Buckeridge, D.L., Emam, K.E., Ng, R. and Strome, E. 2022. Synthetic data as an enabler for machine learning applications in medicine. iScience. 25: 105331.

Rashidi, H., Khan, I., Dang, L., Albahra, S., Ratan, U., Chadderwal. N., et al. 2022. Prediction of tuberculosis using an automated machine learning platform for models trained on synthetic data. Journal of Pathology Informatics. 13(1): 100172.

Saherwardi, I.A. 2023. Synthetic data. Accessed at https://www.linkedin.com/ pulse/synthetic-data-irfan-azim-saherwardi/(on January 29, 2024).

Shen, B., Guo, J. and Yang, Y. 2019. MedChain: efficient healthcare data sharing via blockchain. Applied Sciences. 9(6): 1207.

Yale. A., Dash, S., Dutta, R., Guyon, I., Pavao, A. and Bennett, K.P. 2020. Generation and evaluation of privacy preserving synthetic health data. Neurocomputing. 416: 244–255.

Yilmaz, B. and Korn, R. 2022. Synthetic demand data generation for individual electricity consumers: generative adversarial networks (GANs). Energy and AI. 9: 100161.

Zhang, T., Shen, J., Lai, C.F., Ji, S. and Ren, Y. 2023. Multi-server assisted data sharing supporting secure deduplication for metaverse healthcare systems. Future Generation Computer Systems. 140: 299–310.

Zhou, T. and Chiam, K.-H. 2023. Synthetic data generation method for data-free knowledge distillation in regression neural networks. Expert Systems with Applications. 227: 120327.

Chapter 5

Health Big Data Modelling and Analytics

Abdulkadir Hiziroglu[1], Ali Pisirgen[*,2]
and Keziban Seckin Codal[3]

[1]Department of Management Information Systems,
Izmir Bakircay University, Izmir Türkiye
ORCID: 0000-0003-4582-3732; Email: kadir.hiziroglu@bakircay.edu.tr

[2]Department of Management and Organization,
Karamanoğlu Mehmetbey University, Karaman, Türkiye
ORCID: 0000-0001-7257-2938; Email: alipisirgen@gmail.com

[3]Department of Management Information Systems,
Ankara Yıldırım Beyazıt University, Ankara, Türkiye
ORCID: 0000-0003-1967-7751; Email: kseckin.codal@aybu.edu.tr

INTRODUCTION

Proliferation of digitalization has triggered the need for understanding the creation and storing of a colossal volume of data in modern life. Gaining an edge to follow this vast increase of data requires adequate attention to being capable of extracting meaningful conclusions from the data. In this regard, decision-makers benefit greatly from data modelling and analytics solutions that can mine both structured and unstructured data. The development of the concept of "big data" has thus become central to this paradigm shift (Kambatla et al. 2014).

*For Correspondence: Ali Pisirgen (alipisirgen@gmail.com)

Nevertheless, this rapid evolution of big data terminology has led to some misconceptions, especially with regard to its dimensions. It is obvious that volume is the first dimension that comes to mind. Oussous et al. (2018) suggested the five Vs as "volume, variety, velocity, veracity and value". Therefore, big data means high-volume, high-variety, high-velocity, high veracity and invaluable datasets and requires novel approaches to data modelling and analytics while it is to offer useful insights and sound decisions. Starting with volume, data sizes for big data projects are typically quoted in the terabyte and petabyte range, referring to the magnitude of data.

Furthermore, big data is characterized by a great deal of variation. Both internal (such as sales data) and external (such as social media) sources have been accumulating large datasets. Moreover, the term "velocity" is used to describe the rate at which data is produced and the speed at which it should be examined and acted upon.

The unprecedented rate at which data is being generated by digital devices has become a rising demand. This triggers the emergence of new data management systems, data modelling, and analytics solutions that allow decision-makers facilitate from big data. In the healthcare industry, large volumes of healthcare and medical data relating to inpatient/outpatient registration, patient care, billing, payroll, budget, medical treatment, and so on, are generated each day by healthcare information systems (Philip Chen and Zhang 2014).

Taking this fact into account, this chapter intends to shed light on health big data concept per se while focusing on its modelling and analytics. The next section proposes a health data modelling and analytics framework, expressing health big data, data preprocessing, and modelling, visualization, and interpretation of health data while concluding with users of health data for decision-making. The third section presents health big data applications. The section thereafter highlights the significance of artificial intelligence (AI) in health industry. The chapter ends with conclusions and future research directions.

HEALTH DATA MODELLING AND ANALYTICS FRAMEWORK

Health data modelling involves the development of structured frameworks and systems for organizing and managing healthcare data. It serves as the foundation for efficient data storage, retrieval, and analysis within healthcare systems. With the ever-increasing volume and complexity of healthcare data, effective data modelling becomes crucial for optimizing decision-making, improving patient outcomes, and enhancing overall healthcare operations.

Moreover, health data modelling frameworks play a crucial role in storing and organizing diverse healthcare information, such as patient medical records, insurance claims, and research data. These models are vital for the smooth and productive functioning of healthcare systems. Various types of health data models exist, each with its own advantages and limitations. The choice of the most suitable data model for a specific healthcare system depends on several factors, including the system's scale and complexity, the nature of the data being stored, and the requirements of system users.

A formal framework is necessary to encompass as well as analyse these healthcare data while facilitating machine learning algorithms. This framework encompasses the goals of understanding, diagnosis, and refinement, and highlights the interactive nature of visualization as the primary interface between human cognition and algorithmic learning. It is specifically designed as a human-centred framework. The strength of this framework lies in its thoroughness, which allows it to follow a straightforward approach. In Figure 5.1, we provide a graphical summary of the framework.

Health Big Data

The concept of "big data" in health is derived from the original concept. The term "health data" is often used for personal health records of patients; nevertheless, health big data is a broader term that includes the vast amount of information produced by the health sector. The next sub-section details the classification of health big data.

Classification of Health Big Data

Health big data focusing on patients' data is nascent since the term has evolved with the digitalization of the health industry (Dash et al. 2019). Taking this into account, to improve the knowledge generation from health big data, classification presents an opportunity to address the various data types including records of individual patients' diagnoses, outcomes, and other information gathered during their care (Li et al. 2019). Starting with clinical data, information gathered through hospitals' regular clinical diagnosis and treatment systems includes data from electronic medical record (EMR) systems, medical imaging, clinical diagnosis, patient behaviour, and other sources. Furthermore, health data includes the diagnosis processes and outcome of treatment. Mostly, health data is often generated with the help of clinical data. Moreover, biological data can be referred to as information gathered using many omics techniques, including genomes, transcriptomics, proteomics, and metabolomics. This data is often used for research and

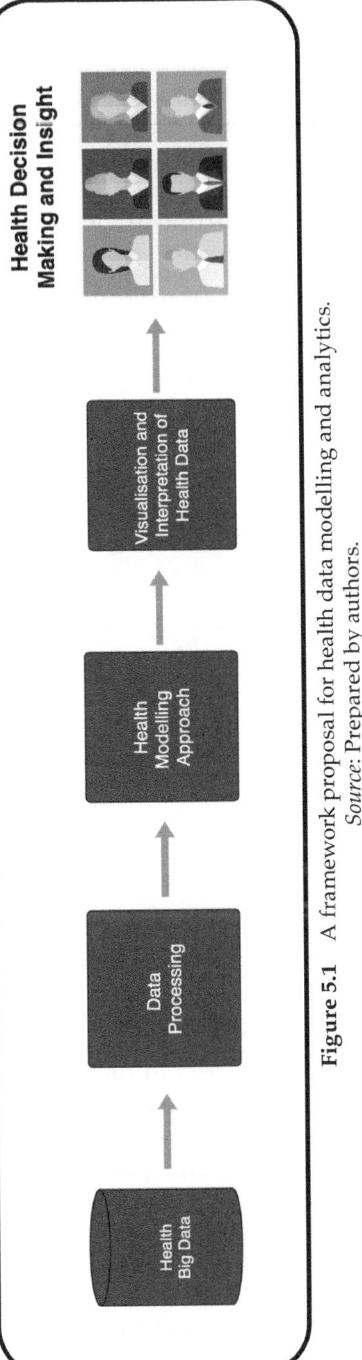

Figure 5.1   A framework proposal for health data modelling and analytics.
Source: Prepared by authors.

development purposes to cure a disease without focusing on patient-level treatment. This then helps treatment procedures to be developed so that practitioners can follow them during their treatment practice. Continuing with operational data, number of patients treated and discharged, average time for patients' appointments, surgery durations, and so on, are included in operational data for health industry. Finally, average costs of treatments for each specific disease, number of support staff working in various departments, etc., can be grouped under business-oriented data.

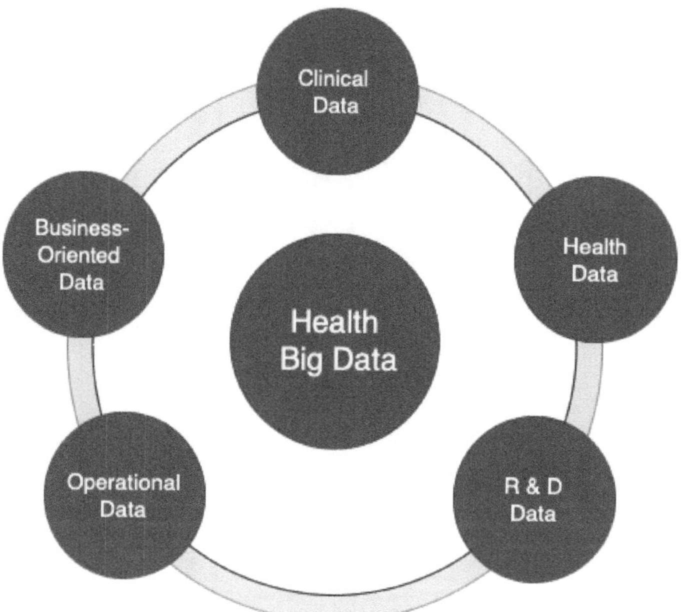

Figure 5.2   Health big data.
Source: Prepared by authors.

Opportunities and Challenges

The application of big data analytics in the healthcare industry has the potential to bring numerous benefits, akin to various other industries. Health big data encompasses a wide array of applications, ranging from clinical treatment to operational and policy-based enhancements. The digitization of medical records has revolutionized the data landscape in healthcare, resulting in an exponential increase in data volume and accentuating the importance of data analytics.

Health big data modelling and analytics offer an array of opportunities, including improvements in the quality of health services, population health management, early disease detection, enhanced decision-making, cost reduction, patient-centric care, personalized medicine, globalization of health services, and fraud detection (Kruse et al. 2016). However, despite the potential advantages, researchers and professionals face notable challenges when attempting to harness the insights from big datasets. These challenges encompass data management complexities, necessitating the collection and storage of vast datasets from diverse sources with minimal technology and software.

The sheer volume and intricacy of patient data, including medical records, lab reports, and imaging scans, presents formidable challenges for healthcare professionals. To address these challenges, efficient data management systems and robust analytical tools are imperative to streamline the analysis process and derive meaningful insights. Furthermore, the complexity of health big data poses another hurdle as data analysis necessitates handling data from distributed environments through a mix of applications. This complexity also imposes a demand for high system capacities to effectively analyse the rapidly growing volume of health big data. Moreover, the issue of imbalanced data hinders knowledge extraction as missing data in health is not easily improvised during the analysis process, potentially limiting the scope of data-driven insights (Assunção et al. 2015).

On the other hand, health big data management offers promising opportunities through the adoption of specific technologies. The EMRs facilitate quick and easy access to comprehensive patient data, enabling more informed decision-making and reducing analysis time and effort. Additionally, the integration of AI and machine learning algorithms empowers healthcare professionals to identify patterns and correlations in patient data, leading to more accurate and timely diagnoses, personalized treatment plans, and improved patient outcomes (Noorbakhsh-Sabet et al. 2019).

Moreover, in this regard, telemedicine emerges as a transformative opportunity, providing remote access to healthcare professionals, particularly advantageous in rural areas or during crisis situations. Remote consultations, monitoring, and diagnosis foster enhanced accessibility to healthcare, cost reduction, and reduced infection risk during pandemics. To fully realize the potential of telemedicine, robust infrastructure, secure communication channels, and strict adherence to privacy regulations are essential (Kumar et al. 2023).

Health Big Data Preprocessing

Data preprocessing plays a vital role in health data modelling by converting raw data into a well-organized and appropriate format for analysis. This essential step involves various procedures aimed at cleaning and refining the data.

Data Cleaning: This step involves identifying and handling missing data, outliers, and inconsistencies in the dataset. Missing data can be imputed or removed based on the specific situation and the impact on the analysis. Outliers, which are extreme values that deviate significantly from the typical patterns, can be detected and either corrected, removed, or treated separately. Inconsistencies, such as conflicting or erroneous entries, are resolved to ensure data integrity (Prakash et al. 2019). One example of health data cleaning is removing duplicate entries from a patient dataset. In healthcare, it is common for multiple records to exist for the same patient due to different visits, departments, or systems. By identifying and removing these duplicates, the dataset becomes more accurate and prevents biases or errors in subsequent analysis (Misra and Yadav 2019).

Data Integration: Health data often comes from multiple sources and may be stored in different formats or databases. Data integration involves combining data from various sources into a unified dataset. This step requires careful matching and merging of records based on common identifiers or data attributes. An example of data integration in health data modelling is combining electronic health records (EHRs) from different healthcare providers or systems (Pandey et al. 2020). In many cases, patients receive care from multiple providers, and each provider may maintain their own separate EHR system. Data integration involves merging and harmonizing these disparate sources of data to create a comprehensive and unified view of a patient's medical history. This process allows researchers or healthcare professionals to access a complete and holistic picture of a patient's health, enabling more accurate analysis and decision-making (Zarour et al. 2021).

Data Transformation: In this step, data is transformed to improve its quality and facilitate analysis. Common transformations include normalization, where numerical data is rescaled to a standard range (e.g., between 0 and 1) to ensure fairness in model training, and log or power transformations to address data skewness or heteroscedasticity (Singh and Singh 2020). Categorical data may be encoded into numerical values using techniques like one-hot encoding or label encoding. One example of health data transformation is converting raw physiological measurements into standardized units or formats. For instance, blood pressure data is collected from various sources, where the measurements are recorded in different formats such as mmHg (millimetres of mercury) or kPa (kilopascals) (Ali et al. 2020). To ensure consistency and comparability, the data can be transformed by converting all the measurements to a standardized unit, such as mmHg. This transformation allows researchers or healthcare professionals to analyse and interpret the data consistently across different sources, facilitating meaningful comparisons and insights. Additionally, data transformation may involve applying mathematical or statistical operations, such as normalizing data to a specific range or applying logarithmic transformations, to make the data more suitable for specific modelling or analysis techniques (Dash et al. 2019).

Missing Value Treatment: A missing value (MV) is a data point that is absent in the cell of a corresponding column. In the healthcare context, MVs can arise due to various reasons such as human errors, instances where the data is not applicable, failure to electronically record information by sensors, medical decisions leading to patients not being present on ventilators, irrelevant patient conditions for specific variables, electricity failures, and database synchronization issues. Conducting statistical analyses or machine learning tasks on datasets containing MVs can yield undesirable or biased results, and mishandling missing data may lead to misleading conclusions. Properly addressing missing data is crucial to ensure accurate and reliable findings in healthcare research and decision-making processes. As a method to overcome MV, statisticians employed the probabilistic method to approximate the MVs (Misra and Yadav 2019).

The most common approach to handle MVs is to discard them, but this may lead to biased results if the training data contains a large number of MVs. Deletion of MVs can be done through list-wise deletion (deleting rows with more than one MV), which works well for a small number of missing cases but is limited by the dataset having the Missing Completely at Random (MCAR) missing pattern. Another method is pairwise deletion, which minimizes errors compared to list-wise deletion by deleting attributes with MVs if they are not used as a case for analysing other attributes. A third approach involves dropping the attribute completely, which is rare but may be considered when the attribute has more than 60% missing observations and is deemed insignificant for the analysis, while relevant attributes with MVs should be retained due to their high relevance.

Data Normalization/Standardization: Normalization and standardization are techniques used to scale data to a common range. Normalization scales data to a specific range, often between 0 and 1, while standardization transforms data to have zero mean and unit variance. These techniques ensure that different features are on a similar scale, preventing certain features from dominating the modelling process (Patro and Sahu 2015).

One example of health data normalization is the normalization of body mass index (BMI) values. BMI is a commonly used measure to assess an individual's body weight in relation to their height. However, BMI values can vary widely depending on the units of measurement used for height and weight, as well as the reference standards employed.

To normalize BMI values, a common approach is to convert them into a standardized scale. For instance, the World Health Organization (WHO) has established standard BMI categories such as underweight, normal weight, overweight, and obesity. The normalization process involves mapping individual BMI values to these predefined categories.

To illustrate, imagine we possess a dataset comprising the heights and weights of individuals, and our goal is to compute and standardize their BMI values. Initially, we would determine the BMI for everyone by dividing their weight in kilograms by the square of their height in meters. This computation yields a collection of BMI values in their original form.

Next, we would apply normalization by categorizing the BMI values according to the WHO standards. For instance, we might assign a BMI value below 18.5 as "underweight", a value between 18.5 and 24.9 as "normal weight", a value between 25 and 29.9 as "overweight", and a value of 30 or above as "obese". By assigning these categories to the raw BMI values, we can normalize the data and make it more standardized and comparable across different individuals (World Health Organization, 2000).

Normalization of health data, such as BMI values, allows for better understanding, comparison, and analysis of individuals' weight status within a population. It enables researchers, healthcare professionals, and policymakers to make informed decisions, identify trends, and develop interventions related to weight management and related health conditions.

Feature Selection/Extraction: Feature selection involves identifying the most relevant and informative features (variables) from the dataset. This step helps reduce dimensionality, improve model efficiency, and mitigate the risk of overfitting. Feature extraction, on the other hand, involves creating new features from the existing ones using techniques like principal component analysis (PCA) or dimensionality reduction methods.

One example of feature extraction in health data is extracting relevant features from electrocardiogram (ECG) signals for cardiovascular disease classification. ECG signals provide information about the electrical activity of the heart, but the raw signal itself can be complex and difficult to analyze directly. Feature extraction techniques are used to extract meaningful characteristics or patterns from the ECG signals that can be used as input for disease classification algorithms (Mazomenos et al. 2012).

For example, features such as heart rate variability (HRV), QRS*
complex duration, and ST** segment deviation can be extracted from
the ECG signal. HRV measures the variation in time intervals between
consecutive heartbeats and is associated with autonomic nervous
system function. QRS complex duration represents the time taken for
electrical depolarization and repolarization of the ventricles, which can
be indicative of certain heart conditions. ST segment deviation refers to
the elevation or depression of the ST segment relative to the baseline,
which can indicate ischemia or myocardial infarction (Mahmoodabadi
et al. 2005).

By extracting these features from the ECG signal, a feature vector
can be constructed for each individual, representing their specific
characteristics. These feature vectors can then be used as input for
machine learning algorithms to classify individuals as healthy or having
specific cardiovascular conditions, such as arrhythmias or myocardial
infarction. Feature extraction plays a crucial role in reducing the
dimensionality of the data and capturing the most relevant information
for accurate classification and decision-making in health data analysis.

Each of these preprocessing steps requires careful consideration
and domain knowledge to ensure that the resulting dataset is accurate,
representative, and suitable for health data modelling. Effective data
preprocessing helps improve the performance and reliability of
models, enhances interpretability, and enables meaningful insights and
predictions from health data.

Health Modelling Approach

Healthcare data analytics has emerged as a transformative field, utilizing
various modelling approaches to analyse and interpret vast volumes of
healthcare data. The application of these modelling techniques facilitates
a better understanding of medical conditions, patient outcomes, treatment
effectiveness, and healthcare system performance. Various modelling
approaches are employed in healthcare data analytics, outlining their
specific applications, advantages, and challenges.

Predictive modelling in healthcare involves the use of machine
learning algorithms to analyse historical patient data and identify

---

*The QRS complex is the combination of Q,R and S waves and represents the
depolarization of the right and left ventricles of the heart. This is a crucial part
of the heart's electrical cycle as it initiates the contraction of the ventricles,
pumping blood out of the heart.

**The ST Segment extends from the end of the S wave to the start of the T wave and
represents he interval between ventricular depolarization and repolarization.

patterns that can predict future outcomes. These models are trained on labelled datasets with patient demographics, medical history, and diagnostic test results, enabling predictions such as readmission likelihood, disease progression, or adverse event probability. Predictive models offer valuable insights to support clinical decision-making and optimize patient care by tailoring personalized treatment plans (Axelrod and Vogel 2003, Becker et al. 2018).

Time series analysis is instrumental in studying data collected over time, including patient vital signs, disease incidence, and hospital admission rates. By identifying temporal patterns and trends, time series analysis aids in forecasting disease seasonality, evaluating interventions' impact, and optimizing resource allocation in healthcare settings. Techniques such as autoregressive integrated moving average (ARIMA) and seasonal-trend decomposition method (STL) are applied to handle temporal data and uncover valuable insights from time-dependent healthcare information (Kaushik et al. 2020, Penfold and Zhang 2013).

Survival analysis is widely used in healthcare to examine the time to an event of interest, such as patient recovery, disease recurrence, or mortality. This approach facilitates disease prognosis, treatment effectiveness assessment, and survival rate estimation. Kaplan-Meier survival curves and Cox proportional hazards models are employed to account for censoring and variations in follow-up times in survival analysis.

Epidemiological models utilize mathematical techniques to simulate disease spread and dynamics in a population. These models help predict disease transmission rates, evaluate intervention strategies, and inform public health policies during outbreaks. The susceptible, infectious, or recovered (SIR) and susceptible, exposed, infectious, then susceptible (SEIR) models are prominent examples that factor in parameters such as the basic reproduction number (R0) and the incubation period to model disease transmission over time (Alanazi et al. 2020).

Natural language processing (NLP) techniques are employed to extract valuable information from unstructured data sources like EHRs and clinical notes. NLP enables automatic identification of medical concepts, detection of adverse drug reactions, and extraction of patient information for clinical decision support. Named entity recognition, sentiment analysis, and text classification are commonly used NLP methods in healthcare data analytics (Zhou et al. 2022).

Clustering and segmentation techniques group patients with similar characteristics or health profiles to enable personalized treatment plans and interventions. Cluster analysis methods like k-means and hierarchical clustering partition patients based on shared attributes such as age, comorbidities, or response to treatment. This approach enhances patient-centric care and improves treatment outcomes (Haraty et al. 2015).

Risk stratification involves assigning risk scores to patients based on their health status and relevant factors. This enables healthcare providers to identify individuals at higher risk of specific health conditions or adverse events, facilitating targeted preventive measures and interventions. Risk prediction models, such as logistic regression and random forest, estimate the likelihood of a patient experiencing certain health outcomes based on their individual characteristics and medical history (Molassiotis et al. 2012).

In conclusion, modelling approaches in healthcare data analytics play a pivotal role in improving patient care, optimizing healthcare operations, and advancing medical research. These techniques enable healthcare professionals to make informed decisions, personalize treatment plans, and allocate resources more efficiently. As healthcare data continues to grow in volume and complexity, the application of diverse modelling approaches will be crucial in harnessing the transformative potential of data-driven insights for better patient outcomes and enhanced healthcare delivery.

Health Data Visualization

Visualization can help in health data analytics by providing a way to understand complex models generated by algorithms, and it can also serve as a valuable tool for exploratory data analysis. It can help facilitate natural inductive reasoning and guide the analyst from observed outcomes to potential hypotheses, making it a source of knowledge (Park et al. 2022).

In the context of health data analytics, visualization can significantly enhance the transparency of machine learning and computational intelligence, making it easier for researchers and practitioners to understand and interpret the results of their models. This can be especially important in areas such as deep learning, where the models can be highly complex and difficult to interpret.

By using visual analytics to improve interpretability, researchers can explore different ways of visualizing the data and models and can use these visualizations to guide the development and refinement of their models (Sopan et al. 2012). This can involve modifying the data sample, dealing with visually detected outliers, implementing alternative forms of feature selection, or guiding model selection and building. Through interactive exploration, visualization can provide the decision-makers with insights that can help evaluate the quality, usability, and adequacy of their own visualization technique.

Interpretability of Health Data

Interpretability plays a crucial role in health data modelling (Stiglic et al. 2020). Here we discuss some ways in which interpretability affects health data modelling.

Model Transparency: Interpretability allows researchers, clinicians, and stakeholders to understand how a health data model makes predictions or decisions. Transparent models provide insights into the underlying factors and variables that influence the model's outputs. This transparency helps build trust and confidence in the model's results and enables stakeholders to understand and validate the model's predictions.

Model Validation: Interpretability enables researchers and clinicians to validate the performance and accuracy of health data models. By understanding the factors considered by the model, they can assess whether the model aligns with existing medical knowledge, clinical guidelines, and domain expertise. This validation process ensures that the model's outputs are reliable and clinically relevant (Tantithamthavorn et al. 2017).

Clinical Interpretation: In healthcare, interpretability is crucial for clinicians to understand and interpret the predictions or recommendations made by health data models. Clinicians need to make informed decisions based on the model's outputs, and interpretability helps them understand the reasoning behind those predictions. It allows clinicians to consider the model's recommendations in the context of their clinical expertise and patient-specific factors.

Compliance with Guidelines: Health data models need to adhere to clinical guidelines and best practices. Interpretability helps ensure that the model's outputs align with these guidelines. By understanding how the model reaches its conclusions, clinicians can assess whether the model's recommendations are consistent with established protocols. This compliance is essential for the safe and effective integration of health data models into clinical decision-making processes (Gurses et al. 2008).

Error Detection and Bias Mitigation: Interpretability enables the identification of errors or biases in health data models. By understanding the model's internal workings, researchers and clinicians can identify potential sources of error such as data quality issues, feature biases, or model limitations. Interpretability allows for the detection and correction of these issues, leading to more accurate and fairer health data models (Gopal et al. 2021).

Communication and Collaboration: Interpretability facilitates communication and collaboration between data scientists, clinicians, and other stakeholders involved in health data modelling. It provides a common language and understanding of the model's operation, allowing for effective discussions about the model's strengths, limitations, and potential improvements. This collaboration leads to better-informed decisions and the development of more effective health data models.

Health Decision-making and Insight

Healthcare decision-makers encompass a diverse group of stakeholders who play essential roles in shaping healthcare policies, strategies, and patient care. These decision-makers can include healthcare executives, administrators, clinicians, researchers, public health officials, and policymakers.

In the context of health big data analytics, these individuals rely on data-driven insights to make informed decisions, improve patient outcomes, and optimize healthcare processes. Healthcare executives and administrators use big data analytics to assess operational efficiency, allocate resources effectively, and streamline workflows. Clinicians leverage data analytics to gain deeper insights into patient populations, identify patterns, and tailor personalized treatment plans. Researchers utilize health big data analytics to conduct studies, identify potential breakthroughs, and contribute to evidence-based medicine. Public health officials rely on data-driven analytics to monitor population health trends, manage disease outbreaks, and design effective health interventions (Dash et al. 2019). Policymakers use health big data analytics to inform healthcare policy decisions, identify areas of improvement, and enhance the overall healthcare system. With the increasing availability and complexity of health big data, the collaboration and alignment of healthcare decision-makers with data analytics experts are crucial to harness the full potential of data-driven decision-making in healthcare (Hızıroğlu et al. 2022).

Health decision-making and insight are therefore essential aspects of healthcare delivery and management. Informed decision-making is the process of choosing the most suitable treatment options, interventions, or healthcare policies based on evidence, patient preferences, and clinical expertise. It involves critically evaluating available information, such as medical research findings, patient data, and best practices, to ensure optimal patient outcomes. Health professionals rely on their expertise, experience, and the latest evidence-based guidelines to make well-informed decisions that align with individual patient needs and preferences. Moreover, gaining valuable insights from healthcare data plays a crucial role in improving healthcare practices, resource allocation, and public health strategies. Analysing and interpreting health data from EHRs, clinical trials, and epidemiological studies offer valuable insights into disease patterns, treatment effectiveness, and population health trends. By integrating evidence-based decision-making with data-driven insights, health professionals can enhance the quality of care, reduce health costs, and ultimately improve the overall health and well-being of individuals and communities.

APPLICATIONS OF HEALTH BIG DATA ANALYTICS

Health big data analytics have been presented in the literature in three categories. From a macro to micro level, these three groups can be listed as (i) government health policy determination and healthcare decision support system development; (ii) analytical business process management–style work towards a more efficient hospital management system; and (iii) analytics on medical diagnostics and disease/treatment monitoring (Cebeci and Hızıroğlu 2016).

Enhancing Healthcare with Data Analytics

Health technocrats at the national level can leverage the insights gained from analysing and mining health big data using modelling and analytics to enhance the standard of service provided nationwide (Herland et al. 2014). In fact, recent efforts have concentrated on the application of data analytics to improve health management and policy generally, with a particular focus on issues such as increasing patient service and satisfaction, and enhancing the efficiency of healthcare operations and policies in terms of finance, marketing, and human resource development.

To enhance the efficiency, accessibility, and affordability of healthcare, it is imperative for each country to establish a comprehensive national AI strategy. This strategy aims to develop a widespread AI-driven digital healthcare ecosystem, benefiting both healthcare organizations and patients. The development of various AI technologies required for these improvements is complex and costly. Presently, a significant portion of funding is allocated towards the development of machine learning on extensive EHR data, primarily for the benefit of healthcare professionals. However, attaining comprehensive health conditions necessitates a collaborative effort between healthcare professionals and patients. Therefore, patients also need access to AI-powered tools that enable self-monitoring and self-management of their chronic conditions. By empowering patients with such tools, the goal of achieving comprehensive healthcare can be realized (Chen and Decary 2019).

Health economics in this regard prioritizes the distribution and utilization of healthcare resources to optimize health-related results. Its scope encompasses assessing the effectiveness and fairness of healthcare systems and evaluating the cost-effectiveness of medical interventions and therapies. Given the significance of business-oriented health data such as cost of investment for medical equipment, or treatment costs per patient of each particular diseases, this information becomes crucial for health economics. Health data, in this regard, plays a vital role in forming healthcare policies and efficiently allocating resources, with the goal of achieving the best possible health outcomes for populations.

Additionally, the healthcare industry has experienced a significant increase in data volume, requiring a robust customer relationship management (CRM) system to effectively interpret and analyse real-time data. To address various healthcare needs such as emergency situations, remote patient monitoring, early diagnosis, fertility prediction for women, and wearable devices for the visually impaired, companies are integrating AI and the Internet of Things (IoT) (Wu et al. 2016). Consequently, AI-CRM is being acknowledged as an essential technique for collecting accurate patient data, enabling comprehensive patient engagement (Gao et al. 2015).

By utilizing AI-CRM capabilities, organizations can develop customer-centric systems that enhance the overall customer experience (Sung et al. 2021). These capabilities include accelerating content management through the integration of natural languages, allowing for personalized emails, reviews, and customer reports. Additionally, AI-CRM capabilities improve the identification of potential customers, enhance relationship management, and aim to leverage these relationships for profitability by automating AI resources and capabilities (Chatterjee et al. 2021, Mostafa and Kasamani 2022). Key activities supported by AI-CRM capabilities include AI-based customer interaction management, leveraging AI expertise to re-establish relationships, and providing flexible AI infrastructure to enhance customer relationships (Wamba-Taguimdje et al. 2020).

Health Operation Management

Improvements in health service quality may result from the use of data modelling and analytics tools applied to health big data. A review of the relevant literature demonstrates the promise of data analytics in this setting, and it shows the ways in which data analytics is being used to improve patient needs assessment, outcome ideas, service operation, and the discovery of associations between interventions and outcomes in operation level. For instance, the main operational concerns are resolved by performing analytics on health big data, including the placement of hospitals and hospital units, the scheduling of staff, and the management of supplies like blood (Choi et al. 2018).

Health Medical Diagnosis Management

Healthcare decision-makers are facing the challenge of increasing patient demand and limited resources, which necessitates greater efficiency in their decision-making processes. In this context, health big data has emerged as a valuable resource for improving decision-making, and data analytics applications serve as supportive tools that not only aid in patients' diagnosis but also enhance their overall health (Paton Shinji 2019). This analysis explores the key focus areas of research in data modelling and analytics for medical diagnosis and treatment, along with the challenges and opportunities associated with health medical diagnosis management (Amann et al. 2020).

There are three main focus areas of research in the use of data analytics in medical diagnosis and treatment:

- *Data mining for hidden rule extraction:* Numerous studies concentrate on developing data mining systems to extract hidden rules related to diseases such as tumours and cancer. These studies take advantage of large health datasets, including health and clinical data, to identify patterns and correlations that can assist in accurate diagnoses.

- *Treatment management and recommendation systems:* Research in this area investigates the effectiveness of various aspects of treatment management, including the creation of recommender systems for nursing diagnoses and the detection of diseases through the examination of tissue samples. By leveraging analytics applications, healthcare professionals can make informed decisions regarding treatment strategies.

- *Theoretical studies on analytics applications:* Theoretical research is being conducted to explore how different analytics applications influence medical diagnoses. These studies aim to enhance our understanding of the potential benefits and limitations of data analytics in healthcare decision-making.

Health medical diagnosis management is a complex and challenging process that requires a balanced integration of technology and human expertise. Leveraging EMRs, AI, and telemedicine presents significant opportunities for improving the accuracy, efficiency, and accessibility of healthcare services. However, it is crucial to implement these technologies responsibly and ethically, with appropriate safeguards to protect patient privacy and data security. By embracing these opportunities and leveraging technological advancements, healthcare professionals can provide more accurate diagnoses, improve patient outcomes, and enhance the overall quality of healthcare delivery.

AI FOR HEALTH DATA MODELLING AND ANALYTICS

Machine learning has emerged as a significant asset across diverse sectors, notably healthcare, where the proliferation of data necessitates effective analysis and interpretation. Healthcare practitioners can capitalize on machine learning algorithms to diagnose illnesses, forecast patient outcomes, and tailor personalized treatment strategies. Consequently, this section delves into the applications of machine learning in healthcare, elucidating its transformative impact on patient care. In the context of health data analytics, the judicious selection of an appropriate AI model assumes critical importance (Chen and Decary 2019, Kuo et al. 2014).

The selection of an appropriate AI model is imperative in healthcare, given the varying levels of accuracy and performance exhibited by different models on distinct types of health data. Opting for the right model guarantees the reliability and precision of predictions or outcomes it produces. In healthcare, achieving high accuracy holds vital significance as erroneous predictions or decisions can significantly impact patients' well-being and treatment outcomes.

Interpretability and explainability hold crucial importance in the healthcare domain as they contribute to building trust and acceptance among healthcare professionals. AI models like decision trees offer interpretable results, enabling clinicians to comprehend the rationale behind the model's predictions. This transparency is instrumental in supporting informed decision-making by physicians and facilitating the explanation of the model's reasoning to patients and other stakeholders.

The availability and complexity of healthcare data pose challenges due to its heterogeneous and intricate nature. AI models exhibit varying requirements concerning data format, size, and quality. Hence, selecting a model that aligns with the available data and its characteristics assumes critical significance to effectively utilize the data and mitigate potential concerns like underfitting or overfitting.

Scalability and efficiency are paramount considerations concerning the mounting volumes of health data driven by the widespread implementation of EHRs, wearable devices, and related healthcare technologies. Opting for a scalable AI model becomes imperative to facilitate the efficient handling of large datasets by the modelling process. Scalability assumes heightened importance particularly in real-time applications, where prompt predictions or decisions hold critical significance.

Ethical and legal considerations are vital when dealing with health data as it is highly sensitive and subject to stringent privacy regulations like Health Insurance Portability and Accountability Act (HIPAA) in the United States or General Data Protection Regulation (GDPR) in the European Union. Selecting an AI model that respects privacy and complies with legal requirements becomes imperative to safeguard patients' confidential information. Data anonymization emerges as a critical aspect of addressing ethical concerns in health data due to its sensitive nature. Through anonymization techniques, personal data is transformed into a modified format without identifiable elements such as names or social security numbers. This process plays a pivotal role in protecting patients' privacy, mitigating potential harm, and ensuring adherence to data protection regulations. Simultaneously, it enables researchers to access valuable health information while upholding ethical principles and maintaining transparency.

Moreover, in the context of healthcare, domain-specific considerations assume significant importance as the field encompasses diverse subdomains, including radiology, genomics, clinical decision support, and drug discovery. Each of these subdomains exhibits distinct characteristics and necessitates specific requirements, which may render certain AI models more suitable for particular tasks within these domains.

A comprehensive understanding of the unique needs and constraints associated with the specific healthcare subdomain being addressed is crucial in facilitating the informed selection of the most appropriate AI model for optimal performance and effective application.

Machine learning plays a significant role in healthcare, aiding in disease diagnosis, outcome prediction, and personalized treatments. Careful selection of appropriate AI models is vital due to variations in accuracy and performance across different health data types. Transparent and interpretable models, like decision trees, foster trust among healthcare professionals by enabling comprehension of model reasoning. Scalable AI models are necessary to efficiently process large and complex healthcare datasets. Ethical and legal considerations must be taken into account to protect patient privacy and confidentiality during AI model selection and implementation.

CONCLUSION AND FUTURE RESEARCH

In conclusion, the rapid evolution of big data in the context of healthcare has presented both opportunities and challenges for decision-makers and researchers. The concept of health big data encompasses vast amounts of information produced by the health sector, including clinical, biological, operational, and business-oriented data. Leveraging health big data through modelling and analytics holds great potential for improving the quality of healthcare services, managing population health, early detection of diseases, enhancing decision-making, reducing costs, and enabling personalized medicine.

However, several challenges need to be addressed to fully exploit the benefits of health big data. These challenges include managing the volume and complexity of patient data, ensuring data quality and integrity, addressing the imbalanced nature of health data, and developing efficient data management systems and analytical tools. Additionally, the integration of AI and machine learning technologies, along with the implementation of telemedicine, EMRs, and AI-centric CRM systems, offers significant opportunities for improving health policy management, health operation management, and health medical diagnosis management.

To effectively leverage health big data, a robust health data modelling framework is necessary. This framework should include data preprocessing steps such as cleaning, integration, and transformation to ensure data quality and usability. Furthermore, the framework should support the application of data mining, treatment management and recommendation systems, and theoretical studies on analytics applications to enhance medical diagnosis and treatment.

Therefore, health big data modelling and analytics have the potential to revolutionize the healthcare industry by improving decision-making, patient outcomes, and the overall quality of healthcare services. However, addressing the challenges and implementing effective data modelling frameworks are crucial for realizing the full potential of health big data in improving healthcare delivery and patient care. Future research should focus on developing advanced data management systems, analytical tools, and ethical guidelines to harness the power of health big data for the benefit of individuals and society. The future research in health data modelling is likely to focus on several key areas:

Improved Model Interpretability: Enhancing the interpretability of AI models in healthcare will remain an important research direction. Developing techniques to provide transparent and understandable explanations for the decisions made by complex models, such as deep learning models, will be crucial for gaining trust and acceptance from healthcare professionals.

Explainable Deep Learning: Deep learning has shown great potential in healthcare, but its black-box nature poses challenges for interpretability. Future research will likely explore methods to make deep learning models more explainable, such as designing model architectures that produce interpretable representations or developing post-hoc explanation techniques specifically tailored to deep learning models.

Personalized and Precision Medicine: The advancement of health data modelling analytics will support the transition towards personalized and precision medicine. Future research will focus on developing models that can effectively utilize large-scale genomic data, EHRs, wearable device data, and other relevant sources to provide individualized treatment recommendations, disease risk assessments, and prognostic predictions.

Real-time and Continuous Monitoring: With the increasing availability of wearable devices and sensors, there is a growing interest in real-time and continuous monitoring of health data. Future research will focus on developing models that can analyse streaming health data in real time, enabling early detection of abnormalities, timely interventions, and personalized feedback to individuals for maintaining their health and well-being.

Integration of Multiple Data Sources: Health big data is diverse and comes from various sources, including EHRs, imaging data, genomics, environmental data, and patient-generated data. Future research will explore methods to effectively integrate and analyse these heterogeneous data sources, enabling comprehensive and holistic health data modelling.

Unsupervised Learning and Privacy Preservation: Privacy concerns are significant in health data modelling and analytics. Federated learning, a distributed machine learning approach, allows models to be trained across multiple institutions while preserving data privacy. Future research will focus on developing robust federated learning frameworks that can effectively utilize distributed health data for modelling while ensuring privacy and security.

Causal Inference and Outcome Prediction: Causal inference techniques play a crucial role in understanding the causal relationships between interventions and health outcomes. Future research will focus on developing models and methods that can better capture causal relationships in health data, enabling more accurate outcome prediction and supporting evidence-based decision-making in healthcare.

Ethical Considerations and Bias Mitigation: As health data modelling and analytics become more pervasive, addressing ethical considerations and mitigating biases in the data and models will be critical. Future research will explore approaches to identify and mitigate biases, ensure fairness in healthcare predictions and decision-making, and address the ethical implications of AI applications in healthcare.

Overall, future research in health data modelling and analytics will aim to advance interpretability, personalization, real-time monitoring, integration of diverse data sources, privacy preservation, causal inference, ethical considerations, and bias mitigation. These areas of research will contribute to the development of more effective and reliable AI models for improving healthcare outcomes.

REFERENCES

Alanazi, S.A., Kamruzzaman, M.M., Alruwaili, M., Alshammari, N., Alqahtani, S.A. and Karime, A. 2020. Measuring and preventing COVID-19 using the SIR model and machine learning in smart health care. Journal of Healthcare Engineering. 8857346.

Ali, F., El-Sappagh, S., Islam, S.M.R., Kwak, D., Ali, A., Imran, M., et al. 2020. A smart healthcare monitoring system for heart disease prediction based on ensemble deep learning and feature fusion. Information Fusion. 63: 208–222.

Amann, J., Blasimme, A., Vayena, E., Frey, D. and Madai, V.I. 2020. Explainability for artificial intelligence in healthcare: a multidisciplinary perspective. BMC Medical Informatics and Decision Making. 20(1): 310.

Assunção, M.D., Calheiros, R.N., Bianchi, S., Netto, M.A.S. and Buyya, R. 2015. Big data computing and clouds: trends and future directions. Journal of Parallel and Distributed Computing. 79–80: 3–15.

Axelrod, R.C. and Vogel, D. 2003. Predictive modeling in health plans. Disease Management and Health Outcomes. 11(12): 779–787.

Becker, D., van Breda, W., Funk, B., Hoogendoorn, M., Ruwaard, J. and Riper, H. 2018. Predictive modeling in e-mental health: a common language framework. Internet Interventions. 12: 57–67.

Cebeci, H.I. and Hızıroğlu, A. 2016. Review of business intelligence and intelligent systems in healthcare domain. pp. 192–206. *In:* Celebi, N. (ed.). Intelligent Techniques for Data Analysis in Diverse Settings. IGI Global.

Chatterjee, S., Chaudhuri, R., Vrontis, D., Thrassou, A. and Ghosh, S.K. 2021. Adoption of artificial intelligence-integrated CRM systems in agile organizations in India. Technological Forecasting and Social Change. 168: 120783.

Chen, M. and Decary, M. 2019. Artificial intelligence in healthcare: an essential guide for health leaders. Healthcare Management Forum. 33(1): 10–18.

Choi, T.-M., Wallace, S.W. and Wang, Y. 2018. Big data analytics in operations management. Production and Operations Management. 27(10): 1868–1883.

Dash, S., Shakyawar, S.K., Sharma, M. and Kaushik, S. 2019. Big data in healthcare: management, analysis and future prospects. Journal of Big Data. 6(1): 54.

Gao, Y., Li, H. and Luo, Y. 2015. An empirical study of wearable technology acceptance in healthcare. Industrial Management and Data Systems. 115(9): 1704–1723.

Gopal, D.P., Chetty, U., O'Donnell, P., Gajria, C. and Blackadder-Weinstein, J. 2021. Implicit bias in healthcare: clinical practice, research and decision making. Future Healthcare Journal. 8(1): 40–48.

Gurses, A.P., Seidl, K.L., Vaidya, V., Bochicchio, G., Harris, A.D., Hebden, J., et al. 2008. Systems ambiguity and guideline compliance: a qualitative study of how intensive care units follow evidence-based guidelines to reduce healthcare-associated infections. Quality and Safety in Health Care. 17(5). 351–359.

Haraty, R.A., Dimishkieh, M. and Masud, M. 2015. An enhanced k-means clustering algorithm for pattern discovery in healthcare data. International Journal of Distributed Sensor Networks. 11(6): 615740.

Herland, M., Khoshgoftaar, T.M. and Wald, R. 2014. A review of data mining using big data in health informatics. Journal of Big Data. 1(1): 2.

Hızıroğlu, A., Pişirgen, A., Özcan, M. and İlter, H.K. 2022. Artificial intelligence in healthcare industry: a transformation from model-driven to knowledge-driven DSS. Artificial Intelligence Theory and Applications. 2(1): 41–58.

Kambatla, K., Kollias, G., Kumar, V. and Grama, A. 2014. Trends in big data analytics. Journal of Parallel and Distributed Computing. 74(7): 2561–2573.

Kaushik, S., Choudhury, A., Sheron, P.K., Dasgupta, N., Natarajan, S., Pickett, L.A., et al. 2020. AI in healthcare: time-series forecasting using statistical, neural and ensemble architectures. Frontiers in Big Data. 3: 4.

Kruse, C.S., Goswamy, R., Raval, Y. and Marawi, S. 2016. Challenges and opportunities of big data in health care: a systematic review. JMIR Medical Informatics. 4(4): e38.

Kumar, P., Sharma, S.K. and Dutot, V. 2023. Artificial intelligence (AI)-enabled CRM capability in healthcare: the impact on service innovation. International Journal of Information Management. 69: 102598.

Kuo, M.-H., Sahama, T., Kushniruk, A.W., Borycki, E.M. and Grunwell, D.K. 2014. Health big data analytics: current perspectives, challenges and potential solutions. International Journal of Big Data Intelligence. 1(1–2): 114–126.

Li, M., Wang, C., Yan, L. and Wei, S. 2019. Research on the application of medical big data. 2019 14th International Conference on Computer Science and Education (ICCSE). 478–482.

Mahmoodabadi, S.Z., Ahmadian, A., Abolhasani, M.D., Eslami, M. and Bidgoli, J.H. 2005. ECG feature extraction based on multiresolution wavelet transform. 2005 IEEE Engineering in Medicine and Biology 27th Annual Conference. 3902–3905.

Mazomenos, E.B., Chen, T., Acharyya, A., Bhattacharya, A., Rosengarten, J. and Maharatna, K. 2012. A time-domain morphology and gradient based algorithm for ECG feature extraction. 2012 IEEE International Conference on Industrial Technology. 117–122.

Misra, P. and Yadav, A.S. 2019. Impact of preprocessing methods on healthcare predictions. Proceedings of 2nd International Conference on Advanced Computing and Software Engineering (ICACSE).

Molassiotis, A., Farrell, C., Bourne, K., Brearley, S.G. and Pilling, M. 2012. An exploratory study to clarify the cluster of symptoms predictive of chemotherapy-related nausea using random forest modeling. Journal of Pain and Symptom Management. 44(5): 692–703.

Mostafa, R.B. and Kasamani, T. 2022. Antecedents and consequences of chatbot initial trust. European Journal of Marketing. 56(6): 1748–1771.

Noorbakhsh-Sabet, N., Zand, R., Zhang, Y. and Abedi, V. 2019. Artificial intelligence transforms the future of health care. The American Journal of Medicine. 132(7). 795–801.

Oussous, A., Benjelloun, F.-Z., Ait Lahcen, A. and Belfkih, S. 2018. Big data technologies: a survey. Journal of King Saud University—Computer and Information Sciences. 30(4): 431–448.

Pandey, A.K., Khan, A.I., Abushark, Y.B., Alam, M.M., Agrawal, A., Kumar, R., et al. 2020. Key issues in healthcare data integrity: analysis and recommendations. IEEE Access. 8: 40612–40628.

Park, S., Bekemeier, B., Flaxman, A. and Schultz, M. 2022. Impact of data visualization on decision-making and its implications for public health practice: a systematic literature review. Informatics for Health and Social Care. 47(2): 175–193.

Paton Shinji, C.K. 2019. An open science approach to artificial intelligence in healthcare. A Contribution from the International Medical Informatics Association Open Source Working Group. 28(1): 47–51.

Patro, S. and Sahu, K.K. 2015. Normalization: A preprocessing stage. International Advanced Research Journal in Science, Engineering and Technology. 2(3): 20–22.

Penfold, R.B. and Zhang, F. 2013. Use of interrupted time series analysis in evaluating health care quality improvements. Academic Pediatrics, 13(6, Supplement): S38–S44.

Philip Chen, C.L. and Zhang, C.-Y. 2014. Data-intensive applications, challenges, techniques and technologies: a survey on big data. Information Sciences. 275: 314–347.

Prakash, A., Navya, N. and Natarajan, J. 2019. Big data preprocessing for modern world: opportunities and challenges. pp. 335–343. *In:* Hemanth, J., Fernando, X., Lafata, P. and Baig, Z. (eds). International Conference on Intelligent Data Communication Technologies and Internet of Things (ICICI) 2018. Springer International Publishing.

Singh, D. and Singh, B. 2020. Investigating the impact of data normalization on classification performance. Applied Soft Computing. 97: 105524.

Sopan, A., Noh, A.S.-I., Karol, S., Rosenfeld, P., Lee, G. and Shneiderman, B. 2012. Community health map: a geospatial and multivariate data visualization tool for public health datasets. Government Information Quarterly. 29(2): 223–234.

Stiglic, G., Kocbek, P., Fijacko, N., Zitnik, M., Verbert, K. and Cilar, L. 2020. Interpretability of machine learning-based prediction models in healthcare. WIREs Data Mining and Knowledge Discovery. 10(5): e1379.

Sung, E. (Christine), Bae, S., Han, D.-I.D. and Kwon, O. 2021. Consumer engagement via interactive artificial intelligence and mixed reality. International Journal of Information Management. 60: 102382.

Tantithamthavorn, C., McIntosh, S., Hassan, A.E. and Matsumoto, K. 2017. An empirical comparison of model validation techniques for defect prediction models. IEEE Transactions on Software Engineering. 43(1): 1–18.

Wamba-Taguimdje, S.-L., Wamba, S.F., Kamdjoug, J.R.K. and Wanko, C.E.T. 2020. Impact of artificial intelligence on firm performance: exploring the mediating effect of process-oriented dynamic capabilities. pp. 3–18. *In*: Agrifoglio, R., Lamboglia, R., Mancini, D. and Ricciardi, F. (eds). Digital Business Transformation. Springer International Publishing.

World Health Organization. 2000. Obesity: preventing and managing the global epidemic: report of a WHO consultation. https://pubmed.ncbi.nlm.nih.gov/11234459 4

Wu, J., Li, H., Cheng, S. and Lin, Z. 2016. The promising future of healthcare services: when big data analytics meets wearable technology. Information and Management. 53(8): 1020–1033.

Zarour, M., Alenezi, M., Ansari, M.T.J., Pandey, A.K., Ahmad, M., Agrawal, A., et al. 2021. Ensuring data integrity of healthcare information in the era of digital health. Healthcare Technology Letters. 8(3): 66–77.

Zhou, B., Yang, G., Shi, Z. and Ma, S. 2022. Natural language processing for smart healthcare. IEEE Reviews in Biomedical Engineering. 17: 4–18.

Chapter 6

Intelligent Diagnosis and Treatment Systems

Cosku Oksuz[1,*], Betul Yurdem[2] and
Mehmet Kemal Gullu[3]

[1]Department of Electrical and Electronics Engineering,
Izmir Bakircay University, Izmir Türkiye
ORCID: 0000-0001-7116-2734; Email: cosku.oksuz@bakircay.edu.tr

[2]Department of Electrical and Electronics Engineering,
Izmir Bakircay University, Izmir Türkiye
ORCID: 0000-0002-0626-9946; Email: betul.yurdem@bakircay.edu.tr

[3]Department of Electrical and Electronics Engineering,
Izmir Bakircay University, Izmir Türkiye
ORCID: 0000-0003-2310-2985; Email: kemal.gullu@bakircay.edu.tr

INTRODUCTION

Precision medicine is one of the recently emerging concepts aiming at uncovering better the underlying causes of diseases by integrating multi-modal data from several resources (MacEachern and Forkert 2021). The multi-modal data from several resources forms big data that should be further analyzed to explore signals inside it. Thus, it has become necessary to develop powerful methods that make inferences by processing these extremely large datasets generated in line with precision medicine. Fortunately, advances in computer science have

*For Correspondence: Cosku Oksuz (cosku.oksuz@bakircay.edu.tr;
coskuoksuz@gmail.com)

allowed the development of precise techniques for analyzing complex big data that cannot be handled properly with traditional statistics. Machine learning as an artificial intelligence (AI) subfield is a set of computer science methodologies aiming at exploring hidden signals (or patterns) inside data for inference, which has great potential for understanding human health. Using machine learning techniques also has the potential to save time and effort and enable more efficient use of resources. Therefore, machine learning–based techniques have been long proposed in the medical field for aiding physicians' decisions. On the other hand, the current study focuses on the subfield of machine learning, namely deep learning, as it allows the learning of task-related features by developing effective architectures.

In order to expedite the process of interpreting the information obtained as a result of the analyses in medical research, the detection and treatment of diseases by using various intelligent diagnosis methods have increased in the recent period. The disorder and treatment studies utilizing AI methods cover a wide field in the literature. Among them, the most studied fields of medicine, are as follows:

- **Cancer:** In addition to the existence of many different types of cancer, many different intelligent methods have been used for the diagnosis of cancer (Huang et al. 2020). For example, when the studies conducted between 2010 and 2020 for the detection of breast cancer were examined, it was observed that many AI methods such as machine learning (ML), decision trees (DT), naïve Bayes (NB), random forest (RF), artificial neural network (ANN), back propagation neural network (BPNN), deep learning (DL), and convolutional neural networks (CNN) were used with the aim of classification of breast cancer (Nassif et al. 2022). Among these studies, 98.3% accuracy was obtained as a result of a study in which Zhang et al. (2013) used feed forward neural network (FFNN) to detect breast cancer with plasma samples. Mostavi et al. (2020), on the other hand, used the CNN method to classify breast cancer by using tumor samples and obtained an accuracy of 95.6% for 33 different subtypes.

- **Nervous system diseases:** Intelligent diagnosis and treatment methods are also used in the detection of diseases that occur in the neurological system such as Alzheimer's, Parkinson's, and epilepsy. Kannan et al. (2022) proposed a long short-term memory network model in which they trained their model using electroencephalography (EEG) signals for predicting epileptic seizures. Geniş and Aydin (2022) also tried to detect epilepsy seizures by using EEG signals. They developed a CNN method, and 94.17% of accuracy was achieved. In a study by Thurmann et al. (2022), the development of speech therapies for Parkinson's disease was carried out using intelligent treatment methods.

- **Mental disorder:** Angelyn and Putri (2021) achieved an intelligent depression and anxiety diagnosis system using the NB method. As a result, they achieved 90% accuracy with the system they constructed. Detection of schizophrenia, which is another mental disorder, can also be performed with intelligent methods. Different features extracted in the time or frequency domain of the dataset obtained by using magnetic resonance imaging (MRI) modalities can be used. Wang et al. (2018) calculated the mean regional homogeneity values from the resting state functional MRI data and detected schizophrenia with 90.14% accuracy by the support vector machine (SVM) classification method, which is a type of ML. Using task-based functional MRI data, Juneja et al. (2018) used a nonlinear feature, generalized discriminant analysis. Then, they detected schizophrenia by obtaining 98% accuracy with the SVM method after reducing the feature with the novel fuzzy rough set.

- **Cardiovascular disease:** Using methods such as electrocardiogram (ECG), echocardiography, and cardiac imaging, data is recorded for the detection of diseases in this field (Itchhaporia 2022). For the prediction of cardiovascular diseases, Mhamdi et al. (2022) used ECG signals, and they obtained the highest validation accuracy of 95% using algorithms of the CNN method. Potter et al. (2021) obtained energy waveforms of ECG signals after applying continuous wave transform to ECG signals, and they obtained 72% specificity and 85% sensitivity with 0.83 AUC for heart disease risk by classifying these energy waves with RF method. Zreik et al. (2018) performed a study with cardiac imaging for the diagnosis of plaque and stenosis. After recording the coronary computed tomography angiography (CCTA) data, the recurrent neural network (RNN) model was trained. As a result, 77% accuracy was obtained for the diagnosis of plaque and 80% for the diagnosis of stenosis. On the other hand, Shao et al. (2018) tried to diagnose dilated cardiomyopathy with another imaging method which was MRI. Then, the detection was performed with 85% accuracy using the SVM method.

As can be inferred from here, similar intelligent diagnosis and treatment methods have been followed on different subjects in the literature. In addition to the exemplary cases given here, intelligent methods are also used for detection and treatment in many medical fields such as diabetes, pathology, dermatology, infection, and flu (Nichols et al. 2019). The ability of an AI method developed for disease detection to be used in a clinical setting is related to the degree of its errors. When the error rate is sufficiently minimized, AI can be used to assist physicians in clinical settings. For example, it is stated by Kumar et al. (2022) that a developed AI system for detecting hazardous lung tumors is in use to assist physicians in China, which makes possible early disease detection, without taking specimens for lab tests. This reveals the potential of intelligent diagnosis and treatment systems. Within the scope of this study, intelligent methods developed in this aspect were examined, taking into account the Covid-19 disease, which has significantly affected human life in the last three years. It is aimed to examine the studies in the literature aimed at detecting this disease, especially using medical imaging features.

The Covid-19 disease has had many devastating effects around the world. The fact that SARS-CoV-2 has become more contagious, especially with new mutations, has caused the disease to spread at an unprecedented rate. Many lives have been lost because of the disease. The capacity of health institutions has remained insufficient due to the increased cases. As a result, a public health crisis has emerged. To prevent the virus spread, border closures and lockdowns were implemented by countries. The protracted pandemic also affected the world's business due to border closures, triggering the economic crisis. With millions of businesses facing an existential threat, nearly half of the world's global workforce has remained at risk of losing their livelihoods. Many breadwinners have lost their livelihoods due to the decimated jobs, especially in countries with low-income (World Health Organization 2020). The Covid-19 pandemic still goes on. As of October 1, deaths on a global scale reached 6.5 million people, according to the WHO's dashboard. Currently, the confirmed cases are around 614.5 million (WHO Coronavirus (Covid-19) Dashboard, n.d.).

The RT-PCR (Reverse Transcription Polymerase Chain Reaction) testing is accepted as the standard test for determination of Covid-19 disease by the World Health Organization (WHO). However, its false negative rate (FNR) has been discussed many times. In Mayers and Baker (2020), it is stated that the even if the RT-PCR assays are highly accurate tools by yielding over 95% of sensitivity and specificity, this is valid only in laboratory conditions. For this reason, they are ideal scores, and are referred to as analytical sensitivity and specificity. In clinical or community setting, there may be many errors that stem from factors such as inefficient sampling, contamination, and sample degradation. Estimating the operational false positives and false negatives from the clinical or community setting is more important in the way to determine how to respond to the Covid-19 pandemic.

Pecoraro et al. (2022) aimed to estimate the FNR of RT-PCR test through a systematic review of the literature. By reviewing Pubmed, Embase, and CENTRAL, more than 18,000 patients infected with SARS-

CoV-2 were included in the analysis. Their systematic review revealed that about 58% of Covid-19 patients might have false negative RT-PCR results at the initial phase. In the study, it was stated that correct diagnosis strategies should be developed in order to identify suspected Covid-19 cases. Kanji et al. (2021) analyzed the FNR of the RT-PCR test by reviewing the samples collected from January 21 to April 18, 2020, at the Public Health Laboratory (Alberta, Canada). The collected 100,001 samples from 99,919 patients during the specified time period were analyzed. The test results of 49 patients in the study were inconsistent with 49 positive and 52 negative swabs. Then, it was determined after re-test that 5 of 52 negative swabs were actually positive. In this study, it is stated that low concentrations of the SARS-CoV-2 virus affect false negatives in patients with multiple samples at different stages of infection.

These studies point that the RT-PCR test may have a high potential to miss cases that are actually positive yet asymptomatic at the onset of the disease. This was one of the factors that made it challenging to control the spread of the disease. For this reason, there has been a great research interest in the development of highly sensitive as well as the fast-resulting alternative methods by researchers.

Table 6.1   Imaging features as the sign of Covid-19 disease.

Image Feature	Brief Explanation
Ground-glass opacity	Hazy gray areas that can be found on both CT and X-ray images (Koo et al. 2018).
Air bronchi sign	This symptom, which is commonly seen in pneumonia, indicates that the pathology is in the lung parenchyma (Algin et al. 2011).
Consolidation	When the fluid fills the lungs, this situation occurs.
Paving stone sign	It is one of the important signs of the disease, which indicates that the virus has settled in the interlobular septum (Wu et al. 2020).
Vascular thickening	It is a result of the inflammation which can cause the thickening as well as increased vascular permeability (Wu et al. 2020).
Halo sign	It is circular region covering the pulmonary nodules that are seen as ground glass shadow at CT image. It is commonly associated with pulmonary hemorrhage, but it may be indicator any other disease (Parrón et al. 2008).

While computed tomography (CT) is the main technique in pulmonary imaging, chest X-ray may also be used for supportive purposes (Lu et al. 2020). However, CT imaging has been the main tool for diagnosing Covid-19 disease. Intensity changes of the image may provide substantial information about several pathological processes such as proliferation, metamorphism, and tissue exudation (Koo et al. 2018). As a result of the intensity changes, some visible imaging features may occur within the CT or X-ray image, which are the potential indicators of Covid-19 disease for medical experts. These are given in Table 6.1 and are briefly described.

There were many situations encountered in clinical setting in which nucleic acid test, that is, RT-PCR test, resulted in negative, but CT imaging suggested that the case was positive for Covid-19. In Chen et al. (2020), while CT examinations of male patient aged 60 years revealed lesions inside the lungs, the nucleic acid test resulted in negative. The nucleic acid test resulted in positive five days later. According to the preliminary data from the virus hospital in Wuhan, China, the true positive rate of CT imaging for Covid-19 detection is over 90%, it is about 40% for nucleic acid tests (Chen et al. 2020).

The fact that imaging features provide powerful patterns has been the motivation for developing intelligent methods that use machine learning for Covid-19 detection based on imagery. It is worth mentioning that recently some researchers focused on a detection method using one-dimensional signals such as cough data collected from patients. However, considerable effort has been made to detect the disease from the imagery during the pandemic. In this study, proposed intelligent diagnosis systems regarding Covid-19 detection using imagery during the pandemic are summarized in a systematic manner.

The organization of this study is as follows: the methods utilizing imagery for Covid-19 detection are presented in the next section. A brief discussion follows thereafter. Finally, the conclusions are presented in the last section.

INTELLIGENT COVID-19 DIAGNOSIS

The methods mainly aim to explore decisive features using the medical imagery. During the pandemic, medical images such as the CT and the X-ray have been widely utilized for feature extraction by the researchers.

After some studies showed that X-ray images can carry some signatures of the disease, many methods have been developed for recognizing Covid-19 disease over X-ray images. Because it is one of the oldest and simplest imaging methods, X-ray imaging machines are available in almost every healthcare facility. Exposure of patients to lower radiation doses, compared to CT imaging, is another source of motivation behind developing X-ray-based Covid-19 detection systems (Rehani and Berry 2000).

While the methods following classical hand-crafted feature extraction with the machine learning classifiers are still available, most of the methods proposed in the published studies are based on CNN. Even if there may be some minor variations, all these methods may be conceptualized as given in Figure 6.1.

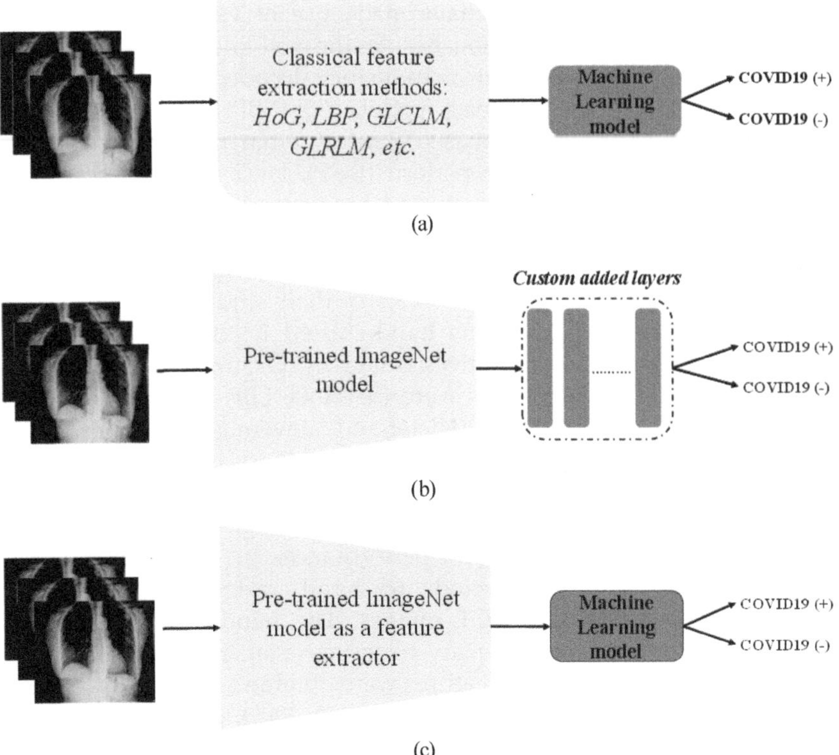

Figure 6.1   Intelligent Covid-19 diagnosis using classical feature extraction methods and the pre-trained ImageNet models. The X-ray image is taken from the COVIDGR-1.0 dataset introduced by Tabik et al. (2020). (a) Classification scheme based on classical feature extraction methods. (b) Classification scheme based on custom layers added to the pre-trained network for learning the downstream task (i.e. Covid-19 detection). (c) Classification scheme based on classical machine learning models in which the pre-trained network behaves like a feature extractor to feed features for the training of machine learning model.

HAND-CRAFTED RADIOMICS FOR DETECTION OF COVID-19 DISEASE

Some of the well-known feature extraction methods including Histogram of Oriented Gradients (HoG) (Dalal and Triggs 2005), gray level co-occurrence matrix (GLCM) (Haralick et al. 1973), gray-level run-length (GLRLM) (Galloway 1975), and local binary patterns (LBP) (Ojala et al. 2002) are used by some researchers for Covid-19 detection. The features extracted by these methods are used to train classical machine learning models such as SVM, k-nearest neighbor (k-NN), neural networks (NN), and RF.

Ismael and Şengür (2021) have made use of various local texture descriptors for Covid-19 detection. Besides the well-known LBP descriptor, other BP-based descriptors such as frequency decoded LBP (FD-LBP) and quaternionic local ranking binary pattern (QLR-BP) have been utilized in the study. In addition to BP-based features, binarized statistical image features (BSIF), binary Gabor pattern (BGP), local phase quantization (LPQ), pyramid histogram of oriented gradients (PHOG), and CENsus Transform hISTogram (CENTRIST) were the descriptors considered in the study. The BSIF was found as the best feature descriptor for Covid-19 detection with an accuracy of 90.5% in their study.

The effectiveness of various hand-crafted feature descriptors for Covid-19 detection was also investigated by Öksüz et al. (2022). The investigated feature descriptors were the HoG, LBP, GLCM, maximally stable extremal regions (MSER) (Nistér and Stewénius 2008), speeded up robust features (SURF) (Bay et al. 2008), and binary robust independent elementary features (BRIEF) (Calonder et al. 2010) within the study. When LBP features were combined with the SVM classifier, 69.01% of accuracy was attained as the best performance.

Guiot et al. (2021) extracted 166 hand-crafted radiomics from segmented lung regions in CT images. The hand-crafted radiomics were first order statistics, intensity histogram statistics, shape features, and texture features. Texture features were obtained by GLCM, GLRLM, gray-level size-zone (GLSZM) (Thibault et al. 2009), gray-level distance-zone (GLDZM) (Thibault et al. 2014), neighborhood gray-tone difference (NGTDM) (Amadasun and King 1989) and neighboring gray-level dependence matrix (NGLDM) (Sun and Wee 1983). The authors reduced the size to 45 after using a feature analysis in which highly correlated feature pairs were removed. The top 5 features aligned based on their importance scores were *complexity* feature of NGTDM, *maximal correlation coefficient* of GLCM, *large distance emphasis feature* of GLDZM, *the median image intensity within the lungs*, and *strength* feature of NGTDM. The performance was 88.2% in terms of area under the ROC curve (AUC) score.

Hussain et al. (2020) extracted texture features and morphological features from X-ray images for the recognition of Covid-19 disease. The texture features, obtained using GLCM, were *contrast, correlation, dissimilarity, energy, entropy, homogeneity, mean, variance, standard deviation (SD), skewness, kurtosis,* and *root-mean-square.* The extracted morphological features were *area, perimeter, max. radius, min. radius, eccentricity, equidiameter, elongatedness, entropy, circulatory I, circulatory II, compactness, dispersion, SD of image,* and *shape index.* All these extracted features were used to train the classifiers, i.e., eXtreme Gradient Boosting–Linear (XGBoost–Linear), eXtreme Gradient Boosting–Tree (XGBoost–Tree), k-NN, classification and regression tree (CART), and naïve Bayes. The performance of each model with the extracted features was investigated both for binary (Covid-19/bacterial pneumonia, Covid-19/normal, Covid-19/viral pneumonia) and multi-class classification (Covid-19, normal, viral pneumonia, and bacterial pneumonia). One of the interesting findings in this work is that the *perimeter* (total count of pixel at the boundary) is the key decisive feature which discriminates Covid-19 disease from the bacterial and the viral infections. An accuracy of 79.52% was achieved with the XGBoost–Linear model for multi-class classification in the study.

COVID-19 DETECTION BASED ON DEEP LEARNING

The proposed methods are basically divided into two categories: using pre-trained networks and developing a new architecture from scratch.

Pre-trained Networks

At the beginning of the Covid-19 pandemic, there was insufficient data to properly train a deep convolutional network. Therefore, the ImageNet models trained with millions of data have been widely utilized with the fine-tuning strategy. Fine-tuning is a strategy that allows an already trained model (i.e., pre-trained) to be fitted to a downstream task. This is carried out by removing the layers specifically assigned for the previous task and adding a series of layers for the new task, as given in Figure 6.1(b). Since the general features common to many tasks have already been gained by the pre-trained network (or primitive model), weights of the primitive model are either frozen or trained only at a fairly low learning rate for the new task. On the other hand, the weights of custom added layers are updated with a higher learn rate.

The other method is based on the direct use of a trained model for feature extraction purposes, as depicted in Figure 6.1(c). The best layer of the pre-trained network yielding optimal feature set should be carefully determined by analyzing representative power of each layer features on a separated validation set.

The available data largely determines which methods should be used. Nevertheless, some published papers have observed performance using both methods. The pre-trained models, i.e., VGG16 (Simonyan and Zisserman 2015), VGG19 (Simonyan and Zisserman 2015), ResNet18 (He et al. 2016), ResNet50 (He et al. 2016), and ResNet101 (He et al. 2016), were fine-tuned by Ismael and Şengür (2021). The outperforming model in the study is ResNet50 with 92.63% of accuracy. On the other hand, 94.7% of accuracy was attained when the deep features obtained by ResNet50 model were combined with SVM model.

Öksüz et al. (2022) used the pre-trained models, GoogLeNet (Szegedy et al. 2015), SqueezeNet (Iandola et al. 2016), ShuffleNet (Zhang et al. 2017), ResNet18 (He et al. 2016), EfficientNetB0 (Tan and Le 2020), and Xceptions (Chollet 2017), directly as feature extractors in accordance with Figure 6.1(c). The layers aligned from the beginning to the end of each network are carefully analyzed to attain the best feature set giving the best performance. Then, the obtained features were aligned for their importance in terms of Laplacian scores, which is an unsupervised feature selection technique (He et al. 2006). Finally, it was investigated how many of these aligned features maximized the performance. This wrapper-based feature selection strategy proposed by Öksüz et al. (2022) yielded 76.06% of accuracy when 605-dimensional feature set extracted by Xception model was used.

Ahsan et al. (2021) also made use of pre-trained networks. However, their study differed from the studies outlined earlier in that they used a combined dataset including both CT and X-ray images. The pre-trained models, i.e., VGG16 (Simonyan and Zisserman 2015), MobileNetV2 (Sandler et al. 2019), InceptionResNetV2 (Szegedy et al. 2017), ResNet50 (He et al. 2016), ResNet101 (He et al. 2016), and VGG19 (Simonyan and Zisserman 2015), were fine-tuned in the study. The fined-tuned MobileNetV2 model yielded 95% of accuracy on the mixed dataset.

Custom-designed Models

Throughout the pandemic, many datasets have been released from different sources around the world. Thus, the scarcity of Covid-19 related data at the beginning of the pandemic has been reduced in a manner. As a result, custom CNN architectures have also been designed for Covid-19 detection. Custom CNN architectures are designed to be trained from the scratch. The main points (or hyper-parameters) to be considered in custom-designed CNN architectures are as follows:

- **Finding proper network architecture:** It is known that when the network depth is increased, more abstract features that may have more representative power can be obtained. However, some discerning features may be weakened with network depth. Therefore, the network depth is one of the hyper-parameters that should be adjusted carefully.

- **Number of the kernels in convolutional layers:** Kernels used in convolutional layers are related with the number of features that are desired to be detected.

- **Determining the suitable kernel size:** Kernel size directly affects the receptive field which has significance for capturing contextual information.

Fortunately, all these hyper-parameters may be optimized by using the optimization methods such as Bayesian and Grid search. However, most of the studies presented experimental results without explaining the rationale behind the designed architectures.

While a CNN has the ability to learn powerful feature representations for the task at hand, this ability will not be revealed in the devoid of a large dataset. When there is not enough data to train a CNN effectively, a particular object in different positions and orientations within an image may not be recognized by the CNN. The reason for this is that the features related to the spatial relationship cannot be learned as a result of the pooling operations. Yet, this issue may be tackled properly when the appearances of an object in different spatial locations and orientations are included in the training data. Beyond that, a capsule network proposed by Sabour et al. (2017), which is nothing but an ANN, is an architecture specifically designed to solve this issue by adding special layers called capsules to the CNN. Unlike an artificial neuron, which produces only a scalar value, a capsule consists of neurons and produces an activity vector. Another difference with capsule network against a CNN is the replacement of pooling operation with the rooting-by-agreement scheme (Sabour et al. 2017). Because capsules consist of neurons, the connection between layers requires fewer learnable parameters, which makes capsule network effectively trainable compared to the CNN.

Toraman et al. (2020) proposed an algorithm for Covid-19 detection based on capsule network and X-ray images. The ability of the capsule network regarding Covid-19 detection was examined. For this purpose, a model was constructed, inspired by the original capsule network model proposed by Sabour et al. (2017). The proposed model included five convolutional blocks followed by a primary capsule layer and label capsule layer. The performance was 84.22% in terms of accuracy. As a result, it has been shown in the study that the capsule network can be effective in recognizing Covid-19 disease.

Afshar et al. (2020) proposed a capsule network framework including four convolutional layers and three capsule layers for detecting disease over X-ray images. First, the designed framework was pre-trained on an external X-ray dataset, which consisted of 94.32k images including the categories such as no findings, tumors, pleural diseases, lung infection, and others. Then, the framework was trained for Covid-19 detection. The performance attained in terms of accuracy was 95.7% without pre-training the model, and it improved to 98.3% after the model was pre-trained. Another point worth mentioning is that the proposed model achieves this accuracy with only 295k trainable parameters, while its CNN counterparts trained on the same dataset underperform with 20M trainable parameters.

Fusion

Feature fusion can be roughly defined as combining the information obtained by different feature extraction methods. The belief that combining features obtained via different methods will have higher representative power is the main motivation behind feature fusion. Alongside many medical image analysis tasks, this simple yet effective strategy has been also used for Covid-19 detection. Fusion strategy has been employed for Covid-19 detection in several different ways as discussed in the following.

Fusion of hand-crafted features: In this way of feature fusion, only the outputs of the different hand-crafted feature extraction methods are combined. Hand-crafted feature fusion is usually performed by connecting the feature vector returned by a method in series with the feature vector returned by another method. After the fusion, similar features are removed from the fused feature vector using a feature selection method, while the remaining features are fed to the machine learning model for training. This process is roughly summarized in Figure 6.2.

Öztürk et al. (2021) fused the feature vectors obtained by the methods GLCM, local binary gray level co-occurance (LBGLCM), segmentation-based fractal texture analysis (SFTA), and GLRLM. In total, 78 features (GLCM: 22, LBGLCM: 22, SFTA: 27, GLRLM: 7) were collected. Due to the scarcity of data, the authors aimed for data augmentation by utilizing the synthetic minority oversampling technique (SMOTE). Then, fused feature vector dimensionality was diminished by using stacked AutoEncoder (sAE) and the principal component analysis (PCA). While the SVM classification with 20 features and a sample size of 260 provided 88.46% accuracy, the accuracy increased to 94.23% for 495 sample sizes in the study.

Shankar et al. (2022) extracted the GLCM, GLRLM, and LBP features from Wiener filtered X-ray images for noise reduction. Then, the salp swarm optimization algorithm (SSA) was used to determine optimal feature set after the extracted features by each method were fused. In the work, while the optimal set of fused features combined with ANN model yielded 95.91% of accuracy for binary classification, the accuracy for the multi-class classification was 95.70%.

Usage of hand-crafted features along with deep learning features: This kind of fusion strategy aims to combine hand-crafted features and deep learning–based features, as given in Figure 6.3. As described earlier, some methods proposed at the beginning of the pandemic focused on hand-crafted feature extraction methods due to data scarcity. Some of these methods performed remarkably well. For this reason, some researchers have aimed to increase the representation power by combining hand-crafted features with local spatial features (i.e., deep learning features).

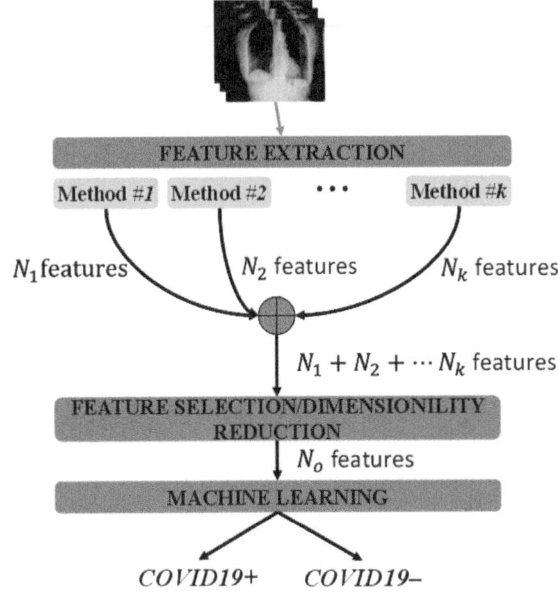

Figure 6.2 Hand-crafted feature fusion. The X-ray image is taken from the COVIDGR-1.0 dataset introduced by Tabik et al. (2020).

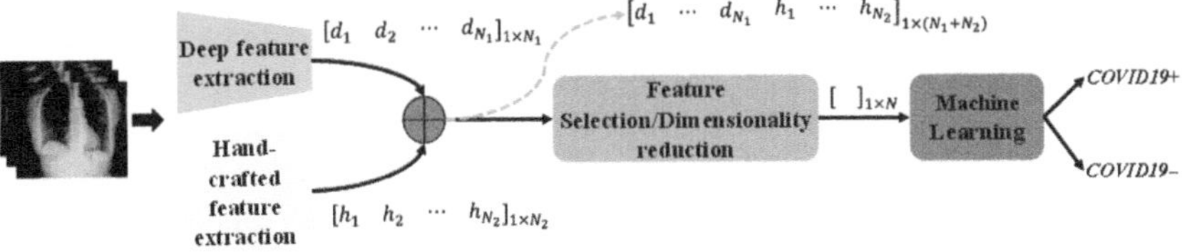

Figure 6.3 Fusion of hand-crafted features with deep features.

Dubey and Agrawal (2021) combined HoG features and fine-tuned VGG19 model features, each derived from X-ray images. While only the HoG features–based SVM classification yielded 72% of accuracy, fine-tuned VGG19 model alone yielded 97% of accuracy. On the other hand, fusing HoG features with VGG19 features increased the accuracy to 99%.

Shankar and Perumal (2020) fused the deep features obtained from the InceptionV3 with the LBP features after performing a preprocessing to eliminate the noise found in X-ray images. An accuracy of 94.08% was attained with the multi-layer perceptron (MLP) model in this study.

Alam et al. (2021) serially fused the HoG (3,780 features) and fine-tuned VGG19 (4,096 features) model features extracted from X-ray images. The fused vector dimension was reduced to 1186 from 7876 using maximum entropy-based feature selection. While the performance with HoG features alone was 87.34% of accuracy, it was 93.64% for CNN features. Indeed, the fused features–based classification improved the performance to 98.36% of accuracy.

Jamil et al. (2021) proposed another feature fusion strategy in which the spatial features are combined with the hand-crafted ones. While the spatial features are extracted by CNN (AlexNet, ResNet50, GoogLeNet, InceptionV3, VGG19), the hand-crafted features are extracted by the methods HoG, LBP, Oriented FAST and Rotated BRIEF (ORB). By integrating all the extracted features, the Bag of Features (BoF) vector was obtained. An accuracy of 77.7% was achieved with ORB feature–based SVM classification, which performed the best compared to HoG and LBP-based classification. On the other hand, the AlexNet features+SVM classification performance yielded 96.2% of accuracy and was the best performing one compared to other pre-trained network features. The best performance in the study was obtained using the BoF vector–based SVM classification, which provides 99.5% of accuracy.

Mostafiz et al. (2022) performed a preprocessing using anisotropic diffusion filtering and histogram equalization methods, respectively, before classification. The watershed segmentation was then performed to separate the lung regions. By performing the discrete wavelet transform (DWT) on the segmented image, it was concluded that the textural information found in the detail coefficients at the second-level of decomposition was more prominent compared to the preceding and subsequent levels. Therefore, GLCM features (computed in four directions 0°, 45°, 90°, 135°) such as energy, entropy, correlation, contrast, and homogeneity, and some statistical features (i.e., mean, standard deviation, skewness, variance, kurtosis) were extracted from three detail coefficients of the second-level of decomposition. The extracted 120 features hand-crafted features were fused with the 1,024 features obtained by the pre-trained ResNet50 model. The 1144-dimensional feature vector was reduced to 100 by minimum redundancy and maximum relevance algorithm (mRMR) combined with recursive feature elimination (RFE). For 4-class classification, while the DWT features–based RF classification alone yielded 81.53% of accuracy, using CNN features alone yielded 96.18% of accuracy. On the other hand, the accuracy improved to 98.48%, when feature fusion was conducted.

Fusion of deep learning features: In this category, different deep learning model features are fused generally before a feature selection stage to avoid the redundant features. Beyond that, features obtained from various layers of a CNN model can be fused with the motivation of combining high- and low-level details. To perform this, the custom designed end-to-end trainable architectures can be designed in accordance with Figure 6.4(a) and Figure 6.4(b), or following a similar fusion strategy. Furthermore, features of different deep learning models are fused in some papers where the end-to-end trainable models are proposed in accordance with Figure 6.5(a).

The pre-trained models, namely, VGG16, GoogLeNet, and ResNet50, were used as feature generator networks by Özkaya et al. (2020). Thus, a 1000-dimensional feature vector was obtained from each pre-trained model. Since there might be similar spatial-local features among the features of each network, fusion was conducted using the method called canonical correlation analysis. Then, the features were ranked according to the t-test method, and correlated features removed based on feature frequency. The accuracy scores attained for the models VGG16, GoogLeNet, and ResNet50 were 96.93%, 97.33%, and 97.87%, respectively. On the other hand, the proposed fusion method increased the performance to 98.27%.

Sitaula et al. (2021) used 4th max-pooling layer of pre-trained VGG16 model to extract features in three different scales. For this purpose, the activation maps obtained by the pooling layer were scaled using three different stride settings to be 1×1, 2×2, and 3×3. In the study, a well-known bag of visual words (BoW) method was used with the input features being deep features. Then the BoW features extracted in three different scales were fused to make final prediction with the SVM classifier. The performance was evaluated on publicly available X-ray datasets.

Fang et al. (2022) proposed a method called MSRCovXNet, which used the ResNet18 as the basis since it is one of the shallow yet effective models. First, the low-level details received from the preceding convolutional layer (named as C4 in the paper), which has $30 \times 30 \times 512$ in resolution, were enhanced via designed single-stage feature enhancement module (SSFM). The output of SSFM module, which was the half of C4 in resolution, was fused with the subsequent convolutional layer (named as C5 in the paper) output via designed multi-stage fusion module.

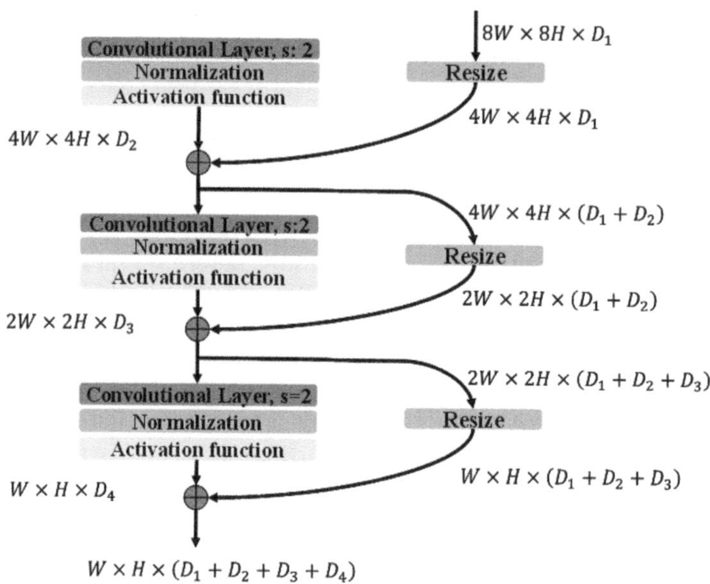

(a)

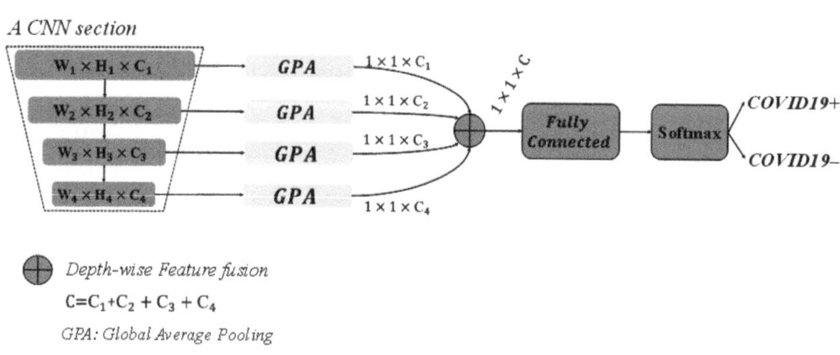

(b)

Figure 6.4 Different fusion methods that can be used in an end-to-end trainable deep learning model. **(a)** Fusion of various layers feature maps. **(b)** Depth-wise (or channel) feature fusion.

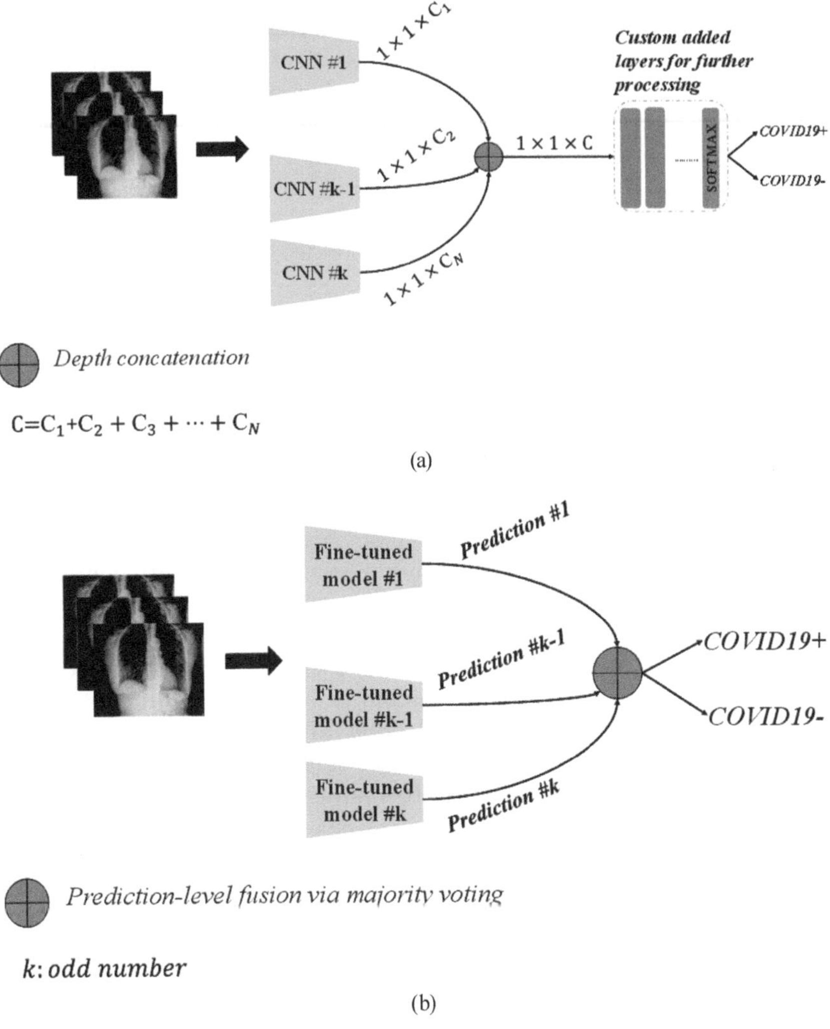

Figure 6.5 Fusing different deep learning model features. **(a)** Fusion of different deep learning model features in end-to-end trainable network. **(b)** Prediction level fusion with deep learning models.

Performance with the proposed methodology was revealed on two publicly available X-ray datasets, namely, the COVIDGR-1.0 and the COVIDx dataset. The performance in terms of accuracy on COVIDGR-1.0 dataset was 82.2%. For the COVIDx dataset, it was 94% in terms of recall metric.

In many methods developed in the literature, either X-ray or CT images are processed. In this sense, a different study was proposed by Muhammad and Shamim Hossain (2021). They proposed a fusion-based classification scheme that uses lung ultrasound (LUS) images for processing. The proposed scheme consisted of five successive blocks, each one including two successive convolution and batch normalization layers, and a skip connection. Then, a pooling operation was performed on the outputs of each block to be fused. The fused output was further processed by a fully connected layer, and softmax classification was then carried out. With this network with a total parameter load of approximately 0.4M, the performance obtained with fusion was 92.5% while it was 86.6% without fusion.

Öksüz et al. (2020) proposed a feature fusion method that assembles the feature maps of three lightweight fine-tuned models, i.e., SqueezeNet, ShuffleNet, and EfficientNetB0, running in parallel. The motivation behind such a fusion was to consolidate the feature map with high-level and low-level details. Accordingly, combining of deeper model EfficientNetB0 with a shallower model SqueezeNet model made an increase about 0.5% in performance, compared to the performance of EfficientNetB0. Moreover, integration of ShuffleNet to the framework, which is deeper than SqueezeNet yet shallow than EfficientNetB0, made an additional increase in performance by about 0.64%. The total performance attained with this end-to-end trainable framework was 98.30% in terms of accuracy. They also used their fusion strategy in Oksuz et al. (2021) for the segmentation of lung regions including the symptoms of Covid-19 disease and other kinds of lung diseases. The performance of the proposed model was improved by 13.87% in terms of Boundary F_1 score owing to the fusion of the feature maps obtained by each encoder.

Prediction-level fusion: In order to consolidate the final result, this fusion strategy aims to combine the predictions generated by different machine learning models. The majority voting scheme is one such technique used for this purpose. The model of the prediction-level fusion with deep learning methods is given in Figure 6.5(b).

Zebari et al. (2020) extracted LBP, Fractal Dimension (FD), and GLCM texture features from CT images, which are obtained from a standard dataset. Then, machine learning models, i.e., k-NN, SVM, and ANN, were trained with each texture feature to determine which model yielded the best performance for a particular textural feature set. The outperforming model for the LBP and the GLCM feature sets was SVM with 89.87% of accuracy and 90.98% of accuracy, respectively. On the other hand, the ANN model was the best-performing one for the FD feature set with 87.84% of accuracy. Finally, fusing ANN and SVM model predictions for corresponding feature sets using majority voting improved the performance to 96.91% of accuracy.

The residual networks, i.e., ResNet18, ResNet50, and ResNet101, were fine-tuned by Kaur and Gandhi (2022). In the study, the fine-tuned ResNet50 model provided the best performance against the other two models with 98.35% of accuracy. Beyond that, the performance with the different activation layer of ResNet50 model was further analyzed using the k-NN, Logistic Regression (LR), and SVM models. As a result, using the features of the layer called *res5b_branch2c*, the predictions of SVM, k-NN, and LR were fused with a majority voting scheme. The accuracy achieved in this work was 99.38%.

Kundu et al. (2021) utilized three transfer learning–based CNN models, namely, VGG11, InceptionV3, Wide ResNet50-2. The decision scores obtained by each model were fused with the help of Gombertz function that have an exponential growth. This kind of fusion was named as fuzzy-rank–based fusion as the adaptive weights were used according to the prediction scores returned by each classifier. The proposed classification scheme was validated on two publicly available CT datasets, the SARS-CoV-2 and the Harvard Dataverse. Performances in terms of accuracy for the SARS-CoV-2 and Harvard Dataverse datasets were 98.93% and 98.80%, respectively.

NEW ASPECTS

Attention-guided Frameworks

While the attention mechanism (Wang et al. 2017, Xiao et al. 2015) was first seen in the natural language processing field, it has now taken its place in the field of medical image analysis. Attention mechanisms allow the model to give more weight to important parts of the input data, allowing it to focus. Thus, more critical part of the data is taken into consideration by the model. Attention mechanisms, which are given in Figure 6.6(a) and 6.6(b), can be easily embedded into a CNN and impose almost no computational burden. Therefore, it is one of the new aspects also for intelligent diagnosis systems regarding Covid-19 detection or segmentation.

The attention mechanism is utilized in several studies regarding Covid-19 detection. Sitaula and Hossain (2021) preferred to use pretrained VGG16 as it yields low-level features due to its shallow nature against the VGG19 model. They modified the VGG16 module by inserting only the spatial attention mechanism after 4th pooling layer. Accordingly, average pooling and max pooling operations were first conducted on the output of this pooling layer. Then, the resultant 2D tensors were concatenated to perform a convolutional operation by the filter in size 7 × 7. Eventually, the sigmoid function was applied to the obtained map. In the study, while the performance was 75.25% in terms of accuracy with the fine-tuned VGG16 model, it was increased to 79.58% with the proposed framework.

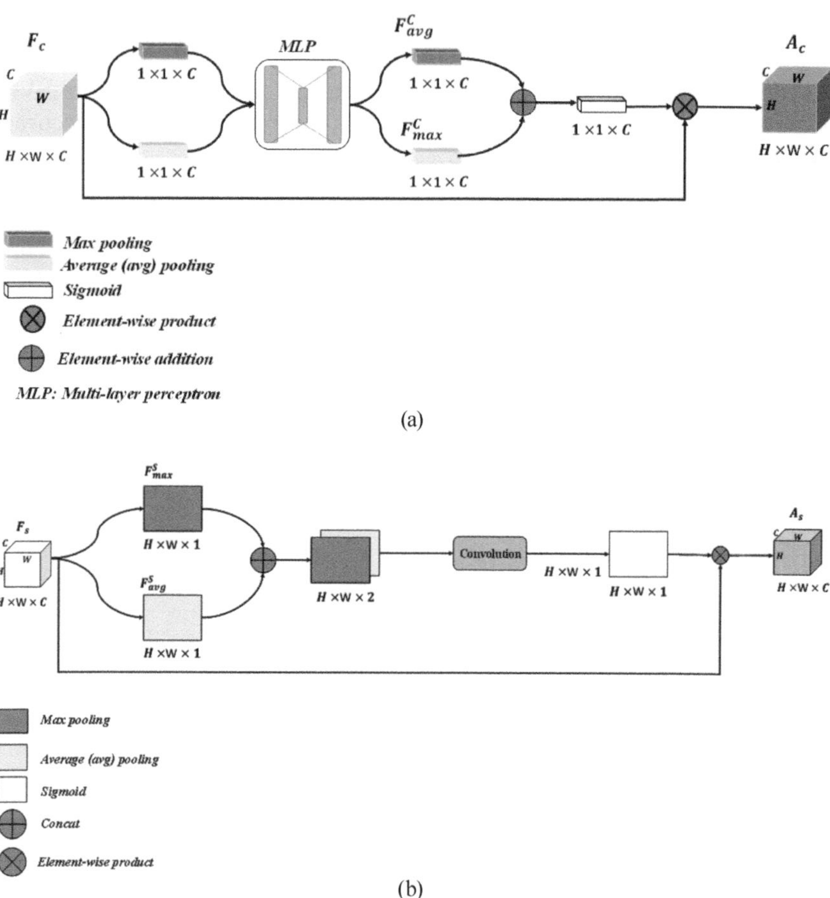

Figure 6.6   Attention mechanisms **(a)** Channel attention mechanism. **(b)** Spatial attention mechanism.

Zhou et al. (2021) used attention mechanisms within the U-Net model for the segmentation of lesions stemming from the Covid-19 disease using CT images. They utilized both the spatial and channel attention mechanism to enrich the contextual information. The main motivation behind their work was to explore a more efficient way of feature fusion to improve the performance of the U-Net model. For this purpose, the attention mechanisms were placed at each layer of the U-Net model in the work. The performance in terms of dice score was 82.2%, while it was 80.7% for the standard U-Net model.

Budak et al. (2021) proposed a SegNet-based framework with the attention mechanism for segmentation of regions affected by Covid-19 disease using CT images. The attention mechanism was used at the layers of the decoding path before each concatenation operation, which combines the feature maps (comes via skip connection) from the encoding path with the upstream feature maps. The performance accomplished by the proposed method was 89.61% in terms of dice score, while it was 87.56% for the bare SegNet model.

Nawshad et al. (2021) proposed a framework using X-ray images for Covid-19 detection in which the attention mechanism is used in the ResNet32 model. The attention mechanism was added to each ResNet32 block. The case in which the attention mechanism was placed before the classification stage was also evaluated for experimental purposes. However, the best-performing model was the former one, as expected. In the study, the performance obtained for the fine-tuned ResNet32 model was 96.79% in terms of accuracy, while it increased to 97.69% with the proposed model (ResNet32 with attention mechanism).

Zhang et al. (2021) proposed an end-to-end deep learning framework based on attention mechanisms called convolutional block attention module (CBAM). The proposed architecture was configured with two inputs to feed CT data and X-ray images for a subject. The authors intended to take advantage of this via feature fusion strategy, as each data has its own unique imaging features. Both the data were processed by successive CBAM modules added to the pathway, where the data was first received. Then, the data processed in parallel branches was fused for classification. An accuracy of 98.02% was achieved with the proposed framework in the study.

Afifi et al. (2021) adopted the Region of Interest (ROI)-based classification scheme in order to remove pertinent tissues that are lying outside the lung region. For this purpose, the lung region was first localized using RetinaNet, then lung tissues in localized regions were segmented after cropping. The classification process was carried out using two-parallel branches in which one was responsible for extracting global features while the other branch was responsible for extracting local features. Each branch commenced with a pre-trained CNN. While a pre-trained CNN was followed by a global average pooling layer for the branch responsible for generating global features, attention mechanism was used after the pre-trained CNN at the other branch. Then the generated class probabilities by each branch were averaged to get final results. An accuracy of 91.2% was achieved in this work.

Siddiqui et al. (2021) proposed a Covid-19 classification scheme in which the multi-attention mechanism was used. First, a generative adversarial network (GAN) was used to produce synthetic images for handling scarcity of Covid-19 data. Then, the generated image by the

GAN was partitioned into patches and also encoded for feeding them to the multi-head attention unit. Thus, attention-weighted features were fed into a CNN for further processing, and finally classification was performed by a dense layer after a simple MLP unit. The accuracy achieved by the proposed method was 83.96%.

Li et al. (2022a) proposed an innovative capsule network architecture by inserting multi-head attention routing unit between the primary capsule and the class capsule. As used in other capsule network–based frameworks related to Covid-19 detection, the proposed framework was commenced with four cascading convolution blocks. Then, the depth-wise convolution operation was performed over the obtained tensor to reduce the number of parameters before feeding it to the primary capsule layer. It was revealed in this work that multi-head attention routing scheme performs better compared to the traditional dynamic routing, and better quantifies the relevancy between capsule layers. The performance obtained with this network, which contained 0.33M of parameters, was 97.28% in terms of accuracy.

Multi-task Convolutional Network

Multi-task learning is an approach that allows learning of different tasks in a parallel way by a shared representation (i.e., the common backbone network). The main assumption behind the multi-task learning is that different tasks share similar feature representations, and so a simultaneous training may be conducted (Amyar et al. 2020). In this approach, learning one task can encourage better learning of other tasks (Caruana 1997). With breakthrough advancements in the deep learning field, multi-task learning approach has taken its place as a multi-task convolutional network. A multi-task convolutional network is a network that is built to perform many tasks like detection, segmentation, and estimation of a score simultaneously. Designing such a network architecture can improve performance, and this is one of the design reasons for researchers. The general structure for a multi-task network is given in Figure 6.7. As seen in Figure 6.7, the encoder is the common backbone network for each task, and its weights are to be optimized based on the losses from these tasks. The total loss is used for gradient updates and the weights of each loss in the total loss function must have a proper value for convergence.

Multi-task networks have also been used for Covid-19 detection during the pandemic. Amyar et al. (2020) proposed a multi-task convolutional network including parallel three branches (or tasks) in accordance with Figure 6.7. The lesion segmentation, Covid-19 disease prediction, and image reconstruction tasks were carried out simultaneously. The motivation behind the image reconstruction task was to improve the feature representations. In this study, the performance achieved with the proposed network was significantly better than networks designed for classification alone or for segmentation alone. While 96% sensitivity was obtained in the classification task, 88% dice score was obtained in the segmentation task. Similar multi-task network architectures have been proposed by Li et al. (2022b) and Bao et al. (2022).

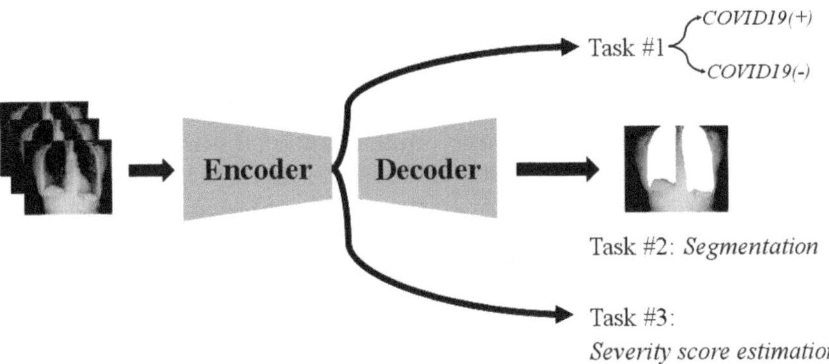

Figure 6.7   General structure of a multi-task network.

While many of the proposed frameworks are focused on detecting the Covid-19 disease, some works aim to propose frameworks that are able to predict the severity level of the disease as it is more informative about the patient's condition. Öksüz et al. (2021) proposed a multi-task network according to Figure 6.7, which predicts two different severity scores, namely, the consolidation extent and the opacity extent. The different ImageNet models, SqueezeNet, ShuffleNet, MobileNetv2, ResNet18, GoogLeNet, and EfficientNetB0, were used as the common backbone models for predicting each score. The superior performance in terms of rmse (root-mean-square-error) for each severity score was achieved when using the ShuffleNet model as the common backbone. The proposed method, which was cross-validated on 76 images, gave a score of 1.39 and 0.98 for lung involvement and opacity, respectively. The pre-trained DenseNet (Huang et al. 2018) model was used in a similar study by Cohen et al. (2020) to predict lung involvement and opacity scores. Performances regarding rmse scores for lung involvement and opacity were 1.43 and 0.92, respectively.

Semi-supervised Learning

Semi-supervised learning (SSL) is a learning approach that falls between supervised and unsupervised learning. In SSL, labeled data, relatively less in amount, is assembled with unlabeled data, which is relatively large compared to labeled data, in the training process. The SSL strategy is based on using the unlabeled data as the regularizer for improving the performance of learner. To do this, some assumptions are needed, namely, smoothness, cluster, and manifold. These assumptions can be realized by using consistency regularization (Berthelot et al. 2019) and entropy regularization (Berthelot et al. 2019) in which the former requires the decision boundary located in a low-density region (the region with a minimum number of samples) and the latter forces the learner to make predictions with low entropy for unlabeled data (Chapelle et al. 2006).

One of the studies adopting SSL in medical image analysis was performed by Liu et al. (2020). They classified 14 different thorax diseases using chest X-ray images. The performance attained was 79.23% in terms of AUC score when 20%-labeled and 80%-unlabeled data was used. On the other hand, performance with the supervised learning was 81.75%, which was slightly higher. This reveals the potential of SSL.

Since the pandemic began, much of what has been done for recognizing Covid-19 disease from medical images has been oriented toward supervised learning, which requires a lot of training data in order to learn the accurate decision boundaries of the model. However, there is not sufficient labeled data in practice, and labeling the data may be laborious and expensive for clinicians. In addition, the privacy of patient data is another issue that states that the model trained with private data cannot be used in any other health center. Accordingly, labeled samples have the potential to remain a minority compared to unlabeled Covid-19 samples. Therefore, recent research predominantly adopts SSL with this motivation.

Zhang et al. (2022) proposed deep SSL method for Covid-19 detection. One of the recent SSL techniques, i.e., MixMatch (Berthelot et al. 2019), was re-arranged to avoid the overfitting risk by following the proposed Training Signal Annealing (TSA) method in this study. The basic principle of the TSA method was to gradually remove labeled data with the increase of unlabeled data in the training process. Instead of the MixUp, which is used as a regularization method with MixMatch, the CAMMix method was proposed as a data enhancement method. In the CAMMix method, the most descriptive region of the medical image was determined by considering the GradCAM responses. Then, this region was cropped for merging it with another image to get the mixed image. The attention module has also been modified for extracting the multi-scale features to be used with the pre-trained architectures, i.e., DenseNet121 and ResNet50. The performances attained for ResNet50, ResNet50+Attention mechanism, ResNet50+SSL, ResNet50+Attention mechanism+SSL were 78.6%, 79.1%, 80.2%, and 90.1%, respectively.

Another challenging issue with deep learning methods is the uneven distribution of the data. Calderon-Ramirez et al. (2021) corrected their imbalanced data by modifying the MixMatch method. The accuracy was improved by up to 18% for multi-class classification. Alizadehsani et al. (2021) proposed a semi-supervised classification using limited labeled data. The output of the GANs discriminator was a probability value in the classification, and the detection was improved with Sobel edge detection. With the proposed methods, 99.60% of accuracy was achieved.

Han et al. (2021) proposed a semi-supervised deep CNN and tried to emphasize the significance of SSL. So, labeled and unlabeled CT datasets were used for supervised and semi-supervised learning methods. Accuracy of 99.83% was accomplished by this method. Khobahi et al. (2020) used a network to extract task-based features together with a Covid-19 identification network in their novel semi-supervised deep learning architecture. The importance of this study is that unrelated datasets can also be trained since autoencoders were used. Obtained accuracy with this study was 93.5%.

DISCUSSION

As can be understood from the studies summarized, the performance revealed by many methods has been reported to be over 90%, which points to the situation that needs to be discussed. The fact that the specified model performances are so high may be closely related to the dataset with bias used in model training and testing. A few factors that can cause bias are mentioned here.

1. **Mismatch of patients' demographics:** One of the Kaggle datasets, namely, the Covid-19 Radiography Dataset (Covid-19 Radiography Database, n.d.), has been largely used in the studies. This is a three-class compilation dataset recorded by combining two different datasets, each with completely different patient demographics. The Covid-19 cases in this dataset, which are collected from another well-known dataset called the Covid-19 Image Data Collection as well as some publications, belong to adults. However, viral pneumonia and normal cases collected from a UCSD-Guangzhou dataset (Chest X-Ray Images (Pneumonia), n.d.; Kermany et al. 2018), shared in Kaggle, belong to pediatric patients.

2. **Imbalance in the number of data on different forms of the disease:** Another thing worth mentioning is that majority of the cases in some datasets include the severe forms of the Covid-19

disease. But the Covid-19 disease may have also asymptomatic, mild, and moderate forms. The Covid-19 disease severe forms can be readily captured by models as the disease-specific patterns are more obvious in images. However, the others, especially the asymptomatic and mild forms, cannot be readily captured since they do not have prominent signatures in medical images.

Tabik et al. (2020) assembled the COVIDGR-1.0 dataset, which is a well-balanced dataset with two-class, by considering the severity forms of Covid-19 disease. About 81% of this dataset is out of severe forms. Their model, namely the COVID-SDNet, was validated on the dataset and yielded about 72.59% of sensitivity. The stated accuracies for mild, moderate, and severe forms were 46%, 85.38%, and 97.22%, respectively. Öksüz et al. (2022) validated their method using the COVIDGR-1.0 dataset, which yielded 78.60% of specificity. The stated accuracies for mild, moderate, and severe forms were 60.51%, 85.95%, and 96.36%, respectively. Lin et al. (2021) also used the COVIDGR-1.0 dataset to develop their method. In this study, which reached 86.05% sensitivity, the accuracies were 73.68%, 91.43%, and 100% for mild, moderate, and severe forms, respectively.

The methods in these studies yielded over 95% performance for severe forms of the disease, which account for 20% of all positive cases in the dataset. On the other hand, performance is significantly lower on mild and moderate forms of the disease, which included 80% of all positive conditions in the dataset. This reveals the difficulty of learning hidden patterns, especially in mild forms of the disease.

3. **Lack of metadata:** Metadata has significance in that it carries information about patients' demographics such as sex, age, weight, height, location, and comorbidity. Metadata also allows for tracking how many images are available for a patient with the given patient ID. Thus, it is possible to partition the data at the patient level, which is important to curb the data leakage issue, and so biased learning of the model.

4. **Uncertainty about training data:** Compilation sets have also been recorded during the pandemic, which do not contain information about what source they came from, what kind of machine they were obtained from, and even how the labeling for the Covid-19 disease was made. This can cause confusion about what models should learn and cause models to focus on unwanted details.

One study that presents interesting findings has been made by Maguolo and Nanni (2021). First, model training was carried out by removing the images from the lung regions of the X-ray image. Then, performance was evaluated by performing a whole image–based classification process without removing the lung regions. For model evaluations performed on one of the datasets commonly used during the pandemic process, a similar performance was obtained in both cases. This situation reveals the model has learned the noise instead of desired features.

Catala et al. (2021) tried to reveal the bias via several tests including network activations, background expansion, and lung exclusion. They have experimented with the datasets, i.e., Covid-19 Image Data Collection (Cohen, Morrison, et al. 2020), CheXpert (Irvin et al. 2019), RSNA pneumonia (RSNA Pneumonia Detection Challenge, n.d.), and BIMCV PadChest (Bustos et al. 2020). Grad-CAM visualizations were utilized to demonstrate the bias via network activations. Accordingly, highly activated regions for images from the BIMCV dataset were outside the lung regions, contrary to expectations. In another experiment, background expansion and lung exclusion were performed to reveal the dataset bias. With background expansion, their rationale was that the gradual incorporation of background regions into the lung region should not increase performance scores for a non-biased dataset. On the other hand, with the lung exclusion experiment, they expected to encounter a situation where performance should decrease as the disease-specific patterns would be lost while the lung region was gradually removed from the entire image. Their findings revealed that the BIMCV dataset contains a high bias as it steadily improves classification performance with background expansion. Moreover, the classification performance was 0.88 in terms of the AUC score (the expected score should be around 0.5) when the whole lung region was occluded. This situation was similar to the RSNA dataset for both tests. However, they encountered an interesting situation in the CheXpert dataset, where the inclusion of background information did not provide any performance improvement, but the performance was around 0.74 in terms of the AUC score when the entire lung region was closed. Again, this was indicative of bias that was not specifically located in the background but was instead embedded in the entire image.

A summary of the studies using intelligent detection methods found in the literature for the detection of Covid-19 disease and included in this study is given in Table 6.2.

Table 6.2   Related literature on intelligent Covid-19 diagnosis.

Authors	Datasets	Used Features and Methods	Best Result(s)
Hand-crafted (Classical) Feature Extraction Methods			
Öksüz et al. (2022)	X-ray images	Investigating feature descriptors: HoG, LBP, GLCM, MSER, SURF, BRIEF	69.01% of accuracy was obtained when LBP features were combined with the SVM classifier.
Guiot et al. (2021)	Lung regions segmented CT images	Used features are first order statistics, intensity histogram statistics, shape features, texture features were obtained by the following methods: GLCM, GLRLM, GLSZM, GLDZM, NGTDM, NGLDM	The performance of the proposed method was 88.2%.
Hussain et al. (2020)	X-ray images	Texture features obtained using GLCM and morphological features were classified with XGBoost–Linear, XGBoost–Tree, k-NN, CART, and naïve Bayes	79.52% of accuracy is achieved with the XGBoost–Linear model for multi-class classification.
Pre-trained Deep Learning Networks			
Ismael and Şengür (2021)	X-ray images	The following pre-trained models were fine-tuned: VGG16, VGG19, ResNet18, ResNet50, ResNet101	94.7% of accuracy was attained when the deep features obtained by ResNet50 model were combined with SVM model.
Öksüz et al. (2022)	X-ray images	Using the following pre-trained models as feature extractors: GoogLeNet, SqueezeNet, ShuffleNet, ResNet18, EfficientNetB0, Xceptions	76.06% of accuracy, feature set extracted by Xception
Ahsan et al. (2021)	CT and X-ray images	Fine-tuning the following pre-trained networks: VGG16, MobileNetV2, InceptionResNetV2, ResNet50, ResNet101, VGG19	MobileNetV2 model yielded 95% of accuracy.
Custom-designed Deep Learning Models			
Toraman et al. (2020)	X-ray images	A capsule network model including five convolutional blocks followed by a primary capsule layer and label capsule layer was constructed.	The performance achieved by the proposed method was 84.22% in terms of accuracy.

Authors	Datasets	Used Features and Methods	Best Result(s)
Afshar et al. (2020)	X-ray images	A capsule network framework designed by including four convolutional layers, and three capsule layers. Firstly trained with other lung diseases data. Then, trained with Covid-19 dataset.	Accuracy was 95.7% without pre-training the model; 98.3% after the model was pre-trained.
Fusion of Hand-crafted Features			
Öztürk et al. (2021)	X-ray images and CT	Fused the feature vectors obtained by the following methods: GLCM, LBGLCM, SFTA, GLRLM. The feature vector dimensionality was reduced by using sAE and PCA.	SVM classification provided 94.23% accuracy by increasing sample sizes.
Shankar et al. (2022)	Wiener filtered X-ray images for noise reduction	Fused featured from GLCM, GLRLM, and LBP	Combined with ANN model, yielded 95.91% of accuracy for binary classification.
Fusion of Hand-crafted and Deep Learning Features			
Dubey and Agrawal (2021)	X-ray images	Combined HoG features and fine-tuned VGG19 model features	99% of accuracy
Shankar and Perumal (2020)	X-ray images	Fused the deep features obtained from the InceptionV3 with the LBP features	94.08% of accuracy was attained with the MLP
Alam et al. (2021)	X-ray images	Fused the HoG features and fine-tuned VGG19 features	98.36% of accuracy
Jamil et al. (2021)	X-ray images	The spatial features extracted by CNN (AlexNet, ResNet50, GoogLeNet, InceptionV3, VGG19) are fused with the hand-crafted features (HoG, LBP, Oriented FAST and Rotated BRIEF [ORB])	BoF vector–based SVM classification provides 99.5% of accuracy.
Mostafiz et al. (2022)	X-ray images	120 features hand-crafted features were fused with the 1,024 features obtained by pre-trained ResNet50 model	98.48% of accuracy when feature fusion was conducted

(Contd...)

Table 6.2 (*Contd.*)   Related literature on intelligent Covid-19 diagnosis.

Authors	Datasets	Used Features and Methods	Best Result(s)
Fusion of Deep Learning Features			
Özkaya et al. (2020)	CT images	Pre-trained models, namely, VGG16, GoogLeNet, and ResNet50 were used as feature extractors	Fusion method increased the performance to 98.27%.
Sitaula et al. (2021)	X-ray datasets	BoW features extracted in three different scales from 4th max-pooling layer of pre-trained VGG16 model	Validated on publicly available X-ray datasets.
Fang et al. (2022)	X-ray images	A method called MSRCovXNet was proposed. It fused the preceding convolutional layer enhanced via SSFM with the subsequent convolutional layer via multi-stage fusion module.	Validated on publicly available X-ray datasets. Accuracy on COVIDGR-1.0 dataset was 82.2%. For the COVIDx dataset, it was 94%.
Muhammad and Shamim Hossain (2021)	Lung ultrasound (LUS) images	Five successive blocks, each one including two successive convolution and batch normalization layer, and a skip connection fused with pooling operation	With fusion accuracy was 92.5%, while it was 86.6% without fusion.
Öksüz et al. (2020)	X-ray images	Fused the feature maps of three fine-tuned models, SqueezeNet, ShuffleNet, and EfficientNetB0	98.30% of accuracy
Attention-guided Frameworks			
Sitaula and Hossain (2021)	X-ray images	Use pre-trained VGG-16 by inserting only the spatial attention mechanism after 4th pooling layer	Improved to 79.58% of accuracy
Zhou et al. (2021)	CT images	Utilized both the spatial and channel attention mechanism within the U-Net model	Improved to 82.2% of accuracy
Budak et al. (2021)	CT images	Attention mechanism was used at the layers of the decoding path	Improved to 89.61% of accuracy
Nawshad et al. (2021)	X-ray images	Attention mechanism was added to each ResNet32 block	Increased to 97.69% of accuracy
Zhang et al. (2021)	CT data and X-ray images	Proposed a CBAM, which is an end-to-end deep learning framework benefitting attention mechanisms	98.02% of accuracy

Authors	Datasets	Used Features and Methods	Best Result(s)
Afifi et al. (2021)	X-ray images	Lung region was first localized using RetinaNet, then lung tissues in localized regions were segmented after cropping	91.2% of accuracy
Siddiqui et al. (2021)	Generated synthetic images	Attention-weighted features were fed into a CNN	With a dense layer after a simple MLP unit, 83.96% of accuracy
Li et al. (2022a)	X-ray images	Capsule network architecture by inserting multi-head attention routing unit between the primary capsule and the class capsule	97.28% accuracy
Öksüz et al. (2024)	X-ray images	CBAM is employed for further processing the feature maps generated by pre-trained encoders which are ensembled in an end-to-end trainable CNN.	85.45% of accuracy
Multi-task Convolutional Networks			
Amyar et al. (2020)	CT images	A multi-task convolutional network including parallel three branches	96% sensitivity was obtained in the classification task, 88% dice score was obtained in the segmentation task.
Öksüz et al. (2021)	X-ray images	Predicts two different severity scores of Covid-19. Different ImageNet models, SqueezeNet, ShuffleNet, MobileNetv2, ResNet18, GoogLeNet, and EfficientNetB0 were used as the common backbone models.	Using the ShuffleNet, a score of 1.39 and 0.98 for lung involvement and opacity was achieved, respectively.
Cohen et al. (2020)	X-ray images	The pre-trained DenseNet model was used.	The rmse scores for lung involvement and opacity were 1.43 and 0.92, respectively.
Semi-supervised Learning			
Zhang et al. (2022)	CT images	Proposed a deep semi-supervised learning method by re-arranging a semi-supervised learning technique, MixMatch regularized with CAMMix. The attention module is modified with the DenseNet121 and ResNet50.	The following accuracies were obtained: 78.6% for ResNet50, 79.1% for ResNet50+Attention mechanism, 80.2% for ResNet50+SSL, 90.1% for ResNet50+Attention mechanism+SSL.

(Contd...)

Table 6.2 (*Contd.*)   Related literature on intelligent Covid-19 diagnosis.

Authors	Datasets	Used Features and Methods	Best Result(s)
Calderon-Ramirez et al. (2021)	X-ray images	Modified the unbalanced data with MixMatch	Accuracy was increased by 18%
Alizadehsani et al. (2021)	CT images	A semi-supervised classification method using limited labeled data was proposed.	Accuracy of 99.60%
Han et al. (2021)	CT images	Proposed a semi-supervised deep CNN	Accuracy of 99.83%
Khobahi et al. (2020)	Chest X-ray image	A deep semi-supervised learning, which is benefitting from two networks, i.e., task-based feature extraction network and Covid-19 identification network.	Accuracy of 93.5%

CONCLUSION

From the literature, it was observed that the use of AI, one of the main intelligent diagnosis and treatment methods, is the most common even for different health issues. Within the scope of this study, the general observation of the working differences of the smart methods developed for the recognition of Covid-19 disease through medical images and the comparison of the results obtained with the use are presented. The highly contagious nature of the Covid-19 disease has prompted the interest of many researchers to develop efficient smart systems to address the global problem. Plenty of methods have been proposed to detect the disease during the pandemic. In this study, we mainly focused on the methods proposed to detect the disease using imaging features. While there are classical strategies using machine learning models with features returned by hand-crafted feature extraction algorithms, the majority of studies adopt innovative strategies using deep learning. As the deep learning models enable the models to learn representations of any given task via weight optimization process, the performance accomplished is superior to traditional methods. However, learning strong representations with a CNN as a deep learning–based method requires a deeper network to extract distinguishing features, which means more trainable parameters and thus more image data. Among the deep learning–based methods, the pre-trained ImageNet models (or CNNs) have been widely utilized with a fine-tuning strategy for handling the scarcity of data, which was an important issue, especially at the beginning of the pandemic.

Now, visual transformer with the self-attention mechanism, which is another deep learning–based method, is among the recent trends for Covid-19 detection. Unlike a CNN that learns features in a hierarchical manner from the local to the global, a global context may be learned even by the first layer of the transformer model owing to the self-attention mechanism. This feature of the attention mechanism has enabled it to be included in CNN architectures to increase focus on important details. The spatial and channel attention mechanisms have been included in well-known models such as VGG16, VGG19, some ResNet family models, and U-Net to optimize the performance.

New developments in the deep learning era make it possible to learn representations effectively even when there is extremely scarce data. Deep SSL is one such advancement utilized for Covid-19 detection as well, as summarized in this study. As stated in the previous sections, even if 20% of the available data is used in deep SSL, the performance achieved when 80% of the data is used in supervised learning can be achieved.

As reviewed in this study, more sophisticated algorithms have more potential to handle the requirements for clinical settings. Nevertheless, the use of an intelligent system in a clinical setting largely depends on the highly minimized false negative rate and false positive rate without biased learning of the models. Only the systems designed for Covid-19 detection in this manner may provide better isolation capability, better observation of disease progression, and better management of the pandemic.

REFERENCES

Afifi, A., Hafsa, N.E., Ali, M.A.S., Alhumam, A. and Alsalman, S. 2021. An ensemble of global and local-attention based convolutional neural networks for Covid-19 diagnosis on chest X-ray images. Symmetry. 13(1): 113.

Afshar, P., Heidarian, S., Naderkhani, F., Oikonomou, A., Plataniotis, K.N. and Mohammadi, A. 2020. COVID-CAPS: a capsule network-based framework for identification of Covid-19 cases from X-ray images. Pattern Recognition Letters. 138: 638–643.

Ahsan, M.M., Nazim, R., Siddique, Z. and Huebner, P. 2021. Detection of Covid-19 patients from CT scan and chest X-ray data using modified MobileNetV2 and LIME. Healthcare. 9(9): 1099.

Alam, N.-A., Ahsan, M., Based, M.A., Haider, J. and Kowalski, M. 2021. Covid-19 detection from chest X-ray images using feature fusion and deep learning. Sensors. 21(4): 1480.

Algin, O., Gökalp, G. and Topal, U. 2011. Signs in chest imaging. Diagnostic and Interventional Radiology (Ankara, Turkey). 17: 18–29.

Alizadehsani, R., Sharifrazi, D., Izadi, N.H., Joloudari, J.H., Shoeibi, A., Gorriz, J.M., et al. 2021. Uncertainty-aware semi-supervised method using large unlabeled and limited labeled Covid-19 data. ACM Transactions on Multimedia Computing, Communication and Applications (TOMM). 17(3s): 1–24.

Amadasun, M. and King, R. 1989. Textural features corresponding to textural properties. IEEE Transactions on Systems, Man, and Cybernetics. 19(5): 1264–1274.

Amyar, A., Modzelewski, R., Li, H. and Ruan, S. 2020. Multi-task deep learning based CT imaging analysis for Covid-19 pneumonia: classification and segmentation. Computers in Biology and Medicine. 126: 104037.

Angelyn, J. and Putri, R.N. 2021. Diagnosis system design of depression and anxiety with naïve Bayes method. Journal of Applied Business and Technology. 2(2): 92–97.

Bao, G., Chen, H., Liu, T., Gong, G., Yin, Y., Wang, L., et al. 2022. COVID-MTL: multitask learning with Shift3D and random-weighted loss for Covid-19 diagnosis and severity assessment. Pattern Recognition. 124: 108499.

Bay, H., Ess, A., Tuytelaars, T. and Van Gool, L. 2008. Speeded-up robust features (SURF). Computer Vision and Image Understanding. 110(3): 346–359.

Berthelot, D., Carlini, N., Goodfellow, I., Papernot, N., Oliver, A. and Raffel, C.A. 2019. MixMatch: a holistic approach to semi-supervised learning. Advances in Neural Information Processing Systems. 32.

Budak, Ü., Çıbuk, M., Cömert, Z. and Şengür, A. 2021. Efficient Covid-19 segmentation from CT slices exploiting semantic segmentation with integrated attention mechanism. Journal of Digital Imaging, 34(2): 263–272.

Bustos, A., Pertusa, A., Salinas, J.-M. and de la Iglesia-Vayá, M. 2020. PadChest: a large chest X-ray image dataset with multi-label annotated reports. Medical Image Analysis. 66, 101797.

Calderon-Ramirez, S., Yang, S., Moemeni, A., Elizondo, D., Colreavy-Donnelly, S., Chavarría-Estrada, L.F., et al. 2021. Correcting data imbalance for semi-supervised covid-19 detection using X-ray chest images. Applied Soft Computing. 111: 107692.

Calonder, M., Lepetit, V., Strecha, C. and Fua, P. 2010. BRIEF: binary robust independent elementary features. pp. 778–792. *In:* Daniilidis, K., Maragos, P. and Paragios, N. (eds). Computer Vision—ECCV 2010. Springer.

Caruana, R. 1997. Multitask learning. Machine Learning. 28(1): 41–75.

Catala, O.D.T., Igual, I.S., Perez-Benito, F.J., Escriva, D.M., Castello, V.O., Llobet, R., et al. 2021. Bias analysis on public x-ray image datasets of pneumonia and Covid-19 patients. IEEE Access. 9: 42370–42383.

Chapelle, O., Schölkopf, B. and Zien, A. (eds). 2006. Semi-supervised Learning. MIT Press.

Chen, H., Ai, L., Lu, H. and Li, H. 2020. Clinical and imaging features of Covid-19. Radiology of Infectious Diseases. 7(2): 43–50.

Chest X-Ray Images (Pneumonia). 2018. Accessed at https://www.kaggle.com/datasets/paultimothymooney/chest-xray-pneumonia (on October 4, 2022).

Chollet, F. 2017. Xception: Deep Learning with Depthwise Separable Convolutions. 1251–1258.

Cohen, J.P., Dao, L., Roth, K., Morrison, P., Bengio, Y., Abbasi, A.F., et al. 2020. Predicting Covid-19 pneumonia severity on chest X-ray with deep learning. Cureus. 12(7): e9448.

Cohen, J.P., Morrison, P., Dao, L., Roth, K., Duong, T.Q. and Ghassemi, M. 2020. Covid-19 image data collection: prospective predictions are the future. arXiv:2006.11988 [Cs, Eess, q-Bio].

Covid-19 Radiography Database. (n.d.). Accessed at https://www.kaggle.com/datasets/tawsifurrahman/covid19-radiography-database (on October 4, 2022).

Dalal, N. and Triggs, B. 2005. Histograms of oriented gradients for human detection. 2005 IEEE Computer Society Conference on Computer Vision and Pattern Recognition (CVPR'05). 1: 886–893. Vol. 1.

Dubey, R. and Agrawal, J. 2021. Fusion of hand-crafted and automatically generated features for improving the performance of Covid-19 X-ray image classification. 2021 IEEE International Conference on Technology, Research and Innovation for Betterment of Society (TRIBES). 1–6.

Fang, Z., Ren, J., MacLellan, C., Li, H., Zhao, H., Hussain, A., et al. 2022. A novel multi-stage residual feature fusion network for detection of Covid-19 in chest x-ray images. IEEE Transactions on Molecular, Biological and Multi-Scale Communications. 8(1): 17–27.

Galloway, M.M. 1975. Texture analysis using gray level run lengths. Computer Graphics and Image Processing. 4(2): 172–179.

Geniş, Y. and Aydin, E.A. 2022. Diagnosis of epilepsy disease with deep learning methods using EEG signals. 2022 30th Signal Processing and Communications Applications Conference (SIU). 1–4.

Guiot, J., Vaidyanathan, A., Deprez, L., Zerka, F., Danthine, D., Frix, A.-N., et al. (2021). Development and validation of an automated radiomic CT signature for detecting Covid-19. Diagnostics. 11(1): 41.

Han, C.H., Kim, M. and Kwak, J.T. 2021. Semi-supervised learning for an improved diagnosis of Covid-19 in CT images. PLoS One. 16(4): e0249450.

Haralick, R.M., Shanmugam, K. and Dinstein, I. 1973. Textural features for image classification. IEEE Transactions on Systems, Man, and Cybernetics, SMC. 3(6): 610–621.

He, X., Cai, D. and Niyogi, P. 2006. Laplacian score for feature selection. pp. 507–514. *In:* Weiss, Y., Schölkopf, B. and Platt, J. (eds). Advances in Neural Information Processing Systems. Vol. 18. MIT Press.

He, K., Zhang, X., Ren, S. and Sun, J. 2016. Deep residual learning for image recognition. Proceedings of the IEEE Conference on Computer Vision and Pattern Recognition. 770–778.

Huang, G., Liu, Z., van der Maaten, L. and Weinberger, K.Q. 2018. Densely connected convolutional networks. arXiv:1608.06993 [Cs].

Huang, S., Yang, J., Fong, S. and Zhao, Q. 2020. Artificial intelligence in cancer diagnosis and prognosis: opportunities and challenges. Cancer Letters, 471: 61–71.

Hussain, L., Nguyen, T., Li, H., Abbasi, A.A., Lone, K.J., Zhao, Z., et al. 2020. Machine-learning classification of texture features of portable chest X-ray accurately classifies Covid-19 lung infection. BioMedical Engineering OnLine, 19(1): 88.

Iandola, F.N., Han, S., Moskewicz, M.W., Ashraf, K., Dally, W.J. and Keutzer, K. 2016. SqueezeNet: AlexNet-level accuracy with 50x fewer parameters and <0.5MB model size. arXiv:1602.07360 [Cs].

Irvin, J., Rajpurkar, P., Ko, M., Yu, Y., Ciurea-Ilcus, S., Chute, C., et al. 2019. CheXpert: a large chest radiograph dataset with uncertainty labels and expert comparison. Proceedings of the AAAI Conference on Artificial Intelligence. 33(01): 590–597.

Ismael, A.M. and Şengür, A. 2021. Deep learning approaches for Covid-19 detection based on chest X-ray images. Expert Systems with Applications. 164: 114054.

Itchhaporia, D. 2022. Artificial intelligence in cardiology. Trends in Cardiovascular Medicine. 32(1): 34–41.

Jamil, S., Abbas, M.S., Ahsan, M. and Ejaz, M.T. 2021. A bag-of-features (BoF) based novel framework for the detection of Covid-19. 2021 15th International Conference on Open Source Systems and Technologies (ICOSST). 1–6.

Juneja, A., Rana, B. and Agrawal, R.K. 2018. A novel fuzzy rough selection of non-linearly extracted features for schizophrenia diagnosis using fMRI. Computer Methods and Programs in Biomedicine. 155: 139–152.

Kanji, J.N., Zelyas, N., MacDonald, C., Pabbaraju, K., Khan, M.N., Prasad, A., et al. 2021. False negative rate of Covid-19 PCR testing: a discordant testing analysis. Virology Journal. 18(1): 13.

Kannan, S., Premalatha, G., Jamuna Rani, M., Jayakumar, D., Senthil, P., Palanivelrajan, S., et al. 2022. Effective evaluation of medical images using artificial intelligence techniques. Computational Intelligence and Neuroscience. 2022, e8419308.

Kaur, T. and Gandhi, T.K. 2022. Classifier fusion for detection of Covid-19 from CT scans. Circuits, System and Signal Processing. 41(6): 3397–3414.

Kermany, D.S., Goldbaum, M., Cai, W., Valentim, C.C.S., Liang, H., Baxter, S.L., et al. 2018. Identifying medical diagnoses and treatable diseases by image-based deep learning. Cell. 172(5): 1122–1131.e9.

Khobahi, S., Agarwal, C. and Soltanalian, M. 2020. CoroNet: a deep network architecture for semi-supervised task-based identification of Covid-19 from chest X-ray images (p. 2020.04.14.20065722). medRxiv. Accessed at https://doi.org/10.1101/2020.04.14.20065722 (on 16 March 2024).

Koo, H.J., Lim, S., Choe, J., Choi, S.-H., Sung, H. and Do, K.-H. 2018. Radiographic and CT features of viral pneumonia. Radiographics: A Review Publication of the Radiological Society of North America, Inc. 38(3): 719–739.

Kumar, Y., Koul, A., Singla, R. and Ijaz, M.F. 2022. Artificial intelligence in disease diagnosis: a systematic literature review, synthesizing framework and future research agenda. Journal of Ambient Intelligence and Humanized Computing, 14, 8459–8486.

Kundu, R., Basak, H., Singh, P.K., Ahmadian, A., Ferrara, M. and Sarkar, R. 2021. Fuzzy rank-based fusion of CNN models using Gompertz function for screening Covid-19 CT-scans. Scientific Reports. 11(1): 14133.

Li, F., Lu, X. and Yuan, J. 2022a. MHA-CoroCapsule: multi-head attention routing-based capsule network for Covid-19 chest x-ray image classification. IEEE Transactions on Medical Imaging. 41(5): 1208–1218.

Li, M., Li, X., Jiang, Y., Zhang, J., Luo, H. and Yin, S. 2022b. Explainable multi-instance and multi-task learning for Covid-19 diagnosis and lesion segmentation in CT images. Knowledge-Based Systems. 252: 109278.

Lin, Z., He, Z., Xie, S., Wang, X., Tan, J., Lu, J., et al. 2021. AANet: adaptive attention network for Covid-19 detection from chest x-ray images. IEEE Transactions on Neural Networks and Learning Systems. 1–12.

Liu, Q., Yu, L., Luo, L., Dou, Q. and Heng, P.A. 2020. Semi-supervised medical image classification with relation-driven self-ensembling model. IEEE Transactions on Medical Imaging. 39(11): 3429–3440.

Lu, H., Stratton, C.W. and Tang, Y.-W. 2020. Outbreak of pneumonia of unknown etiology in Wuhan, China: the mystery and the miracle. Journal of Medical Virology. 92(4): 401–402.

MacEachern, S.J. and Forkert, N.D. 2021. Machine learning for precision medicine. Genome. 64(4): 416–425.

Maguolo, G. and Nanni, L. 2021. A critic evaluation of methods for Covid-19 automatic detection from X-ray images. Information Fusion. 76: 1–7.

Mayers, C. and Baker, K. 2020. Impact of false-positives and false-negatives in the UK's Covid-19 RT-PCR testing programme, 3 June 2020. Accessed at https://www.gov.uk/government/publications/gos-impact-of-false-positives-and-negatives-3-june-2020/impact-of-false-positives-and-false-negatives-in-the-uks-covid-19-rt-pcr-testing-programme-3-june-2020 (on October 2, 2022).

Mhamdi, L., Dammak, O., Cottin, F. and Dhaou, I.B. 2022. Artificial intelligence for cardiac diseases diagnosis and prediction using ECG images on embedded systems. Biomedicines. 10(8): 2013.

Mostafiz, R., Uddin, M.S., Alam, N.-A., Mahfuz Reza, Md. and Rahman, M.M. 2022. Covid-19 detection in chest X-ray through random forest classifier using a hybridization of deep CNN and DWT optimized features. Journal of King Saud University—Computer and Information Sciences. 34(6, Part B: 3226–3235.

Mostavi, M., Chiu, Y.-C., Huang, Y. and Chen, Y. 2020. Convolutional neural network models for cancer type prediction based on gene expression. BMC Medical Genomics. 13(5): 1–13.

Muhammad, G. and Shamim Hossain, M. 2021. Covid-19 and non-Covid-19 classification using multi-layers fusion from lung ultrasound images. Information Fusion. 72: 80–88.

Nassif, A.B., Talib, M.A., Nasir, Q., Afadar, Y. and Elgendy, O. 2022. Breast cancer detection using artificial intelligence techniques: a systematic literature review. Artificial Intelligence in Medicine. 127: 102276.

Nawshad, M.A., Shami, U.A., Sajid, S. and Fraz, M.M. 2021. Attention based residual network for effective detection of Covid-19 and viral pneumonia.

2021 International Conference on Digital Futures and Transformative Technologies (ICoDT2): 1–7.

Nichols, J.A., Herbert Chan, H.W. and Baker, M.A. 2019. Machine learning: applications of artificial intelligence to imaging and diagnosis. Biophysical Reviews. 11(1): 111–118.

Nistér, D. and Stewénius, H. 2008. Linear time maximally stable extremal regions. pp. 183–196. *In:* Forsyth, D., Torr, P. and Zisserman, A. (eds). Computer Vision—ECCV 2008. Springer.

Ojala, T., Pietikainen, M. and Maenpaa, T. 2002. Multiresolution gray-scale and rotation invariant texture classification with local binary patterns. IEEE Transactions on Pattern Analysis and Machine Intelligence. 24(7): 971–987.

Öksüz, C., Urhan, O. and Güllü, M.K. 2020. Ensemble-CVDNet: a deep learning based end-to-end classification framework for Covid-19 detection using ensembles of networks. arXiv:2012.09132 [Eess].

Öksüz, C., Urhan, O. and Güllü, M.K. 2021. A two-headed deep learning framework for predicting severity of Covid-19 disease. Artificial Intelligence Theory and Applications. 1(2): 19–28.

Oksuz, C., Urhan, O. and Gullu, M.K. 2021. Ensemble-LungMaskNet: automated lung segmentation using ensembled deep encoders. 2021 International Conference on INnovations in Intelligent SysTems and Applications (INISTA). 1–8.

Öksüz, C., Urhan, O. and Güllü, M.K. 2022. Covid-19 detection with severity level analysis using the deep feature. and wrapper-based selection of ranked features. Concurrency and Computation: Practice and Experience. 34(20): e6802.

Öksüz, C., Urhan, O. and Güllü, M.K. 2024. An integrated convolutional neural network with attention guidance for improved performance of medical image classification. Neural Computing and Applications. 36(4): 2067–2099.

Özkaya, U., Öztürk, Ş. and Barstugan, M. 2020. Coronavirus (Covid-19) classification using deep features fusion and ranking technique. pp. 281–295. *In:* Hassanien, A.-E., Dey, N. and Elghamrawy, S. (eds). Big Data Analytics and Artificial Intelligence Against Covid-19: Innovation Vision and Approach. Springer International Publishing.

Öztürk, Ş., Özkaya, U. and Barstuğan, M. 2021. Classification of coronavirus (Covid-19) from X-ray and CT images using shrunken features. International Journal of Imaging Systems and Technology. 31(1): 5–15.

Parrón, M., Torres, I., Pardo, M., Morales, C., Navarro, M. and Martínez-Schmizcraft, M. 2008. The halo sign in computed tomography images: differential diagnosis and correlation with pathology findings. Archivos de Bronconeumología. 44(7): 386–392.

Pecoraro, V., Negro, A., Pirotti, T. and Trenti, T. 2022. Estimate false-negative RT-PCR rates for SARS-CoV-2. A systematic review and meta-analysis. European Journal of Clinical Investigation. 52(2): e13706.

Potter, E.L., Rodrigues, C.H., Ascher, D.B., Abhayaratna, W.P., Sengupta, P.P. and Marwick, T.H. 2021. Machine learning of ECG waveforms to improve selection for testing for asymptomatic left ventricular dysfunction. Cardiovascular Imaging. 14(10): 1904–1915.

Rehani, M.M. and Berry, M. 2000. Radiation doses in computed tomography: the increasing doses of radiation need to be controlled. BMJ. 320(7235): 593–594.

RSNA Pneumonia Detection Challenge. 2018. Accessed at https://kaggle.com/competitions/rsna-pneumonia-detection-challenge (on October 15, 2022).

Sabour, S., Frosst, N. and Hinton, G.E. 2017. Dynamic routing between capsules. arXiv:1710.09829.

Sandler, M., Howard, A., Zhu, M., Zhmoginov, A. and Chen, L.-C. 2019. MobileNetV2: inverted residuals and linear bottlenecks. arXiv:1801.04381 [Cs].

Shankar, K. and Perumal, E. 2020. A novel hand-crafted with deep learning features based fusion model for Covid-19 diagnosis and classification using chest X-ray images. Complex & Intelligent Systems, 7: 1277–1293.

Shankar, K., Perumal, E., Tiwari, P., Shorfuzzaman, M. and Gupta, D. 2022. Deep learning and evolutionary intelligence with fusion-based feature extraction for detection of Covid-19 from chest X-ray images. Multimedia Systems. 28(4): 1175–1187.

Shao, X.-N., Sun, Y.-J., Xiao, K.-T., Zhang, Y., Zhang, W.-B., Kou, Z.-F., et al. 2018. Texture analysis of magnetic resonance T1 mapping with dilated cardiomyopathy: a machine learning approach. Medicine. 97(37): e12246.

Siddiqui, A., Ahmed, A., Saleem, A.F., Alvi, Z.K., Alam, T. and Qureshi, R. 2021. Attention based Covid-19 detection using generative adversarial network. 2021 4th International Conference on Computing & Information Sciences (ICCIS). 01–06.

Simonyan, K. and Zisserman, A. 2015. Very deep convolutional networks for large-scale image recognition. arXiv:1409.1556.

Sitaula, C. and Hossain, M.B. 2021. Attention-based VGG-16 model for Covid-19 chest X-ray image classification. Applied Intelligence. 51(5): 2850–2863.

Sitaula, C., Shahi, T.B., Aryal, S. and Marzbanrad, F. 2021. Fusion of multi-scale bag of deep visual words features of chest X-ray images to detect Covid-19 infection. Scientific Reports. 11(1): 23914.

Sun, C. and Wee, W.G. 1983. Neighboring gray level dependence matrix for texture classification. Computer Vision, Graphic and Image Processing. 23(3): 341–352.

Szegedy, C., Ioffe, S., Vanhoucke, V. and Alemi, A. 2017. Inception-v4, Inception-ResNet and the impact of residual connections on learning. Proceedings of the AAAI Conference on Artificial Intelligence. 31(1).

Szegedy, C., Liu, W., Jia, Y., Sermanet, P., Reed, S., Anguelov, D., et al. 2015. Going deeper with convolutions. Proceedings of the IEEE Conference on Computer Vision and Pattern Recognition. 1–9.

Tabik, S., Gomez-Rios, A., Martin-Rodriguez, J.L., Sevillano-Garcia, I., Rey-Area, M., Charte, D., et al. 2020. COVIDGR dataset and COVID-SDNet methodology for predicting Covid-19 based on chest X-ray images. IEEE Journal of Biomedical and Health Informatics. 24(12): 3595–3605.

Tan, M. and Le, Q.V. 2020. EfficientNet: rethinking model scaling for convolutional neural networks. arXiv:1905.11946 [Cs, Stat].

Thibault, G., Angulo, J. and Meyer, F. 2014. Advanced statistical matrices for texture characterization: application to cell classification. IEEE Transactions on Biomedical Engineering. 61(3): 630–637.

Thibault, G., Fertil, B., Navarro, C., Pereira, S., Lévy, N., Sequeira, J., et al. 2009. Texture indexes and gray level size zone matrix application to cell nuclei classification. 10th International Conference on Pattern Recognition and Information Processing. 140–145.

Thurmann, A., Bilda, K. and Dörr, F. 2022. Artificial intelligence solutions in Parkinson therapy. *In*: Tareq Ahram, Waldemar Karwowski, Pepetto Di Bucchianico, Redha Taiar, Luca Casarotto and Pietro Costa (eds). Intelligent Human Systems Integration (IHSI 2022): Integrating People and Intelligent Systems. AHFE (2022) International Conference. AHFE Open Access, vol 22. AHFE International, USA. http://doi.org/10.54941/ahfe1001037.

Toraman, S., Alakus, T.B. and Turkoglu, I. 2020. Convolutional capsnet: a novel artificial neural network approach to detect Covid-19 disease from X-ray images using capsule networks. Chaos, Solitons & Fractals. 140: 110122.

Wang, F., Jiang, M., Qian, C., Yang, S., Li, C., Zhang, H., et al. 2017. Residual attention network for image classification. Proceedings of the IEEE Conference on Computer Vision and Pattern Recognition. 3156–3164.

Wang, S., Zhang, Y., Lv, L., Wu, R., Fan, X., Zhao, J., et al. 2018. Abnormal regional homogeneity as a potential imaging biomarker for adolescent-onset schizophrenia: a resting-state fMRI study and support vector machine analysis. Schizophrenia Research. 192: 179–184.

World Health Organization. 2020. Impact of Covid-19 on people's livelihoods, their health and our food systems. Accessed at https://www.who.int/news/item/13-10-2020-impact-of-covid-19-on-people's-livelihoods-their-health-and-our-food-systems (on October 2, 2022).

WHO Coronavirus (COVID-19) Dashboard. 2022. Accessed at https://covid19.who.int (on October 1, 2022).

Wu, J., Pan, J., Teng, D., Xu, X., Feng, J. and Chen, Y.-C. 2020. Interpretation of CT signs of 2019 novel coronavirus (Covid-19) pneumonia. European Radiology. 30(10): 5455–5462.

Xiao, T., Xu, Y., Yang, K., Zhang, J., Peng, Y. and Zhang, Z. 2015. The application of two-level attention models in deep convolutional neural network for fine-grained image classification. Proceedings of the IEEE Conference on Computer Vision and Pattern Recognition. 842–850.

Zebari, D.A., Abdulazeez, A.M., Zeebaree, D.Q. and Salih, M.S. 2020. A fusion scheme of texture features for Covid-19 detection of CT scan images. 2020 International Conference on Advanced Science and Engineering (ICOASE). 1–6.

Zhang, F., Chen, J., Wang, M. and Drabier, R. 2013. A neural network approach to multi-biomarker panel discovery by high-throughput plasma proteomics profiling of breast cancer. BMC Proceedings. 7(7): 1–8.

Zhang, X., Zhou, X., Lin, M. and Sun, J. 2017. ShuffleNet: an extremely efficient convolutional neural network for mobile devices. arXiv:1707.01083 [Cs].

Zhang, Y., Su, L., Liu, Z., Tan, W., Jiang, Y. and Cheng, C. 2022. A semi-supervised learning approach for Covid-19 detection from chest CT scans. Neurocomputing. 503: 314–324.

Zhang, Y.-D., Zhang, Z., Zhang, X. and Wang, S.-H. 2021. MIDCAN: a multiple input deep convolutional attention network for Covid-19 diagnosis based on chest CT and chest X-ray. Pattern Recognition Letters. 150: 8–16.

Zhou, T., Canu, S. and Ruan, S. 2021. Automatic Covid-19 CT segmentation using U-Net integrated spatial and channel attention mechanism. International Journal of Imaging Systems and Technology. 31(1): 16–27.

Zreik, M., Van Hamersvelt, R.W., Wolterink, J.M., Leiner, T., Viergever, M.A. and Išgum, I. 2018. A recurrent CNN for automatic detection and classification of coronary artery plaque and stenosis in coronary CT angiography. IEEE Transactions on Medical Imaging. 38(7): 1588–1598.

Chapter 7

Smart Health and Artificial Intelligence Applications in Mobile Technologies

Mustafa Furkan Aksu[1] and Mehmet Sagbas[2]

[1]Electrical and Electronics Engineering Department,
Izmir Bakircay University, Izmir Türkiye. ORCID: 0000-0002-9478-7240
Email: mustafafurkan.aksu@bakircay.edu.tr

[2]Electrical and Electronics Engineering Department,
Izmir Bakircay University, Izmir Türkiye. ORCID: 0000-0001-5776-3947
Email: mehmet.sagbas@bakircay.edu.tr

INTRODUCTION

Chronic diseases such as cardiovascular disease, diabetes, and hypertension are becoming more common as the world population grows. As a result, it is becoming increasingly difficult for healthcare providers to manage and monitor patients with these illnesses on a regular basis. Late patient intervention is a serious issue since many of these disorders necessitate early diagnosis and treatment. This is especially important for patients with high-risk illnesses such as cardiac arrhythmias, obstructive sleep apnea syndrome, diabetes, and hypertension. To solve this issue, ubiquitous wireless patient monitoring devices are gaining popularity around the world because they allow

---

*For Correspondence: Mehmet Sagbas (mehmet.sagbas@bakircay.edu.tr)

for early detection and continuous monitoring of patients with chronic diseases (Baig and Gholamhosseini 2013, Mendonca et al. 2018).

Patients with chronic conditions that necessitate continual monitoring must visit hospitals on a regular schedule. This condition raises the load on medical personnel and the density of healthcare institutions. At the same time, this is a really challenging economic scenario. Collecting basic health data in patients' own living areas as well as the capacity to track the patient without having to contact health facilities or personnel will lessen the workload of health facilities and staff. The primary purpose of such monitoring systems is to collect data from biological sensors put on patients inside or outside the hospital and to offer healthcare providers access to this data at any time (Baig et al. 2015, Pantelopoulos and Bourbakis 2009). This method allows for the early detection and treatment of such disorders.

With the advancement of technology, new technological devices are now being employed in the field of medicine for patient monitoring, diagnosis, and therapy. The utilization of smart health services by these gadgets facilitates patient follow-up. The monitoring and treatment of the disease can make use of the data collected from the patient or the surroundings with various sensors. Wearable technologies and the Internet of Things (IoT) play a significant role in data collection.

Wearable patient monitoring applications were first used by the National Aeronautics and Space Administration (NASA) in the 1960s to monitor the vital data of astronauts (Pitts 1985). Then, it started to develop in the area of military with the need to observe the health data of the soldiers in the field. In the following years, these systems started to be used in the follow-up and treatment of patients and became more common day by day. Robots with wearable gloves, which are being used in the field of robotic surgery today, can be given as an example of wearable technology in the field of health that facilitates surgeries by doctors. The advancement in technologies has also led to the development of low-cost, portable, remote access patient monitoring systems (Barfield 2015).

Wearable patient monitoring systems are highly customizable and can incorporate a variety of components, including sensors, smart fabrics, wireless communication devices, power supplies, processor and microcontroller units, and software (Sujith et al. 2022). These systems can record vital data like heart rate, blood pressure, body temperature, blood oxygen levels, electrocardiogram (ECG), electromyogram (EMG), and breathing rate. The collected data can be communicated to healthcare specialists via wireless sensor networks, allowing them to remotely monitor patients without the need for face-to-face engagement. Furthermore, the data can be analyzed using a variety of AI algorithms, assisting in the development of expert decision support systems. Smart devices that can process real-time data and give alerts to healthcare professionals, patients, or athletes are in high demand nowadays. Patients can utilize wearable devices in their regular routine to keep track of their health information and avoid visiting healthcare institutions or hospitals.

In recent years, the healthcare industry has undergone a major transformation with the advent of smart health and AI technologies. The integration of these technologies with mobile devices has further revolutionized the way we access and manage healthcare services. With the increasing use of smartphones and wearables, mobile technologies have become an important tool for monitoring and improving our health and well-being.

This chapter focuses on the applications of smart health and artificial intelligence (AI) in mobile technologies. It begins with an overview of the sensors used in smart health applications followed by the communication protocols used in smart health applications. It then discusses the various applications of these technologies in mobile health, including disease diagnosis, monitoring and management, and wellness and fitness monitoring.

SENSORS USED IN SMART HEALTH APPLICATIONS

Smart health apps are being used by more and more people to promote healthy lifestyles and expand access to healthcare. Thanks to technological advances, individualized health services are increasingly taking the place of hospital care. Smart health applications hold great promise for the healthcare sector as they simplify access to healthcare services and give medical professionals accurate and up-to-date information. Disease management is facilitated by smart health services thanks to the information gathered from the user. And as the collected data is incorporated into AI models, early detection of diseases is now possible. These services should use a variety of sensors attached to the user's body or environment to collect data. These sensors are found in a variety of devices, including smartwatches and phones that are owned by the user. There are also wearable sensors designed for a specific purpose. Data from the user's environment, as well as data obtained from body-worn sensors, is critical for smart health applications. In this chapter, specific information is offered using examples from the literature review on sensors used in smart health applications.

There are several types of sensors commonly used in smart health applications. Some of the most common ones are pulse and oximetry sensors, ECG sensors, temperature sensors, motion sensors (accelerometers and gyroscopes), heart rate sensors, blood pressure sensors, glucose sensors, etc. Overall, sensors play a crucial role in smart health applications as they provide important data that can be used to monitor and improve a person's health and well-being. These sensors can be integrated with various wearable devices and mobile applications to monitor and track health-related data in real time.

PULSE AND OXIMETRY SENSORS

Smart health applications collect a lot of data from users. One of these data is the amount of oxygen in the blood. Oximeters are used to measure the amount of oxygen. They are very popular as they can be found in some smartwatches. Oximeters that can be worn on the finger are also available. Oximeters use light-emitting diodes (LEDs) with two different wavelengths and photodiodes to measure the amount of oxygen in the blood. The LEDs used usually emit light with red and infrared wavelengths. These LEDs enable light to be sent to the veins on the surface of the body. Part of the emitted light is absorbed depending on the oxygen content of the blood and the width of the vessel. After part of the light is absorbed, the photodiode detects the reflected light. The diagram of an oximeter is given in Figure 7.1.

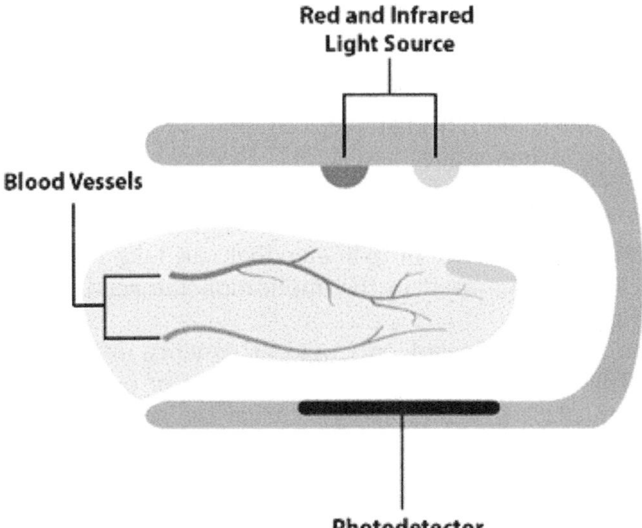

Figure 7.1   Internal structure of an oximeter sensor.

The extent of absorption of the various wavelengths of light sent into the vein depends on the oxygen content of the blood. Infrared light is highly absorbed by oxygenated oxyhemoglobins in the blood, while red wavelength light is highly absorbed by deoxyhemoglobins that have lost their oxygen. Based on the difference in absorption, the amount of oxygen in the blood can be determined. As the vessels expand when blood is pumped through the heart, the absorption of light also increases. The increase in absorption of the transmitted light means that less light falls on the photodiode on the opposite side. Pulse measurement can also be done by the amount of light falling on the photodiode (Sinex 1999). The extent of absorption of light of different wavelengths by oxyhemoglobin and deoxyhemoglobin is shown in Figure 7.2.

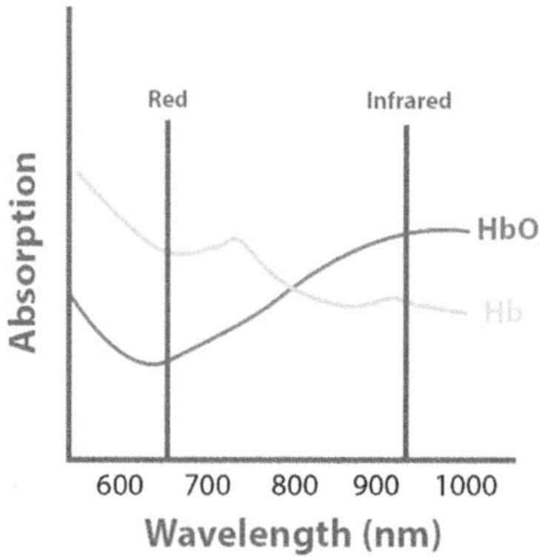

Figure 7.2   Extinction curve of reduced hemoglobin (Hb) and oxyhemoglobin (HbO_2).

Using oximeters in smart health applications is prevalent in many different contexts. As an example, Gay and Leijdekkers implemented a health monitoring application in 2007 that makes use of a variety of sensors (Gay and Leijdekkers 2007). This application used sensors such as ECG, accelerometer, blood pressure meter, global positioning system (GPS), weight meter, and an oximeter that can take measurements on a finger. The sensors used in the application can send data wirelessly to the smartphone.

In the study conducted on Covid-19 patients, an oximetry sensor (MAX30100) was used to measure the amount of oxygen in the blood (Khan et al. 2023). The data received from the sensor was sent to the microcontroller, and then was transmitted wirelessly to the smartphone via Bluetooth.

ECG SENSORS

Electrocardiogram sensors are used to monitor the heart rate and electrical activity of the heart, and the data obtained from these sensors are used in the diagnosis of various heart diseases. During the heartbeat, electrical signals are transmitted to the muscles on the surface of the body. These signals are of very small magnitude and therefore require multiple electrodes to be attached to different parts of the body in order to be observed. The signals received from the electrodes contain a significant amount of noise, including unwanted signals known as common mode noise, which are present in all electrodes due to grounding. To mitigate this common mode noise, one electrode is connected to the right leg and the resulting signal is subtracted from the signals of the other electrodes to reduce the noise level. The resulting signal is then subjected to filtering, where low-pass and high-pass filters can be applied separately. After filtering, the signals are passed to the analog-to-digital converter component (ADC) of the ECG sensor. The ADC converts the analog electrical signal obtained from the muscles into digital data that can be visualized and processed (Gregg et al. 2008). A diagram of the ECG sensor is given in Figure 7.3.

The ADCs convert continuous-time analog signals into discrete-time digital signals. The voltage of the continuous-time signal is measured at specific time intervals, and the number of samples taken per second is called the sampling rate. The obtained samples are rounded to certain values based on the resolution of the ADC. In the case of the ECG sensor, the use of an ADC with high resolution and a large number of samples improves the quality of the digitization process. The digital signals obtained from the ADC are finally processed by a microcontroller and can be displayed on a computer screen.

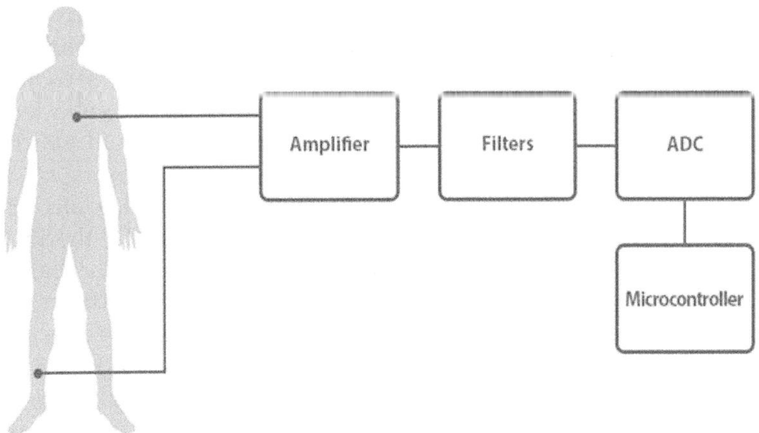

Figure 7.3 Schematic of the ECG sensor.

A wearable medical device was developed for the use of an ECG sensor in a study conducted by Ribeiro et al. (2011). This device is capable of displaying heart rate and ECG signals. The ECG signals were collected from the body surface using ECG electrodes embedded in the garment produced in the study. In addition, blood pressure was measured using a photoplethysmography (PPG) sensor on the earlobe. The data collected by the sensors can be wirelessly transmitted to a computer or mobile device, and the blood pressure information and ECG signals can be displayed via applications on these devices.

In addition to data collection, transferring this data to an IoT-based cloud system is important for accessing the data. In the study proposed by Yang et al. ECG data was acquired using the AD8232 ECG sensor with three electrodes (Yang et al. 2016). The acquired data was transmitted to an IoT cloud via a WiFi module. In the study, a graphical user interface was provided to the user to visualize the data in the cloud.

For wearable sensors to be useful, they should not restrict the user's movements. In the case of ECG sensors, the unit where the data is processed is usually located on circuit boards, which can restrict the user's movement. In such applications, it may be advantageous to place the electronic components on flexible platforms. The study by Poliks et al. (2016) can be cited as an example of this. In the study, flexible electrodes and nanomaterials were used to create contact points with the skin. These capabilities allow for the collection of trustworthy and precise data even while the user is moving.

TEMPERATURE SENSORS

Information regarding the user's body temperature is particularly crucial in smart health apps. Temperature data can be collected from smart devices used daily. In addition, wearable or non-contact sensors can also be used to collect this data. Temperature data can be collected not only from the user's body but also from the environment in which the user is located. Generally, three types of temperature sensors are used in smart health applications to measure temperature. One of them is an NTC (negative temperature coefficient) thermistor. NTC thermistors are made of various materials such as manganese, nickel, cobalt, and copper. These sensors have two poles. When the temperature of NTC thermistors increases, the resistance between these two poles decreases. By measuring the resistance of the known thermistors, a temperature measurement can be made (Chandrasegar and Vutukuri 2019, Patel et al. 2012).

Another type of temperature sensor is infrared thermometer, which measures the infrared radiation emitted from an object. The temperature of the object can be determined by the amount of radiation it emits.

The advantage of this sensors is that it does not need to be touched (Keränen et al. 2010).

Digital temperature sensors are another type of sensors used to measure temperature. These sensors have voltage values on the output pins that change with temperature. The sensed voltage data can be used to measure temperature. Because they are readily available and easy to use with microcontrollers, these sensors are becoming more common in wearable smart devices and smart health applications.

MOTION SENSORS

Motion sensors are mechanical and electronic devices that detect the movements of users. A motion sensor consists of two main sub-sensors. An accelerometer is used to detect linear motion while a gyroscope is used to detect rotational motion (Zeng and Zhao 2011). Sensors such as accelerometers and gyroscopes can be found in most smartphones today, which facilitates the collection of motion data for smart health applications.

Accelerometer

Accelerometers are used to measure the acceleration of a moving object. With the advancement of technology, accelerometers can be manufactured using the principle of micro electromechanical system (MEMS), a combination of electronic and microscopic mechanical systems. MEMS accelerometers can be divided into three main categories. The first is the piezoelectric accelerometer. This type of accelerometer is most commonly used to measure small vibrations. The vibrations are absorbed by a piezoelectric material and converted into an electrical signal. Another category, piezoresistive accelerometers, is used to detect vibrations similar to piezoelectric accelerometers. In these sensors, vibrations cause a change in the resistance in the piezoresistive material so that vibrations can be detected (Albarbar et al. 2009, Zhang et al. 2010). The last type of MEMS accelerometer is capacitive accelerometer. This type of accelerometer is used in many devices such as smartphones, smartwatches, and motion sensors. Capacitive accelerometers have a small mass attached with springs that moves between electrodes. The capacitance between the electrodes changes depending on the movement of this mass. The acceleration data can be measured as a function of this capacitance (Béliveau et al. 1999, Benmessaoud and Nasreddine 2013). The structure of a MEMS capacitive accelerometer is shown in Figure 7.4.

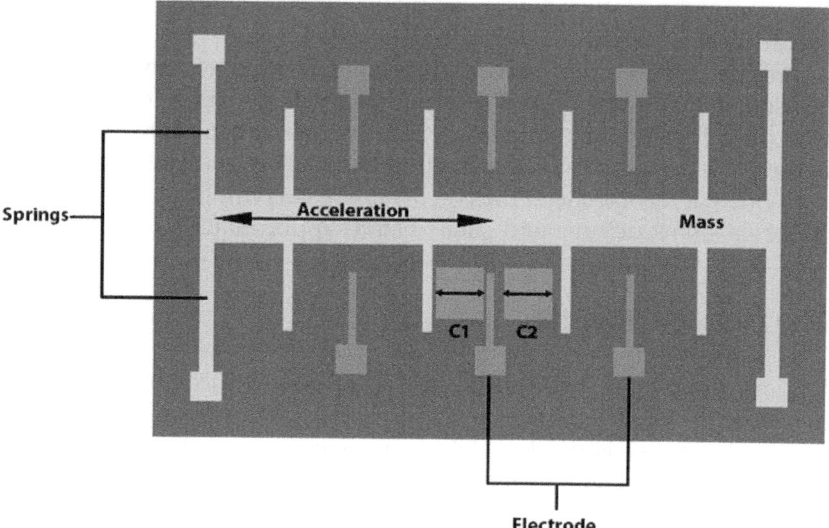

Figure 7.4   The structure of a MEMS capacitive accelerometer.

Gyroscope

Gyroscopes are used to detect the rotational motion of an object. Like accelerometers, MEMS gyroscopes contain a mass that is in constant motion. According to the Coriolis effect, when this mass rotates externally, moving at a certain speed and in a certain direction, a force is created that causes the mass to move in a direction that is perpendicular to its direction of motion. This force is measured using a method similar to that used by accelerometers, which allows the detection of rotational motion (Li et al. 2015, Wang et al. 2018). The forces acting on the mass inside the MEMS are shown in Figure 7.5.

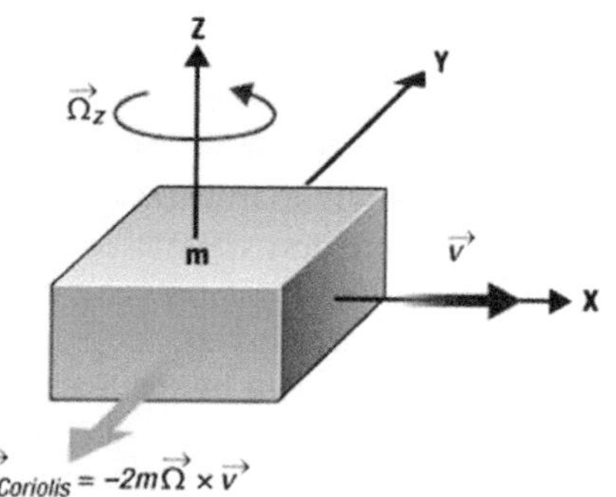

Figure 7.5   Coriolis effect (Esfandyari et al. 2010).

There are several studies on the use of motion sensors in smart health applications. Fall detection was performed using an accelerometer in a study conducted by Gay and Leijdekkers (2007). If a fall was detected in the application, the user's location was transmitted to a healthcare facility, and an emergency call was placed via the GPS and mobile application used in the study. In another study, Hernandez and Cretu (2018) used an accelerometer to measure heart rate. Moreover, the heart rate values measured with the accelerometer were compared with those obtained with an ECG sensor.

OTHER SENSORS

Wireless health monitoring systems can also use blood pressure, glucose, and heart rate sensors. They are all important components of smart health monitoring systems based on wearables and mobile apps that collect a variety of health data. Since they provide real-time data and enable early detection of health problems, these sensors are becoming increasingly popular.

Heart rate sensors measure a person's heart rate, or the number of heart beats per minute. PPG is used by these sensors to measure changes in blood volume in the arteries. PPG sensors provide continuous monitoring of the heart rate throughout the day and are typically worn on the wrist or chest. Applications for heart rate monitors include stress relief, fitness tracking, and cardiovascular health monitoring.

Blood pressure sensors measure the pressure of blood flowing through the arteries. These sensors typically use oscillometric or tonometric methods to measure blood pressure. Oscillometric sensors measure the pressure changes in the arteries caused by the heartbeat while tonometric sensors measure the pulse wave velocity in the arteries. Blood pressure sensors are used to monitor hypertension and cardiovascular health.

Glucose sensors are used to measure glucose levels in the blood. To measure glucose levels, these sensors typically use electrochemical or optical methods. While optical sensors use light to detect changes in glucose levels, electrochemical sensors use enzymes to break down glucose and generate an electrical signal. Glucose sensors are commonly used to monitor diabetes and can provide real-time glucose level data to help individuals manage their disease.

In general, sensors for vital signs such as glucose, blood pressure, and heart rate are important components of smart health monitoring systems. These sensors provide real-time data that can be used to monitor health status and detect potential health problems before they become serious. It is expected that these sensors will be used more frequently in healthcare in the future as wearable technology and smartphone apps become more popular.

COMMUNICATION TECHNOLOGIES

Communication between microcontrollers and sensors used in applications is an important issue for obtaining accurate data. The network structure of the IoT provides a system that enables communication between sensors and microcontrollers. In this structure, sensors are connected to microcontrollers. After the data is sent to the IoT server, various AI algorithms can process the data or mobile applications can be created to use the data.

When the IoT is used for smart health applications, a concept called the Internet of Medical Things (IoMT) emerges. The IoT system that is created by processing the data collected by medical devices or sensors is defined as IoMT. In this system, the data collected from the sensors of the patient or the environment in which the patient is located is aggregated in the IoMT cloud. After the data is processed, the sensors can communicate with each other and request help from a healthcare facility in case of an emergency. Figure 7.6 shows a schematic of an IoT-based smart health application. The data collected by the sensors is interpreted by microcontrollers and sent to the IoMT network. Various communication technologies such as Bluetooth and Wi-Fi are used in this transmission process. This section discusses the communication technologies commonly used in this phase.

RADIO FREQUENCY IDENTIFICATION (RFID)

Radio frequency identification (RFID) is a technology that uses radio waves to read digital data encoded on tags. An RFID system consists of two parts: a reader and an RFID tag. The reader has antennas that can transmit and receive radio waves. It sends a signal to the RFID tags and processes the returning signal. RFID tags can be divided into two categories: active and passive. Active RFID tags have their own power source, so they can send strong signals to the reader from a greater distance than passive tags. Passive RFID tags do not have their own power source. Instead, they store the necessary energy from the electromagnetic signal sent by the reader in a capacitor and then use that energy to transmit the stored information to the reader. Passive tags have a shorter range but are cheaper than active tags (Al-Sarawi et al. 2017, Weinstein 2005).

Four frequency bands are basically used in RFID technology. Depending on the frequency band used, the data transmission rate,

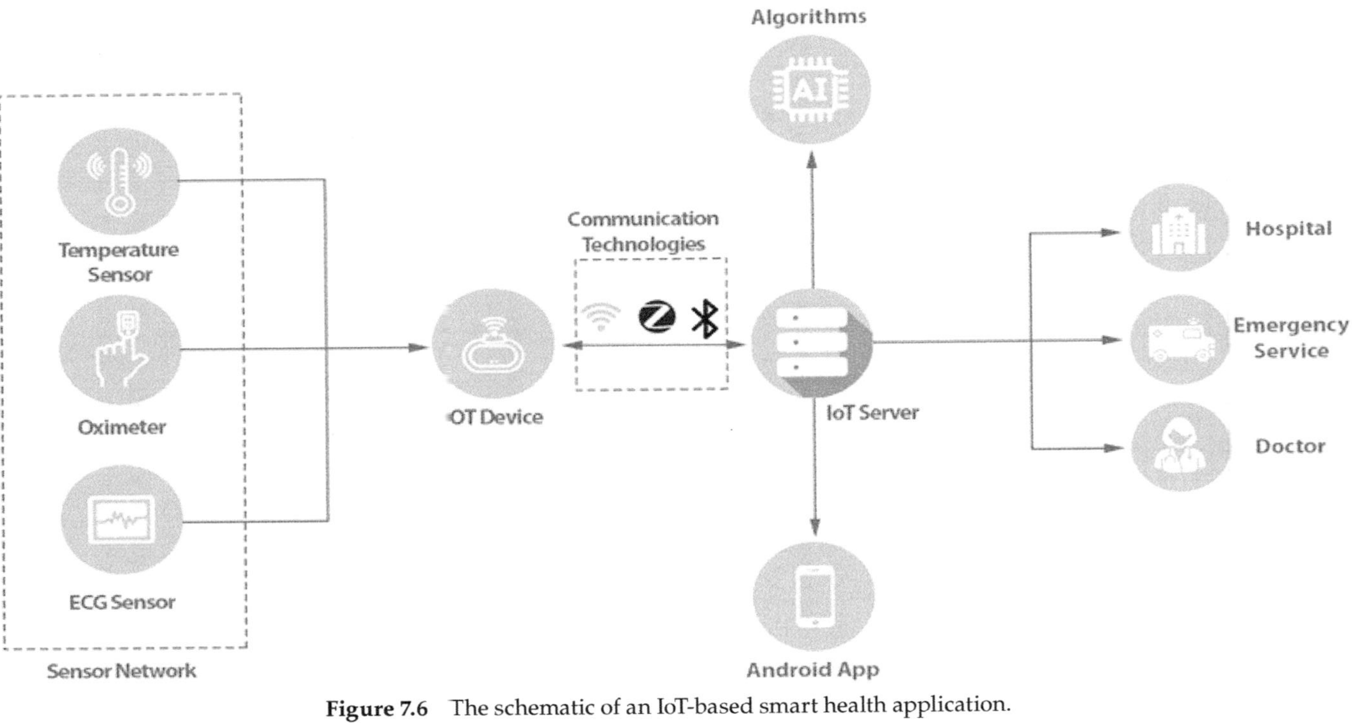

Figure 7.6 The schematic of an IoT-based smart health application.

range, cost, and other features of the RFID system can vary. The frequency bands used in RFID systems and their characteristics are listed in Table 7.1 (Want 2006).

Table 7.1   The frequency bands and features utilized in RFID systems.

Frequency	LF 125–134 KHz	Hf 13.56 MHz	UHF 433, 860–930 MHz	Microwave 2.4, 5.8 GHz
Range	~30 cm	~1 m	~30 m	>100 m
Data Transfer Rate	Low	Medium	High	Highest
Tag Type	Passive	Mainly Passive	Active and Passive	Active and Passive
Cost	Low	Medium	High	Highest

BLUETOOTH

Bluetooth technology is a widely used technology that is now found in many electronic devices such as smartphones, smartwatches, headphones, and computers. It is also included in new generation microprocessors. It operates in the 2.4 GHz frequency band and has an average range of up to 200 meters. As technology advances, so does Bluetooth. Bluetooth LE technology, introduced with Bluetooth 4.0, offers low power consumption. In Bluetooth 5.0, which will be released in 2016, the range and speed have been improved while maintaining low power consumption (Samie et al. 2016, Zeadally et al. 2019). Due to its widespread use in most smart devices and its reasonable range and data speed, Bluetooth is a useful technology for short-distance data transmission in smart health applications.

WI-FI/WI-FI HALOW

Wi-Fi technology is a wireless communication technology that allows electronic devices such as smartphones, laptops, and smart home devices to connect to the Internet or communicate with each other wirelessly using radio waves. Wi-Fi technology is mainly used in the 2.4 GHz and 5 GHz frequency bands. Depending on the frequency band used, it has an average range of 4–20 meters. Its advantages include high bandwidth and data rates. However, conventional Wi-Fi technology has high power consumption, which is a disadvantage for use in low-power IoT devices. Wi-Fi HaLow technology, on the other hand, has a lower data rate compared to conventional Wi-Fi technology. However, it consumes less power, which makes it suitable for use in IoT applications (Karimi and Atkinson 2013, Samie et al. 2016).

ZIGBEE

Zigbee technology is a popular technology used in IoT networks. This technology offers features such as low power consumption, low cost, and long range. Its architecture provides reliability for wireless networks. Since the data rate is not very high, it is well suited for small networks that do not require high data rates. It works in different frequency bands depending on the region where it is used, but the 2.4 GHz frequency band can be used in most countries. The range depends on the output power, but data can be transmitted up to an average of 150 meters (Karimi and Atkinson 2013, Samie et al. 2016, Tomar 2011).

Z-WAVE

The Z-wave technology was developed in 2001. It offers low power consumption and is particularly employed in applications for smart homes. Depending on the area it is utilized in, it uses the 828 MHz and 908 MHz frequency bands to operate. Its low data transfer rate in comparison to other technologies makes it appropriate for applications that call for modest data transfer rates. It has a maximum data transmission range of 30 meters (Marksteiner et al. 2017).

CELLULAR

Cellular technology is used in mobile devices today. These networks use a system of cells, each of which is covered by a tower, to provide coverage over a large geographic area. 3G/4G and the increasingly popular 5G can be cited as examples of cellular communication technology. Cellular technology offers high data rates and long-range communication. However, due to these features, it consumes high power and is not suitable for M2M applications that enable two devices to communicate with each other (Al-Sarawi et al. 2017, Samie et al. 2016).

6LoWPAN

The 6LoWPAN (IPv6 over Low-Power Wireless Personal Area Networks) technology is a wireless communication protocol designed for IoT devices that have limited power, processing, and storage resources. It enables these devices to connect to the Internet using IPv6, the latest version of the Internet protocol, which offers a large address space and better security features. Due to its low power consumption and long range, it is a very suitable communication technology for IoT applications. This technology architecture enables the transmission of IPv6 packets. The frequency band used varies depending on the location, but the 2.4 GHz band is most commonly used. 6LoWPAN technology offers approximately the same data rates as Zigbee but can transmit data over longer distances (Mulligan 2007).

The advantages and disadvantages of different communication technologies make them suitable for different IoT applications. Figure 7.7 shows a diagram depicting the data rate, range, and cost of the communication technologies mentioned in this section.

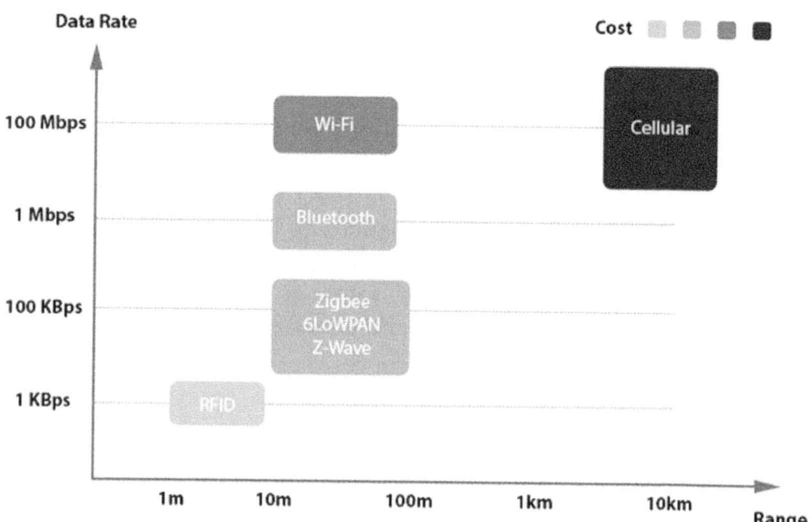

Figure 7.7   The data rate, range, and cost of the communication technologies.

APPLICATIONS

The AI-based smart health apps developed with mobile technology have had a significant impact on the healthcare sector. These apps assist people in tracking their health, communicating with medical professionals, analyzing symptoms, and managing their health. Mobile devices used in smart health apps make data collection easier. The data obtained is analyzed by AI systems, which aids in obtaining more accurate results on the patients' health status.

For example, in the study by Gao et al. (2011), motion tracking was performed using four different accelerometers implanted in eight different participants. The data was collected in the microprocessor and sent wirelessly to the computer via Bluetooth. After the data was collected and the dataset was created, the Naive Bayes classifier was used to predict which of the multiple actions such as walking, sitting, and lying down were performed by the participants. The influence on classification was investigated in the study by varying the number of sensors. The Naive Bayes algorithm achieved 97.66% accuracy in the case of four accelerometers.

In the work of Zhang et al. (2006), data was obtained from the accelerometer sensor in mobile phones for fall detection. The information collected from 32 volunteer participants was classified into five categories: daily activities, low-risk falls, high-risk falls, critical movements, and high-intensity daily activities. The support vector machine (SVM) method was used to assess each category. The study found that the average accuracy of the six different categories was 93.3%.

Gay and Leijdekkers (2007) implemented a multisensor smart health application in their study. Data from ECG sensor, oximeter, pulse sensor, GPS, and electronic scale was collected on a smartphone. The smartphone application has many functions. The application monitors heart rate data and sends information to emergency medical services or medical professionals when the heart rate exceeds or falls below certain thresholds. The method developed by Brown can detect falls using the accelerometer in conjunction with the ECG sensor (Brown 2005). The patient's weight can be linked to various surveys and transmitted to the medical professional. Using GPS, the patient's location, a detected emergency, heart rate, etc., can be transmitted to emergency centers under various defined emergency scenarios, or the patient can be forced to call an ambulance with a single click.

In the study by Bhardwaj et al. (2022), an intelligent health monitoring system was developed for Covid-19 patients. The system uses an oximeter, an infrared temperature sensor, and a heart rate sensor. The Raspberry Pi microcontroller processed the sensor data, and the Wi-Fi module on the board then wirelessly transmitted the results to the server. Oximeters and temperature sensors were used in the study on the same topic by Khan et al. (2023). In the study, a separate microcontroller was used with a Bluetooth sensor and Wi-Fi module, which used Arduino as the microcontroller to transmit the data to the server and smartphone (Khan et al. 2023). When the continuously collected data falls below a certain threshold, the system may sound an audible alarm.

In the study by Yang et al. (2016), an IoT-based smart health application and an ECG sensor were used. The study consisted of four different subsystems. Data was collected by a three-electrode ECG sensor, processed by an STM32 control board, transmitted wirelessly by a Wi-Fi module, and powered by a power supply module that provided the necessary energy to the overall system. The Wi-Fi module was used to transmit the data to the server after the ECG sensor completed data acquisition. It was found that the received ECG signal had some characteristics that typical ECG signals should have, and it was decided that the data was collected in a healthy way.

A finger and wrist wearable device was used by Malhi et al. (2010) in their study. The wrist-mounted portion of the device used an accelerometer and a temperature sensor. A heart rate monitor was located on the finger. The C8051F02 microcontroller collected the sensor data, which was then wirelessly transmitted to the controller's ZigBee module and then to the computer. The device was powered by a 9V battery. The low power consumption of the ZigBee module allowed for 25 hours of continuous operation.

Vippalapalli and Ananthula (2016) investigated blood pressure, body temperature, and heart rate in their study. Since the Arduino Fio microcontroller supports ZigBee, the data was collected in it. The data was transmitted to the server using the ZigBee protocol, and a graphical interface for real-time monitoring was created using the LabView application.

Table 7.2 contains information about the sensors and communication methods used in the analyzed studies.

Table 7.2   Information about the sensors and communication protocols used in the literature.

Authors	Sensors	Communication Technologies	Medical Application
Gay and Leijdekkers (2007)	ECG, accelerometer, oximeter, blood pressure, weight scale	Bluetooth	Cardiac monitoring
Khan et al. (2023)	Temperature, oximeter	Bluetooth, Wi-Fi	Covid-19 patient monitoring
Ribeiro et al. (2011)	ECG, PPG	Bluetooth, Wi-Fi	ECG and continuous blood pressure monitoring
Yang et al. (2016)	ECG	Wi-Fi	ECG monitoring
Poliks et al. (2016)	ECG	Bluetooth	ECG monitoring
Gao et al. (2011)	Accelerometer	Bluetooth	Activity recognition
Zhang et al. (2006)	Accelerometer	Wi-Fi	Fall detection
Bhardwaj et al. (2022)	Blood pressure, temperature, pulse oximeter	Wi-Fi	Covid-19 patient monitoring
Malhi et al. (2010)	Temperature, accelerometer, heart rate	ZigBee	Medical distress detection
Vippalapalli and Ananthula (2016)	Temperature, pulse rate, blood pressure	ZigBee	Patient monitoring

In contrast to natural intelligence, AI refers to the ability of computers to exhibit intelligence similar to that of humans. Machine learning, a subfield of AI, allows computers to learn and improve on their own without being explicitly programmed. This field is concerned with developing algorithms that can collect data and use it to learn on their own. AI has applications in a variety of areas, including the IoT, machine vision, driver assistance, and natural language processing. In healthcare, AI is being used in areas such as cancer research, cardiology, diabetes, mental health, prognosis, Alzheimer's disease, clinical differences, and cardiovascular disease, among others. Given the rapid progress of AI, significant breakthroughs in healthcare are expected in the future.

Hawley et al. (2012) proposed an automated machine application to identify and produce speech communication from people with dysarthria.

To estimate how closely a spoken sentence will resemble a language model, researchers used hidden Markov models unique to each person.

An AI-based health app was presented by Larburu et al. (2018) to help people avoid heart failure. For this purpose, predictive models were developed based on clinical data from 242 patients with heart failure. The most effective model reduced the number of false alarms from 28.64 to 7.8 per patient per year by combining multiple signals using a Naive Bayes classifier. However, detection accuracy is lower in patients who have already undergone cardiac surgery.

In their study, Burns et al. (2011) emphasized the importance of mobile-based multicomponent models of AI, examining various facets of patient behavior such as mood, cognitive state, depression, motivation, activities, environmental behavior, and social behavior. To provide feedback graphs and coaching for self-reflection of behavior, they proposed a system based on regression and decision trees combined with phone sensors. Although the overall prediction accuracy was quite good, ranging from 60% to 91%, the accuracy was relatively low for emotions such as melancholy.

For the diagnosis and prognosis of chronic diseases such as heart disease, cancer, diabetes, epilepsy, respiratory diseases, and chronic kidney disease, there are several studies in the literature on the current machine learning approaches (Chandrasegar and Vutukuri, 2019, Dahiwade et al. 2019, Eke et al. 2020, Rahane et al. 2018, Rohan et al. 2020, Sarwar et al. 2018). SVM, K-nearest neighbor (KNN), random forest, artificial neural network (ANN), and Deep learning (DL) are some of the machine learning methods used in these works. The results of these studies show that the machine learning and DL models provide good predictions for disease detection and diagnosis, and depending on the dataset and condition studied, some models achieve higher accuracy than others. To improve the classification accuracy and speed up the execution of these models, the Relief, Minimal Redundancy Maximal Relevance (mRMR),

Least absolute shrinkage selection operator (LASSO), Local learning-based features selection (LLBFS), Fast conditional mutual information (FCMIM) feature selection algorithms were used. Overall, machine learning and deep learning methods offer hope for better diagnosis and prognosis of chronic diseases. The algorithms and approaches of machine learning for chronic disease diagnosis and prognosis are listed in Table 7.3.

Table 7.3 Comparison of methods and machine learning algorithms used in the literature to diagnose disease.

Reference	ML Model and Method Used	Advantages	Disadvantages	Medical Application
Sarwar et al. (2018)	SVM, KNN, RF, DT, NB	Use of many ML algorithms	Low accuracy	Prediction of diabetes
Rohan et al. (2020)	ANN, XGBoost	High accuracy	No execution time	Epileptic seizure detection
Rahane et al. (2018)	SVM, image processing methods	Requiring less time	Only SVM algorithm is used	Lung cancer detection
Chandrasegar and Vutukuri (2019)	CFS, RF, SVM, ANN, DT	CFS achieves high accuracy with RF	CFS achieves low accuracy with other models	Cancer prediction
Eke et al. (2020)	SVM	High accuracy of 89%	Small sample size	Alzheimer's disease detection
Dahiwade et al. (2019)	KNN	CNN has better time and memory capacity	Low accuracy	General disease prediction
McGinnis et al. (2018)	LR, SVM	Low cost, less time consumption	Low accuracy	Diagnosis of anxiety and depression

In Sarwar et al. (2018), SVM, KNN, logistic regression (LR), decision trees (DT), RF, and Naïve Bayes (NB) algorithms were used for diabetes prediction on the Indian dataset PIMA, which consists of 768 records. The diabetes predictions were developed using Indian dataset of 768 records PIMA. SVM and KNN achieved 77% accuracy in this work. Therefore, it can be concluded that SVM and KNN are suitable for diabetic prediction.

Rohan et al. (2020) proposed a method for classifying epileptic seizures. The dataset consisted of 11,500 instances, each with 178 features. The proposed approach ANN improved accuracy and correctly diagnosed individuals with epileptic seizures. A 10-fold cross validation is used for validation. XGBoost has a test accuracy of 96.6% while ANN has a test accuracy of 98.26%.

The main goal of the test described in Rahane et al. (2018) is to detect lung cancer and its stages using computed tomography (CT) images. When users upload their CT images to the website, the query is created on the client side and sent to the server side. SVM and image processing methods are run on it, and the result is sent back to the clients to tell them whether the patients have cancer or not.

Machine learning classifiers such as CFS, RF, SVM, ANN, and DT have been used to predict breast cancer in Chandrasegar and Vutukuri (2019). The proposed cluster-based feature selection approach (CFS) aims to increase accuracy while reducing the feature dimension.

A strategy to search for possible blood-based non-amyloid biomarkers for early diagnosis of Alzheimer's disease was developed in Eke et al. (2020). The recommended method was based on machine learning techniques, especially SVM, as they are able to build multivariable models by extracting patterns from large amounts of complicated data. The authors discovered five new panels of non-amyloid proteins that have the potential to act as biomarkers for early Alzheimer's disease using feature selection and scoring methods.

In Dahiwade et al. (2019), general disease prediction based on patient's symptoms was proposed. KNN and convolutional neural network (CNN) machine learning algorithms were used to predict diseases with high accuracy. Compared to the KNN algorithm, CNN has an accuracy of 84.5%. In addition, KNN has higher memory and time requirements than CNN.

An approach for detecting depression and anxiety in young children is presented in McGinnis et al. (2018). The study used a 90-second anxiety-inducing task in which participants' activity was monitored with a readily available wearable sensor. A sample of children with and without an internalizing diagnosis was used to predict diagnosis using machine learning data and the clinically optimal 20-second phase of the task.

FUNDING

This work has been supported by Izmir Bakircay University Scientific Research Projects Coordination Unit, under grant number BBAP.2022.008.

CONCLUSION

Day by day, the use of smart health applications and artificial intelligence technologies in the field of health is becoming more widespread. These technologies enable users to monitor their health, receive diagnoses, and even receive treatment, while making healthcare more accessible, personalized, and effective. Artificial intelligence-supported mobile applications, combined with big data analytics, offer significant benefits such as early diagnosis of diseases, optimizing treatment plans and improving health outcomes. In this context, mobile health technologies and artificial intelligence will continue to play a key role in the further development of healthcare services in the future. In this book section, sensors used in smart health applications, artificial intelligence models, and communication technologies used in this field are mentioned

REFERENCES

Al-Sarawi, S., Anbar, M., Alieyan, K. and Alzubaidi, M. 2017. Internet of things (IoT) communication protocols. 2017 8th International Conference on Information Technology (ICIT). 685–690.

Albarbar, A., Badri, A., Sinha, J.K. and Starr, A. 2009. Performance evaluation of MEMS accelerometers. Measurement. 42(5): 790–795.

Baig, M.M. and Gholamhosseini, H. 2013. Smart health monitoring systems: an overview of design and modeling. Journal of Medical Systems. 37: 1–14.

Baig, M.M., Gholam Hosseini, H. and Connolly, M.J. 2015. Mobile healthcare applications: system design review, critical issues and challenges. Australasian Physical and Engineering Sciences in Medicine. 38: 23–38.

Barfield, W. 2015. Fundamentals of wearable computers and augmented reality. CRC Press.

Béliveau, A., Spencer, G.T., Thomas, K.A. and Roberson, S.L. 1999. Evaluation of MEMS capacitive accelerometers. IEEE Design and Test of Computers. 16(4): 48–56.

Benmessaoud, M. and Nasreddine, M.M. 2013. Optimization of MEMS capacitive accelerometer. Microsystem Technologies. 19: 713–720.

Bhardwaj, V., Joshi, R. and Gaur, A.M. 2022. IoT-based smart health monitoring system for COVID-19. SN Computer Science. 3(2): 137.

Brown, G. 2005. An accelerometer based fall detector: development, experimentation and analysis. University of California, Berkeley. 1–9.

Burns, M.N., Begale, M., Duffecy, J., Gergle, D., Karr, C.J., Giangrande, E., et al. 2011. Harnessing context sensing to develop a mobile intervention for depression. Journal of Medical Internet Research. 13(3): e1838.

Chandrasegar, T. and Vutukuri, S.B.N. 2019. Optimized machine learning model using decision tree for cancer prediction. 2019 Innovations in Power and Advanced Computing Technologies (i-PACT). 1–4.

Dahiwade, D., Patle, G. and Meshram, E. 2019. Designing disease prediction model using machine learning approach. 2019 3rd International Conference on Computing Methodologies and Communication (ICCMC). 1211–1215.

Eke, C.S., Jammeh, E., Li, X., Carroll, C., Pearson, S. and Ifeachor, E. 2020. Early detection of Alzheimer's disease with blood plasma proteins using support vector machines. IEEE Journal of Biomedical and Health Informatics. 25(1): 218–226.

Esfandyari, J., De Nuccio, R. and Xu, G. 2010. Introduction to MEMS gyroscopes. Solid State Technology. 31.

Gao, L., Bourke, A.K. and Nelson, J. 2011. A system for activity recognition using multi-sensor fusion. 2011 Annual International Conference of the IEEE Engineering in Medicine and Biology Society. 7869–7872.

Gay, V. and Leijdekkers, P. 2007. A health monitoring system using smart phones and wearable sensors. International Journal of ARM. 8(2): 29–35.

Gregg, R.E., Zhou, S.H., Lindauer, J.M., Helfenbein, E.D. and Giuliano, K.K. 2008. What is inside the electrocardiograph? Journal of Electrocardiology. 41(1): 8–14.

Hawley, M.S., Cunningham, S.P., Green, P.D., Enderby, P., Palmer, R., Sehgal, S., et al. 2012. A voice-input voice-output communication aid for people with severe speech impairment. IEEE Transactions on Neural Systems and Rehabilitation Engineering. 21(1): 23–31.

Hernandez, J.E. and Cretu, E. 2018. Simple heart rate monitoring system with a MEMS gyroscope for sleep studies. 2018 IEEE 9th Annual Information Technology, Electronics and Mobile Communication Conference (IEMCON). 61–67.

Karimi, K. and Atkinson, G. 2013. What the internet of things (IoT) needs to become a reality. White Paper, FreeScale and ARM. 1–16.

Keränen, K., Mäkinen, J.-T., Korhonen, P., Juntunen, E., Heikkinen, V. and Mäkelä, J. 2010. Infrared temperature sensor system for mobile devices. Sensors and Actuators A: Physical. 158(1): 161–167.

Khan, M.M., Mehnaz, S., Shaha, A., Nayem, M. and Bourouis, S. 2023. IoT-based smart health monitoring system for COVID-19 patients. Computational and Mathematical Methods in Medicine. 2023: 9824131. https://doi.org/10.1155/2023/9824131.

Larburu, N., Artetxe, A., Escolar, V., Lozano, A. and Kerexeta, J. 2018. Artificial intelligence to prevent mobile heart failure patients decompensation in real time: monitoring-based predictive model. Mobile Information Systems. 2018: 1–11.

Li, X., Xiao, W. and Fei, Y. 2015. Status quo and developing trend of MEMS-gyroscope technology. 2015 Fifth International Conference on Instrumentation and Measurement, Computer, Communication and Control (IMCCC). 727–730.

Malhi, K., Mukhopadhyay, S.C., Schnepper, J., Haefke, M. and Ewald, H. 2010. A zigbee-based wearable physiological parameters monitoring system. IEEE Sensors Journal. 12(3): 423–430.

Marksteiner, S., Jimenez, V.J.E., Valiant, H. and Zeiner, H. 2017. An overview of wireless IoT protocol security in the smart home domain. 2017 Internet of Things Business Models, Users and Networks. 1–8.

McGinnis, R.S., McGinnis, E.W., Hruschak, J., Lopez-Duran, N.L., Fitzgerald, K., Rosenblum, K.L., et al. 2018. Rapid anxiety and depression diagnosis in young children enabled by wearable sensors and machine learning. 2018

40th Annual International Conference of the IEEE Engineering in Medicine and Biology Society (EMBC). 3983–3986.

Mendonca, F., Mostafa, S.S., Ravelo-Garcia, A.G., Morgado-Dias, F. and Penzel, T. 2018. A review of obstructive sleep apnea detection approaches. IEEE Journal of Biomedical and Health Informatics. 23(2): 825–837.

Mulligan, G. 2007. The 6LoWPAN architecture. Proceedings of the 4th Workshop on Embedded Networked Sensors. 78–82.

Pantelopoulos, A. and Bourbakis, N.G. 2009. A survey on wearable sensor-based systems for health monitoring and prognosis. IEEE Transactions on Systems, Man and Cybernetics, Part C (Applications and Reviews). 40(1): 1–12.

Patel, S., Park, H., Bonato, P., Chan, L. and Rodgers, M. 2012. A review of wearable sensors and systems with application in rehabilitation. Journal of Neuroengineering and Rehabilitation. 9(1): 1–17.

Pitts, J.A. 1985. The human factor: biomedicine in the manned space program to 1980 (Vol. 4213). Scientific and Technical Information Branch, National Aeronautics and Space Administration.

Poliks, M., Turner, J., Ghose, K., Jin, Z., Garg, M., Gui, Q., et al. 2016. A wearable flexible hybrid electronics ECG monitor. 2016 IEEE 66th Electronic Components and Technology Conference (ECTC). 1623–1631.

Rahane, W., Dalvi, H., Magar, Y., Kalane, A. and Jondhale, S. 2018. Lung cancer detection using image processing and machine learning healthcare. 2018 International Conference on Current Trends towards Converging Technologies (ICCTCT). 1–5.

Ribeiro, D.M., Colunas, M.F., Marques, F.A.F., Fernandes, J.M. and Cunha, J.P.S. 2011. A real time, wearable ECG and continous blood pressure monitoring system for first responders. 2011 Annual International Conference of the IEEE Engineering in Medicine and Biology Society. 6894–6898.

Rohan, T.I., Yusuf, M.S.U., Islam, M. and Roy, S. 2020. Efficient approach to detect epileptic seizure using machine learning models for modern healthcare system. 2020 IEEE Region 10 Symposium (TENSYMP). 1783–1786.

Samie, F., Bauer, L. and Henkel, J. 2016. IoT technologies for embedded computing: a survey. Proceedings of the Eleventh IEEE/ACM/IFIP International Conference on Hardware/Software Codesign and System Synthesis. 1–10.

Sarwar, M.A., Kamal, N., Hamid, W. and Shah, M.A. 2018. Prediction of diabetes using machine learning algorithms in healthcare. 2018 24th International Conference on Automation and Computing (ICAC). 1–6.

Sinex, J.E. 1999. Pulse oximetry: principles and limitations. The American Journal of Emergency Medicine. 17(1): 59–66.

Sujith, A., Sajja, G.S., Mahalakshmi, V., Nuhmani, S. and Prasanalakshmi, B. 2022. Systematic review of smart health monitoring using deep learning and artificial intelligence. Neuroscience Informatics. 2(3): 100028.

Tomar, A. 2011. Introduction to ZigBee technology. Global Technology Centre. 1: 1–24.

Vippalapalli, V. and Ananthula, S. 2016. Internet of things (IoT) based smart health care system. 2016 International Conference on Signal Processing, Communication, Power and Embedded System (SCOPES). 1229–1233.

Wang, M., Cao, H., Shen, C. and Chai, J. 2018. A novel self-calibration method and experiment of MEMS gyroscope based on virtual coriolis force. Micromachines. 9(7): 328.

Want, R. 2006. An introduction to RFID technology. IEEE Pervasive Computing. 5(1): 25–33.

Weinstein, R. 2005. RFID: a technical overview and its application to the enterprise. IT Professional. 7(3): 27–33.

Yang, Z., Zhou, Q., Lei, L., Zheng, K. and Xiang, W. 2016. An IoT-cloud based wearable ECG monitoring system for smart healthcare. Journal of Medical Systems. 40: 1–11.

Zeadally, S., Siddiqui, F. and Baig, Z. 2019. 25 years of bluetooth technology. Future Internet. 11(9): 194.

Zeng, H. and Zhao, Y. 2011. Sensing movement: microsensors for body motion measurement. Sensors. 11(1): 638–660.

Zhang, S., Jiang, X., Lapsley, M., Moses, P. and Shrout, T.R. 2010. Piezoelectric accelerometers for ultrahigh temperature application. Applied Physics Letters. 96(1).

Zhang, T., Wang, J., Liu, P. and Hou, J. 2006. Fall detection by embedding an accelerometer in cellphone and using KFD algorithm. International Journal of Computer Science and Network Security. 6(10): 277–284.

Chapter 8

Artificial Intelligence Supported Design of Biomedical Materials and Devices

Kadir Gok

Faculty of Engineering and Architecture,
Biomedical Engineering Department,
Izmir Bakircay University, Izmir Türkiye
ORCID: 0000-0001-5736-1884; Email: kadir.gok@bakircay.edu.tr

INTRODUCTION

Biomedical engineering is a rapidly developing interdisciplinary field that plays a vital role in the development of innovative processes, analyses, devices, and procedures used in the diagnosis and treatment of various medical conditions. It combines engineering principles and problem-solving techniques with knowledge from biology and medical sciences to provide valuable healthcare solutions.

Biomedical engineers collaborate with experts from diverse backgrounds, including mechanical engineering, chemical engineering, material engineering, electrical engineering, mechatronics engineering, computer engineering, as well as professionals from the basic sciences such as physics, chemistry, biology, and medical practitioners such as doctors, nurses, physiotherapists, and technicians. This multidisciplinary approach allows them to tackle complex challenges and develop cutting-edge technologies.

The scope of work for biomedical engineers is broad, ranging from the design of medical devices and software to the integration of information from various technical sources, ultimately aiming to solve clinical problems and enhance patient care. This field encompasses a wide array of devices, such as computed tomography, magnetic resonance, ultrasonic imaging systems, nuclear medicine, Positron Emission Tomography (PET) imaging, and various laser devices, all of which are instrumental in diagnostics, treatment, and research.

One crucial aspect of biomedical engineering revolves around biomaterials—materials with specific properties and applications in contact with biological systems. Biomaterials, including metals, ceramics, polymers, and composite materials, are extensively used in medical applications. Their use spans areas such as the skeletal system, cardiovascular system, dental implants, organs, sensory devices, and support systems.

The study of biomaterials represents a multidisciplinary field encompassing medicine, chemistry, biology, and materials sciences, which has been advancing for over half a century. Initially employed solely in medical applications, biomaterials have found utility in cell culture for reproduction, clinical laboratory analysis of blood proteins, biomolecule processing equipment, and other similar applications. The seamless interaction between biological systems and artificial or modified natural materials has led to the widespread use of these materials across various domains. Biomaterials are often integrated into devices or implants for medical applications rather than used in isolation.

In this chapter, we explore and clarify the definition and working areas of biomedical engineering, biomechanics, biomaterials, biomedical devices, medical imaging systems, and the increasingly important role of Artificial Intelligence (AI) in supporting the design of biomedical materials and devices. By getting into these topics, we hope to provide a comprehensive overview of this fascinating and continuously developing field, shedding light on its contributions to improving healthcare outcomes and enhancing the quality of life for individuals worldwide.

BIOMEDICAL ENGINEERING DEFINITION AND FIELDS OF WORK

Biomedical engineering is a discipline that aims to use engineering principles and technological tools to solve medical problems. Biomedical engineers work in various fields, including the design, development, production, testing, maintenance, and calibration of devices designed for healthcare services.

Biomedical engineering fields of study include:

1. **Design and development of medical devices:** Biomedical engineers are concerned with the design and development of medical devices used in the diagnosis and treatment of diseases. These devices include imaging devices such as magnetic resonance imaging (MRI), computed tomography (CT) and ultrasound, implant devices such as pacemakers, prostheses, and other medical devices.

2. **Bioengineering:** It can be defined as the analysis and design of biological systems using engineering principles and techniques. Biomedical engineers use engineering principles and techniques for the design and manufacture of biological materials and biological systems.

3. **Clinical engineering:** It is a discipline that undertakes the responsibility for planning, implementing, and supervising the maintenance, repair, and calibration processes of medical devices used for diagnosis and treatment in hospitals. Clinical or biomedical engineers are also responsible for the safety testing of these devices.

4. **Biomedical signal processing:** It refers to the process of analysing, interpreting, and processing the signals measured from the body. Biomedical engineers deal with the processing and interpretation of signals used in medical devices such as electrocardiography (ECG), electromyography (EMG), electroencephalography (EEG), electromyography (EMG), and MRI systems.

5. **Health informatics:** It is defined as the use of information technologies for the management, analysis, and processing of health data. Biomedical engineers design and develop computer systems for the collection, storage, and analysis of this health data.

6. **Biomaterials:** Biomedical materials are natural or artificial materials suitable for organs or tissues that cannot perform their function due to any trauma or aging-related factors in the human body. Biomedical engineers are closely involved in the design and production of biomaterials. These materials include implants, prosthetics, orthoses, and materials used for tissue engineering.

Biomedical engineering is a specialized field that bridges healthcare and engineering, contributing to the protection and treatment of human health. Biomedical engineers are responsible for ensuring the quality and safety of medical devices used in diagnosis and treatment, and they actively conduct research to advance health technology through the development of innovative medical devices and biological systems.

Biomedical engineers find the opportunity to work in many different fields related to health. They may work with companies that design and manufacture medical devices, hospitals, pharmaceutical companies, and many healthcare providers. In addition, public institutions, universities, and research centers also offer job opportunities for biomedical engineers.

Biomedical engineering is one of the most important professions that helps make health services more effective and efficient. Therefore, biomedical engineers will continue to play an even more important role in healthcare in the future.

BIOMECHANICS

Biomechanics studies the mechanical functions of biological structures. It is concerned with the application of classical mechanics to various biological problems. It specifically combines the fields of biology and physiology with the fields of engineering mechanics. Basically, biomechanics is about the human body. In biomechanics, the principles of mechanics are applied to the idea, design, development, and analysis of equipment and systems in biology and medicine. In essence, biomechanics is a multidisciplinary science concerned with the application of mechanical principles to man at rest or in motion (Özkaya et al. 2012).

Biomechanics studies the movements of the human body and the mechanical properties of biological systems using the principles of biology and engineering. The scope of biomechanics is quite broad and covers many different fields. For example:

1. **Musculoskeletal system:** Biomechanics examines the functioning and mechanical properties of the musculoskeletal system. This includes the analysis and modeling of movements of bones, joints, muscles, and tendons.

2. **Biomaterials:** Biomechanics deals with the development and use of materials similar to body tissues, called biomaterials. This includes areas such as prostheses, implants, and artificial tissue engineering.

3. **Movement analysis:** Biomechanics objectively measures and analyzes people's movements using a method called movement analysis. In this context, sports performance, gait analysis, physiotherapy, and rehabilitation areas are included.

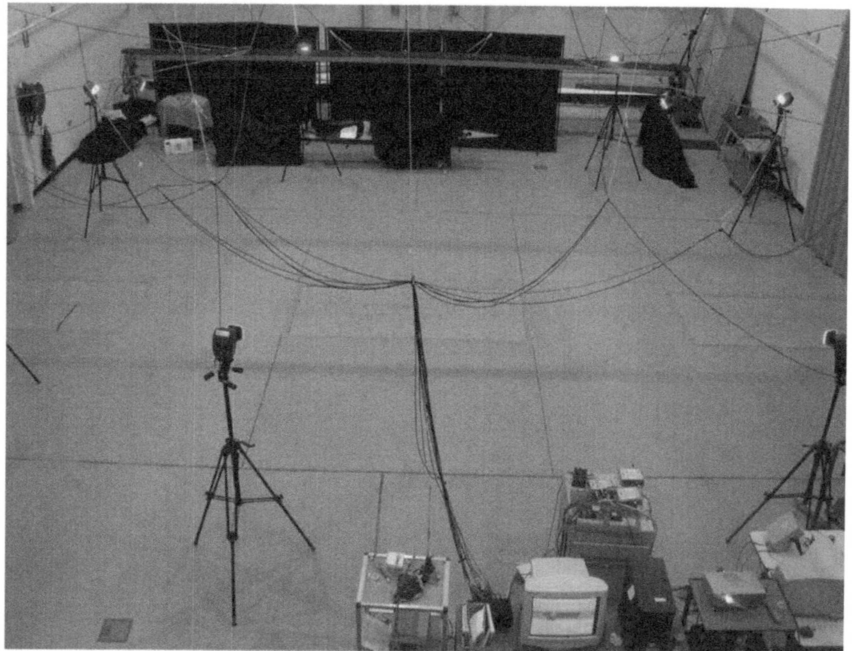

Figure 8.1   Biomechanical gait analysis.
Source: Robertson (2005).

4. **Biological fluids:** Biomechanics deals with the movement of blood and other biological fluids. This includes the study of the functioning of systems such as the heart, vessels, and lymphatic system.

5. **Modeling of biomechanics:** Biomechanics describes biological systems using mathematical and physical models. This includes body mechanics, system dynamics, and control systems.

6. **Biomechanics simulation:** Biomechanics attempts to model the movements of the human body and biological systems using computer simulation. This includes areas such as medical simulation, surgical planning, and medical education.

In general, biomechanics uses the principles of engineering and science to understand and improve the functioning of the human body. Therefore, it can be applied in many fields such as medicine, sports, physiotherapy, rehabilitation, prostheses, and implants.

Throughout history, the popularity of biomechanics, which has been the focus of study by many scientists, has been increasing continuously in the field of medicine and engineering. Arthur Steindler, one of the founders of Iowa Orthopaedics, entered the literature years ago with the words, "I visualize biomechanics as a powerful and indispensible ally of the orthopedic clinician" in 1933 which showed how important the subject is, especially for orthopedic clinicians.

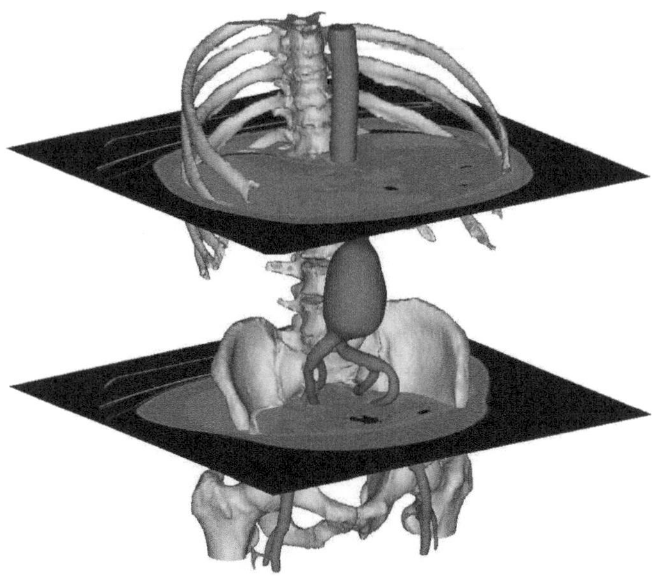

Figure 8.2 3D surface models created in Mimics from CT.
Source: Eboelen (2010).

The roots of the University of Iowa Orthopedic Biomechanics Laboratories (UIOBL) can be traced back to the early collaborations between Dr Arthur Steindler and the faculty of the College of Engineering in the 1930s. These pioneering efforts paved the way for the establishment of the UIOBL in 1969, which has since become a leading center for research in the field of orthopedic biomechanics. Dr Steindler, a prominent orthopedic surgeon, expressed a forward-thinking vision for the field in his presidential address to the American Orthopaedic Association on May 9, 1933. His words continue to inspire and motivate the work of the UIOBL to this day (Iowa Orthopedic Biomechanics Laboratories 1969).

Leonardo da Vinci (1452–1519), Edwin Smith Papyrus (c. 2600–2200 BCE), Hippocrates (c. 460–361 BCE), Aristotle (384–322 BCE), Archimedes (c. 288–212 BCE), Galen (131–201 CE), Ibn Sina (980–1037 CE), Galileo Galilei (1564–1642), Isaac Newton (1642–1727), and Carl Hirsch (1913–1973) have made significant contributions to the historical development of biomechanics.

Biomechanics contributes to understanding the mechanical behaviors of biological systems by investigating various components and functions of the human body. These fields encompass the musculoskeletal system and orthopedics, spinal biomechanics, cell biomechanics, circulatory system biomechanics, artificial organ biomechanics (e.g., prosthetics and implants), dental and jaw biomechanics, tissue biomechanics, and sports biomechanics.

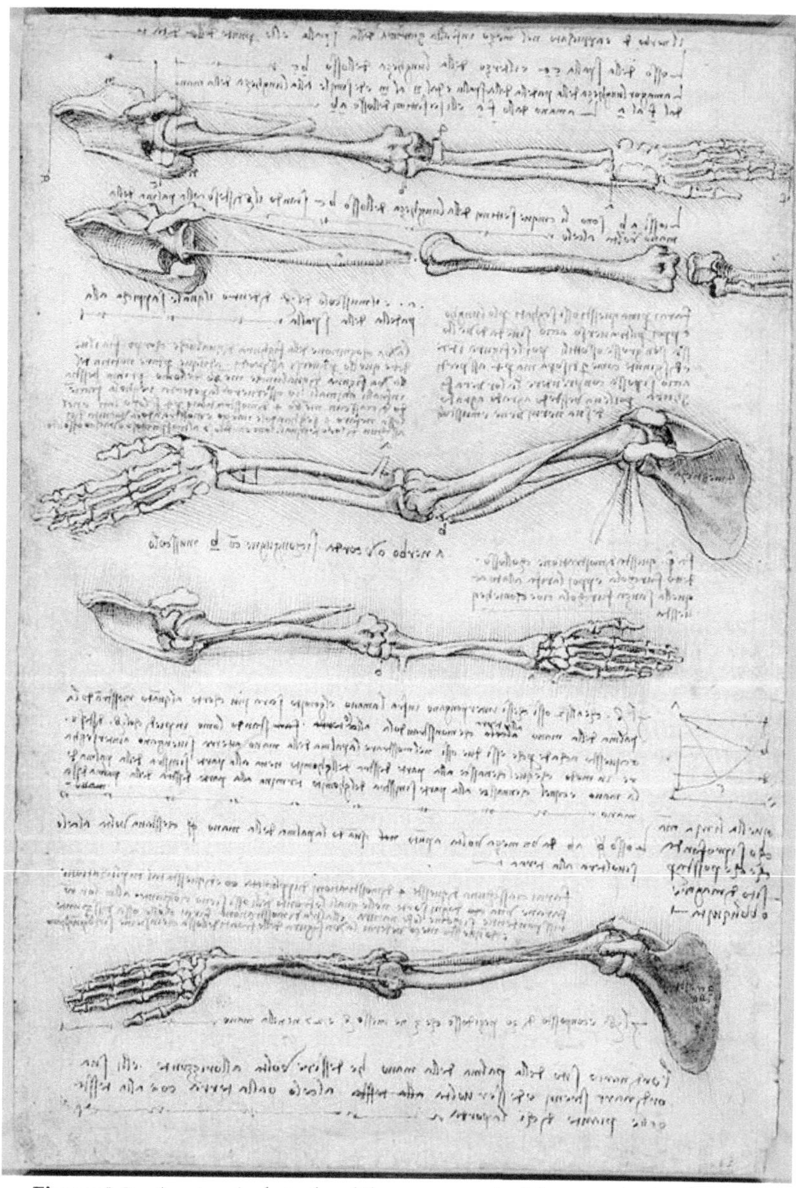

Figure 8.3   Anatomical study of the movement of the muscles in the arm.
Source: VİKİPEDİ (2021).

Using biomechanics, many advances have been made in these different areas, especially in the healthcare industry. For example, prostheses and implants help people regain lost organs or limbs. In another example, musculoskeletal and orthopedic biomechanics have helped develop new treatment modalities and devices for the treatment of conditions such as bone fractures or joint problems.

The use of biomechanics at the cellular level is used to provide greater understanding of cell behavior and differentiation, while sports biomechanics helps athletes develop techniques and equipment to enhance their performance.

These different application areas of biomechanics are very important for human health research and applications, and it is expected that further progress in this field will continue in the future.

The application fields of biomechanics are as follows:

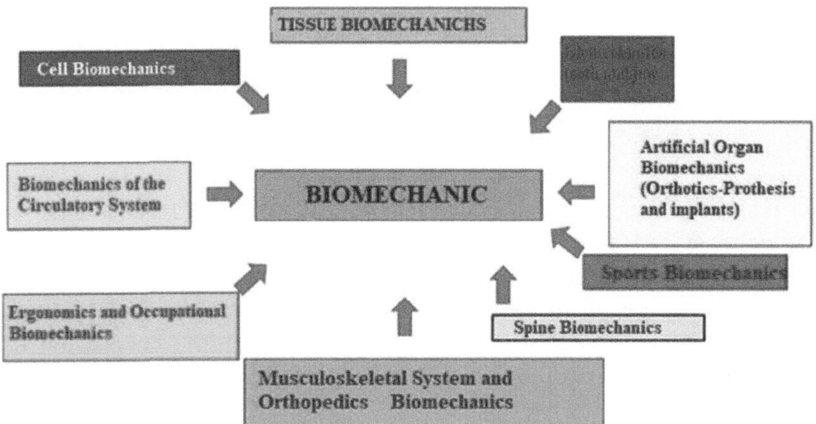

Figure 8.4   Application areas of biomechanics.
Source: Prepared by the authors.

1. Tissue biomechanics
2. Biomechanics of teeth and jaw
3. Artificial organ biomechanics (orthotics-prosthesis and implants)
4. Sports biomechanics
5. Spine biomechanics
6. Musculoskeletal system and orthopedics biomechanics
7. Ergonomics and occupational biomechanics
8. Biomechanics of the circulatory system
9. Cell biomechanics

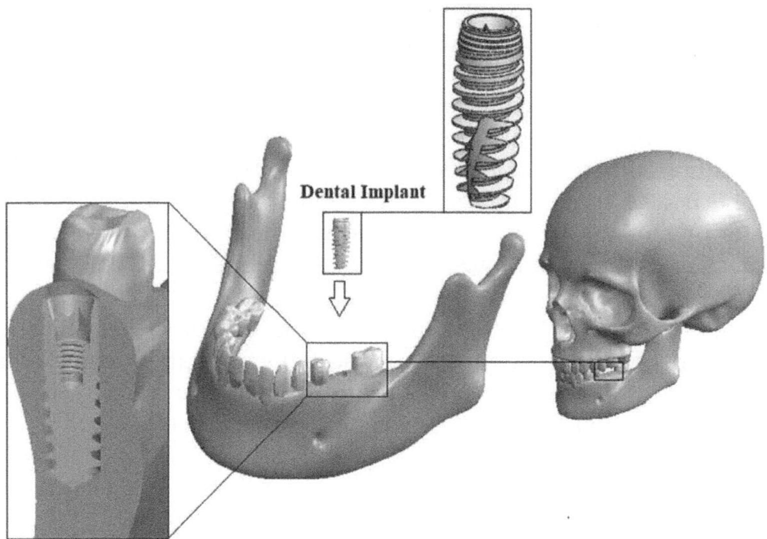

Figure 8.5   Dental implant.
Source: Prepared by the authors.

STRUCTURE AND MECHANICAL BEHAVIOR OF BONE TISSUE

Bones are composed of an organic and inorganic phase. The inorganic phase is a naturally occurring form of impure calcium phosphate called hydroxyapatite, which makes up about 60% of the weight of bone, while water accounts for about 8–10%, and the remaining portion is organic matter (Gong et al. 1964). The organic phase consists of type I collagen and other non-collagenous proteins, and makes up only about 2% of the cells (Einhorn 1994), with cells such as osteocytes, osteoblasts, and osteoclasts also present in the bone structure, along with the extracellular matrix. Bone is one of the hardest tissues in the body and unlike cartilage tissue, it contains blood vessels. Bones are composed of outer cortical or compact bone, and inner cancellous or spongy bone. The cancellous bone is surrounded by cortical bone and is protected by a hard connective tissue called the periosteum. The inner part is called bone marrow. Both periosteum and endosteum contain a vascularized bone system that supplies oxygen and nutrients for bone development and repair. Bone fractures can occur as a result of any trauma, and bone-forming cells are provided by the periosteum and endosteum (Hillery and Shuaib 1999). These tissues on bone are shown in Figure 8.6.

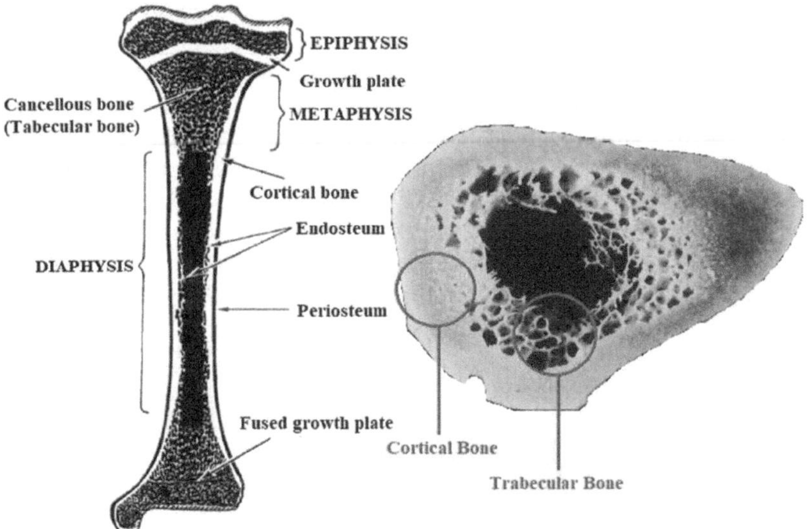

Figure 8.6   Hard and spongy bone structures (tibia bone).
Sources: Morgan et al. (2013), Weiss (1988)

How much strain a bone tissue sample is subjected to in response to an applied stress is dependent on tissue stiffness (strength). This stiffness, which is a material property, is expressed as the modulus of elasticity or Young's modulus. The mechanical properties of the materials are understood with a testing machine called a tensile device (Figure 8.7). The mechanical behavior of bones and soft tissues is determined by tensile, compression, bending, and fatigue tests.

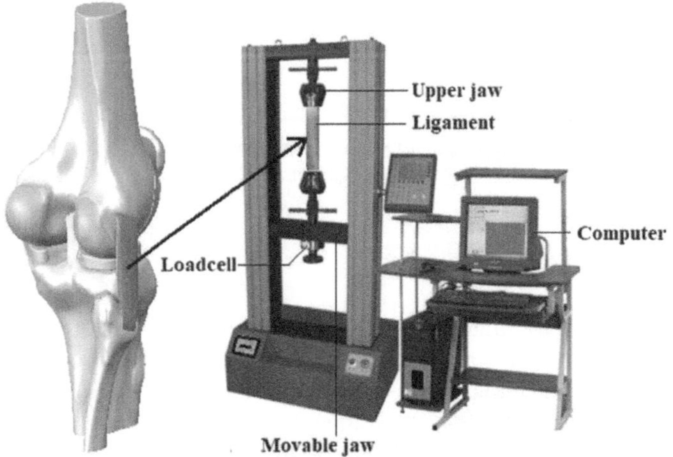

Figure 8.7   Computer servo control universal tensile device.
Source: Prepared by the authors

The stress-strain curves for cortical bone in tension and compression tests are shown in Figure 8.8. This region represents the resistance of the material to permanent deformation under applied load. If the load is applied in the form of shear force, the corresponding material property is the shear modulus. Bone tissue, like many other tissues, exhibits anisotropic properties, where the elastic modulus varies depending on the direction of the applied force. In general, bone tissue shows orthotropic anisotropy (Odgaard et al. 1997, Yang et al. 1998). Unlike metallic materials, bone does not exhibit elastic deformation, and therefore Young's modulus can be determined using the offset rule, similar to brittle materials such as cast iron.

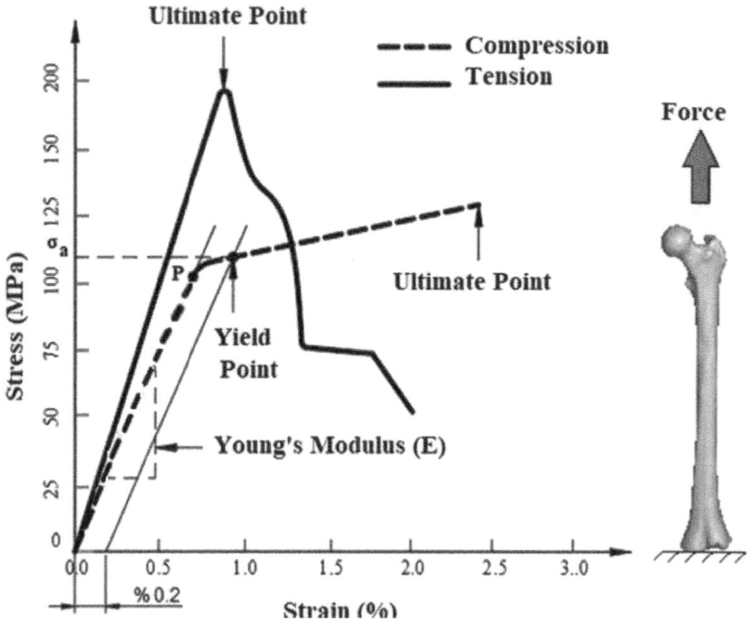

Figure 8.8   Stress-strain curves for cortical bone in compression and tensile testing. *Source*: Morgan et al. (2013).

BIOMATERIALS

When it comes to materials in the field of medicine, the properties and applications of natural or synthetic materials used in contact with biological systems come to mind. These materials are commonly referred to as biomaterials. Biomaterials is a multidisciplinary field that encompasses medicine, chemistry, biology, and materials science, and has been continuously evolving for over half a century. It is rooted in engineering principles and finds applications in both diagnostic and therapeutic areas. While initially used exclusively in medical applications, biomaterials are now utilized in equipment for cell culture, blood protein analysis in clinical laboratories, processing of biomolecules for biotechnological purposes, and other similar fields. The interaction between biological systems and synthetic or modified natural materials has been ensured in the creation of the common use area of these materials used in different fields. In medical applications, biomaterials are rarely used as standalone materials, but rather integrated into devices or implants. However, their effects on both the recipient and the device itself can potentially lead to device failure. Additionally, the evaluation of a biomaterial should always take into consideration its final fabricated and sterilized form (Ratner et al. 2004). Implants are devices that are manufactured using biomaterials or biomaterials that are inserted into a living system (Figure 8.9).

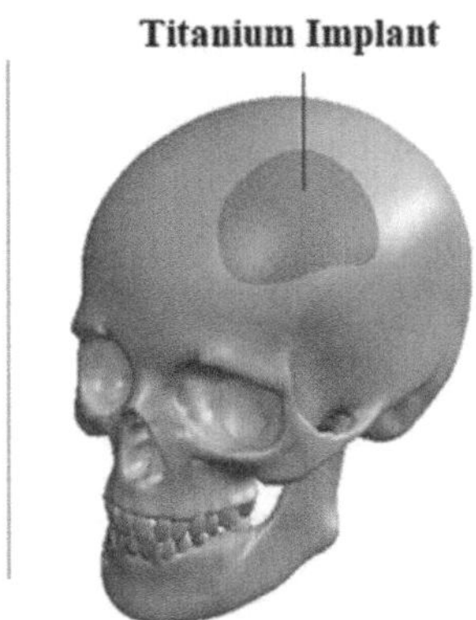

Figure 8.9   Titanium implant placed in a patient's skull as a result of trauma. *Source*: Prepared by the authors.

The features that a permanent implant should have are as follows:

- Biocompatibility
- Corrosion and wear resistance
- Fatigue strength
- Appropriate stiffness
- Damage tolerance

The potential problems of a permanent implant are:

- Allergic reactions
- Stress shielding (elastic modulus difference)
- Inflammation and sterilization loss caused by the rashes caused by abrasion

Recently, the concept of biocompatibility has been expanded to reconstruct functional tissues using in-vitro and in-vivo pathophysiological processes with careful selection of cells, materials, and metabolic and biomechanical conditions, using a broad approach called "tissue engineering" (Burdick and Mauck 2010, Hollinger 2011).

Biomaterials generally include many different materials such as metals, ceramics, polymers, glasses, carbons, and composite materials. In addition to these materials, molded or machined parts, coatings, fibers, films, foams, and fabrics are also among the components of biomaterials (Ratner et al. 2004). Table 8.1 shows some applications of synthetic and modified natural materials used in medicine. This table covers many biomaterials and applications that have become a major commercial market worldwide today. This market covers various fields such as the skeletal system, cardiovascular system, dental implants, organs, senses, and assistive devices.

In light of these explanations, it is evident that biomaterials science requires more open communication than any other field of contemporary technology, bringing together researchers from different backgrounds. It should be noted that this is based on interdisciplinary work.

Table 8.1   Examples of applications of synthetic and modified natural materials. *Source*: Ratner et al. (2004).

Application	Material Type
Skeletal System	
Joint prostheses (hip, knee)	Titanium, Ti—Al—V alloy, stainless
Bone plate fixation for fracture	steel, polyethylene
Bone defect repair	Stainless steel, cobalt-chromium alloy
Artificial tendon and ligament	Hydroxylapatite
Fixing dental implant for tooth	Teflon, Dacron
	Titanium, alumina, calcium phosphate
Cardiovascular system	
Blood vessel prosthesis	Dacron, Teflon, polyurethane
Cardiac valve	Reworked tissue, stainless steel, carbon
Catheter	Silicone rubber, Teflon, Polyurethane
Organs	
Artificial heart	Polyurethane
Skin repair plate	Silicone-collagen composite
Artificial kidney	Cellulose, polyacrylonitrile
Heart-lung machine	Silicone, rubber
Senses	
Intraocular lens	Methyl methacrylate, silicone, rubber,
Contact lens	hydrogel
Corneal bandage	Silicone-acrylate, hydrogel
	Collagen, hydrogel

Especially with the development of technology, custom-made bone grafts, tissues, implants, and prostheses are produced using additive manufacturing technologies. Additive manufacturing or "3D printing" has revolutionized the medical field, bringing with it a wealth of excitement and innovation. The ability to offer customized healthcare solutions has become almost effortless, providing great relief to medical practitioners and patients alike. Beyond its expected uses in customization, prototyping, manufacturing, and research, 3D printing in medicine has a surprisingly wide range of applications. These extend far beyond general medical practice and research, and include the following areas (ALL3DP 2019):

- Surgical preparation
- Prostheses
- Dental
- 3D printing of tissues and organs
- Medication dosage and pharmacology
- Manufacturing of medical tools and devices

Overall, the potential of 3D printing to transform the medical field is vast, and its impact has already been significant. By providing customized healthcare solutions, medical practitioners and patients can both benefit from improved outcomes and quality of care. You can see a knee cartilage produced with additive manufacturing method in Figure 8.10.

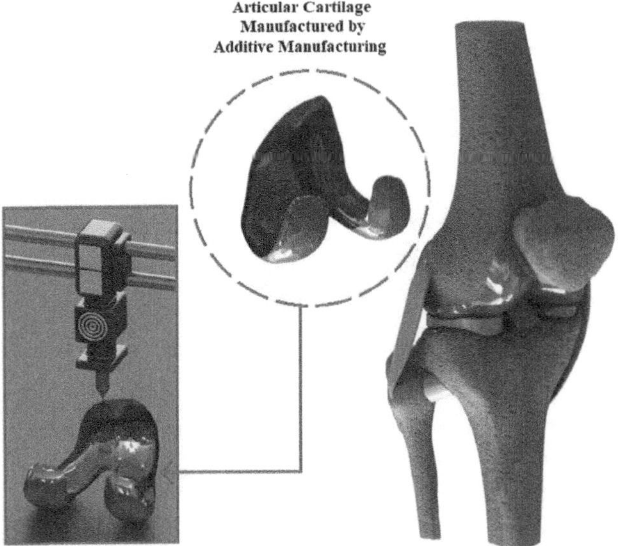

Figure 8.10   Personalized vertical articular cartilage produced by additive manufacturing.
Source: Prepared by the authors.

BIOMEDICAL DEVICES AND MEDICAL IMAGING SYSTEMS

From past to present, biomedical devices have been used in the diagnosis and treatment of many diseases. If we examine the historical development of biomedical devices, the first biomedical device was the stethoscope (Figure 8.12), which was invented in 1816 by René Laennec (Figure 8.11).

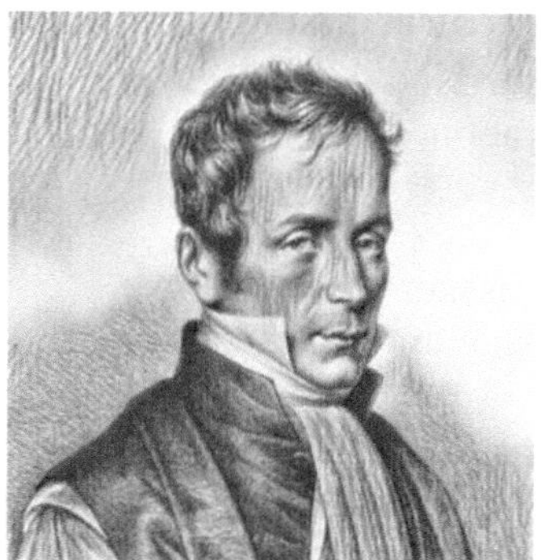

Figure 8.11   Inventor of the stethoscope and French physician René Laennec. *Source*: (Lemelson-MIT 2023).

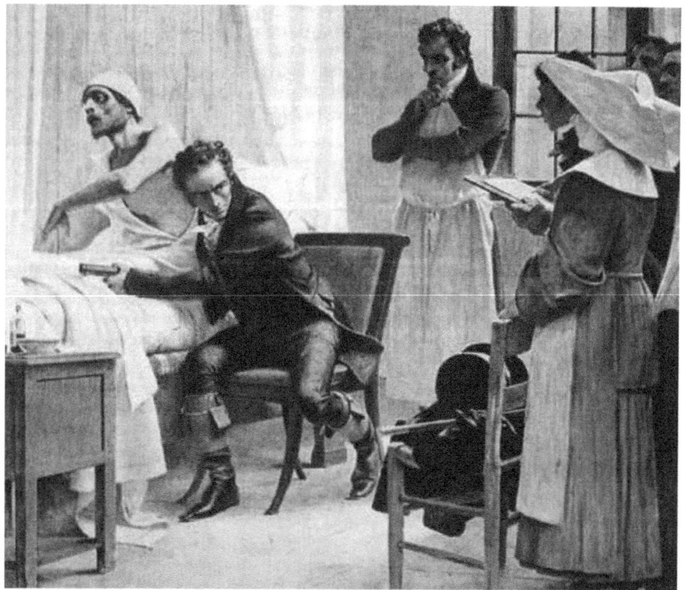

Figure 8.12   Dr Laennec examines a consumptive patient with a stethoscope in front of his students at the Necker Hospital (Théobald Chartran). *Source*: Independent (2016).

Laennec was a French physician and inventor who made significant contributions to the medical field. He is considered a pioneer in the diagnosis and treatment of pulmonary diseases. Additionally, Laennec invented a device called the stethoscope, which revolutionized medical practice. This simple but ingenious invention became an indispensable tool for doctors worldwide, enabling more accurate and non-invasive diagnosis of various medical conditions. Laennec's innovations have made him a visionary and pioneer in the history of medicine (Lemelson-MIT 2023).

Dutch doctor and physiologist William Einthoven (Figure 8.13) invented the first electrocardiography device in 1903 (Figure 8.14). This breakthrough is seen as one of the most important steps in the history of biomedical engineering.

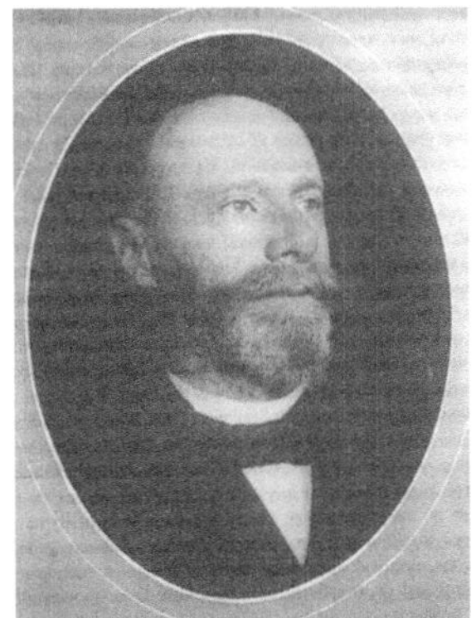

Figure 8.13   Willem Einthoven.
Source: Leiden (2022).

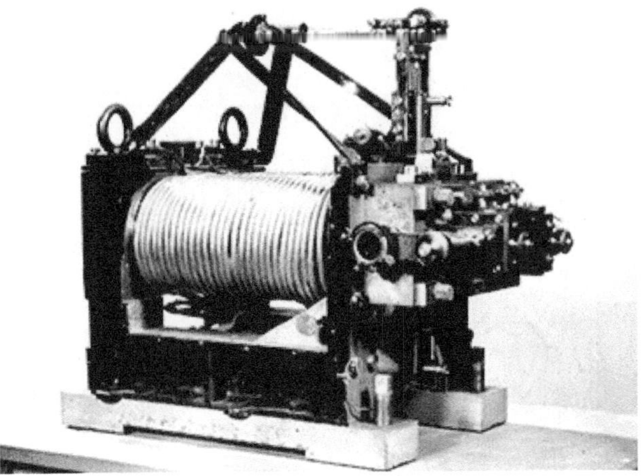

Figure 8.14   Electrocardiography device.
Source: Leiden (2022).

Today, robotic surgery and many technological medical devices supported by AI are widely used in diagnosis and treatment of diseases. These robots, which offer a sensitive solution for many surgical operations, make the work of surgeons easier day by day and come to the fore with low complications.

The Da Vinci surgical system is a revolutionary medical technology that has transformed the way surgeries are performed (Figure 8.15). It is a robotic system that enables surgeons to perform complex surgeries with greater precision and control, using a minimally invasive approach. The system is manufactured by Intuitive Surgical and has gained popularity in recent years for its use in a range of surgeries including

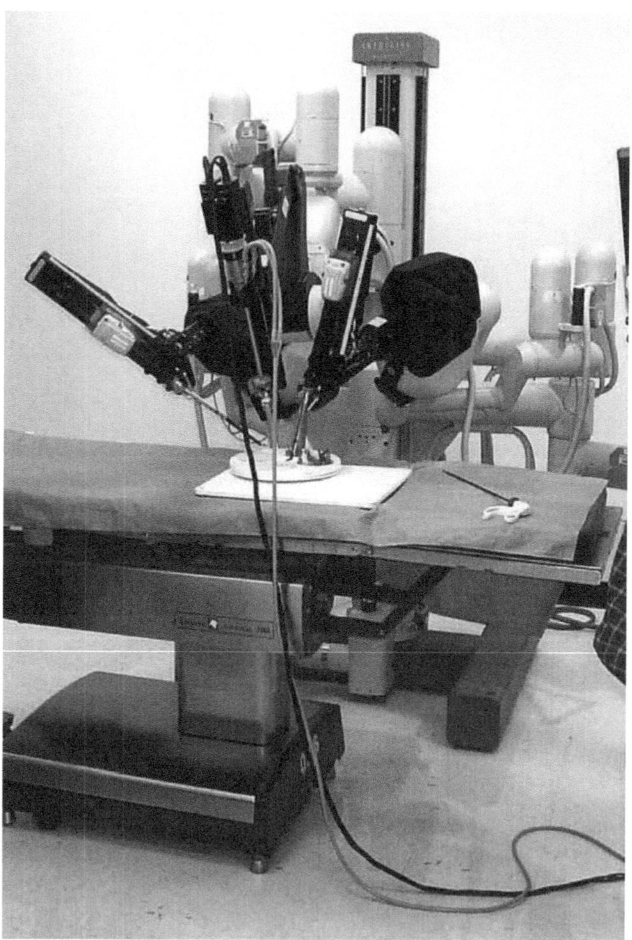

Figure 8.15   Da Vinci surgical system.
Source: Wikipedia 2020.

prostatectomies, cardiac valve repair, and renal and gynecologic procedures. It has been estimated that in 2012, the system was used in around 200,000 surgeries, making it one of the most widely used surgical systems in the world. The system owes its name to Leonardo da Vinci, the renowned artist and inventor, whose study of human anatomy laid the foundation for the development of the first robot in history (Economist 2012, Fatima 2022, Future 2012, MarketWatch 2005, *The New York Times* 2008, Wikipedia 2020).

Medical imaging comprises of the techniques and procedures used to create visual representations of the internal parts of the body or to visually depict the functions of certain organs or tissues. It is also used for medical analysis and intervention.

There are three basic methods in medical imaging systems:

- Transmission of energy (X-Ray, Computed Tomography (CT))
- Diffusion of energy (Magnetic Resonance (MR))
- Reflection of energy (ultrasoundography)

TRANSMISSION OF ENERGY

Energy transmission can be defined as the expression of how the movement of energy in an object or medium occurs. This is seen in many physical processes. In medical imaging systems such as X-rays and CT, the energy generated is absorbed by the living body or object to be imaged. This absorbed energy is transmitted at different rates, especially by different organs or tissues in the living body.

X-rays, a type of electromagnetic radiation, are an imaging method used to view the internal structure of an object (Figure 8.16). In particular, different tissues in the human body absorb X-rays at different rates. Therefore, X-rays show different reactions on objects. X-rays pass, absorb, or scatter depending on the state of the object. The images are detected by the device and captured.

In CT (Figure 8.17), an object is displayed in layers. In fact, CT is performed by scanning many X-rays of the object from different directions and angles. The properties of the scanned object are important. This scan data is processed by computer and 3D data is obtained.

DIFFUSION OF ENERGY

The diffusion of energy refers to the movement of energy in a medium. MRI is a medical imaging technique for the state of diffusion of energy. This medical imaging technique consists of magnetic fields and radio

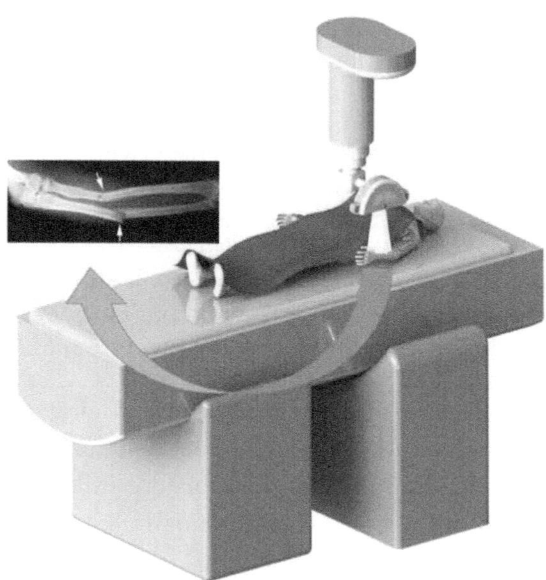

Figure 8.16   X-ray device (illustration and X-ray showing fractures of both the radius and ulna from OrthoInfo [n.d.]).
Source: Prepared by the authors

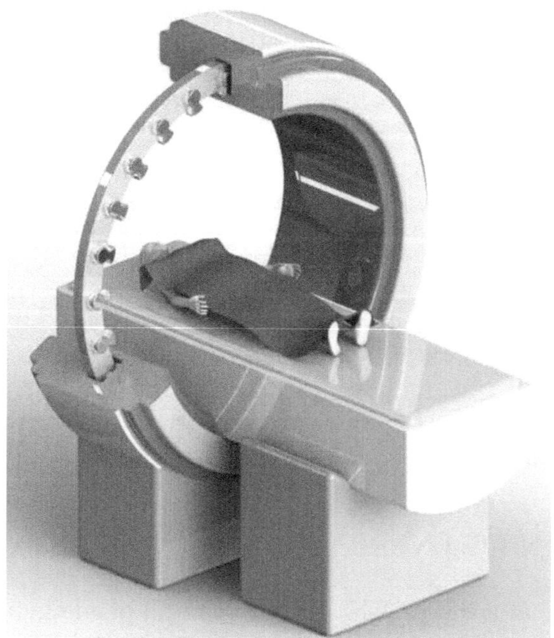

Figure 8.17   CT device.
Source: Prepared by the authors.

waves. It is examined by the effect of the magnetic field created in the human body on the hydrogen atoms in the human body. When these hydrogen atoms in the human body are exposed to a magnetic field, they vibrate and these vibrations received by radio waves are processed in the computer, and images of the desired regions in the human body are obtained. With this medical imaging technique, we can obtain detailed images of soft tissues (heart, muscles, connective tissue, brain), as well as diagnosis of cancer, brain damage, muscle rupture, and other medical conditions. The difference from other imaging techniques is that there is no risk of ionizing radiation.

While the MRI device (Figure 8.18) is preferred because of its high resolution properties, it may have the potential to cause electromagnetic interference in surrounding biological tissues by affecting the structure and function of biomaterials used for medical purposes. This can cause serious health problems. For example, patients who carry an insulin pump, have a neurostimulator, or are treated with pacemakers can have fatal consequences as a result of magnetic interference during MRI. In addition, the presence of ferromagnetic objects in the MR environment can cause hundreds of serious tissue burns and injuries. Therefore,

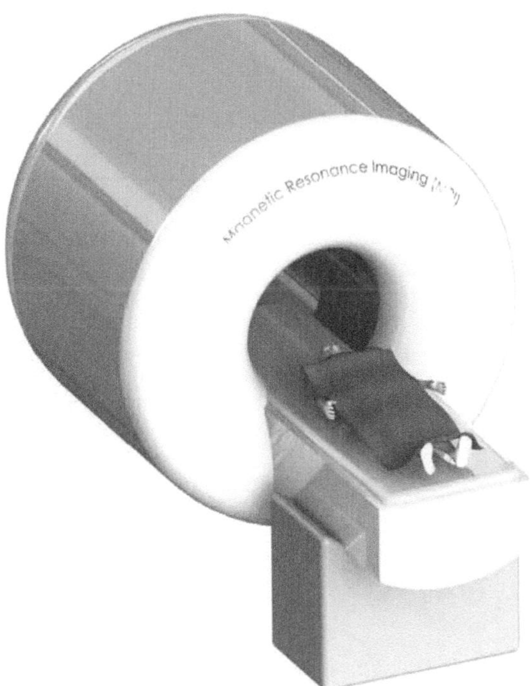

Figure 8.18   MRI device.
Source: Prepared by the authors.

biomaterials to be used in the body should be compatible and reliable with the MRI device (Chen 2001, Dempsey and Condon 2001, Hardy and Weil 2010, Irnich et al. 2005, Klucznik et al. 1993, Shellock 2002).

REFLECTION OF ENERGY

Ultrasonography is an imaging method using high-frequency sound waves to determine the structure and position of organs in the body. The device that performs this operation is called the ultrasound device (Figure 8.19). With this device, high-frequency sound waves are sent to the organs or tissues in the human body to be imaged. High-frequency sound waves are reflected back by hitting organs or tissues. These are detected and processed on the computer to obtain images of organs or tissues. Ultrasound does not contain radiation, and portable types

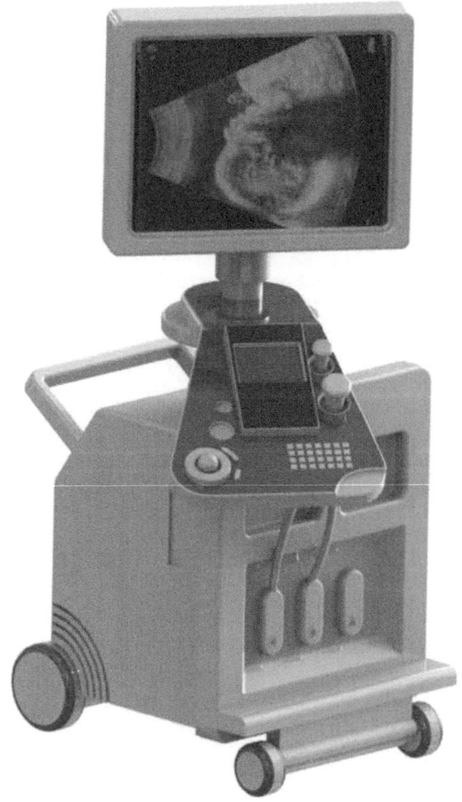

Figure 8.19   Ultrasound device.
Source: Prepared by the authors.

are also available. It is used especially in cases of pregnant women to follow the development of the fetus. Therefore, low-intensity ultrasonic applications are preferred in medical imaging. In addition, it is also used in imaging of the heart, eye, kidney, and the musculoskeletal system.

AI SUPPORTED BIOMEDICAL MATERIAL AND DEVICE DESIGN

Artificial intelligence is intelligence displayed by machines. Natural intelligence includes the consciousness and emotionality exhibited by human intelligence and animal cognition. With the development of computer processors in recent years, AI technology has made great progress in many areas. Especially in the field of biomedical engineering, AI support has a crucial impact on the design and development of biomedical devices and determining the best parameters. The diagnosis of many diseases can be made easily with AI algorithms created by using very large data.

Artificial intelligence especially helps biomedical and medical engineers to analyze using very large data from patients and to develop biomedical materials and devices that measure more sensitively and accurately by obtaining these optimum values. AI improves the performance of life support units, artificial heart devices, or implants and prostheses. In addition, AI can optimize the performance of an MRI device or adjust the insulin dosage level to an insulin pump that continuously delivers insulin to diabetics using vital signs. In particular, with the development of computer processors and the processing of large data accordingly, AI-based devices appear in imaging systems used in imaging any organ or tissue in the human body. One of them is the Artificial Intelligence 3 Tesla Magnetic Resonance Imaging (3 Tesla MR) device (Figure 8.20). With the AI-supported 3 Tesla MR device, the images in the human body can be analyzed and the tissues, organs, or desired regions can be labeled and the images can be evaluated more precisely by the radiologists. The big data obtained from the 3 Tesla MR device is analyzed with machine learning, and the diagnosis of the health status of the patients is made faster and more reliable with the support of AI.

Especially in hospitals, the use of AI-supported imaging, diagnosis, and rehabilitation devices is beneficial. It also facilitates telemedicine applications, which are remote treatment and control processes of patients in some cases. Thus, before the patient goes to the hospital, the doctor can advise on which treatment might be effective or update the treatment program based on MRI or other image results.

There are many different applications of AI in the field of biomedical engineering. The use of AI in the design and manufacture of biomedical materials and devices can help develop higher quality products and provide medical practitioners with more effective devices to treat patients.

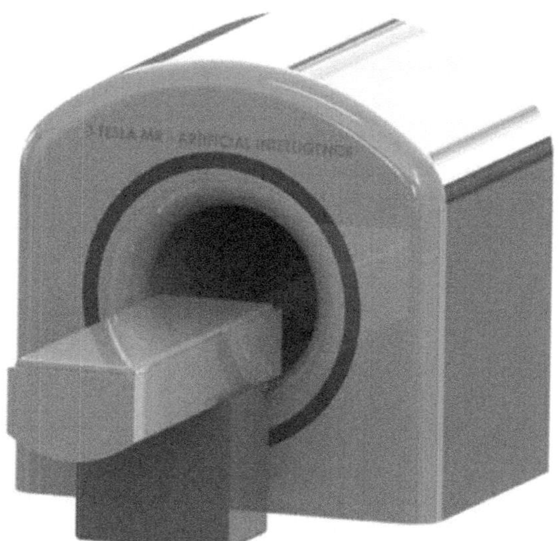

Figure 8.20   Tesla MR device.
Source: Prepared by the authors.

CONCLUSION AND DISCUSSION

In conclusion, biomedical engineering has emerged as a critical field that combines engineering principles, medical sciences, and biology to address healthcare challenges. This interdisciplinary approach has enabled the development of innovative processes, devices, and procedures for diagnosis, treatment, and patient care. By collaborating with professionals from various domains, biomedical engineers have been able to leverage expertise from engineering, basic sciences, and medical practitioners to create impactful solutions.

An important aspect of biomedical engineering is the use of biomaterials, which have revolutionized medical applications. Metals, ceramics, polymers, and composite materials have found utility in implants, diagnostic devices, and tissue engineering. The continuous advancements in biomaterials have significantly contributed to improving the quality of medical devices and enhancing patient outcomes. Furthermore, the integration of AI in the design of biomedical materials and devices holds great promise for further advancements in the field.

The topics covered in this chapter, including biomedical engineering, biomechanics, biomaterials, biomedical devices, medical imaging systems, and the role of AI, provide a comprehensive understanding of the breadth and depth of this rapidly evolving field. By exploring these subjects, we gain insights into the collaborative efforts required to address complex healthcare issues and enhance patient well-being.

The discussion presented in this chapter highlights the importance of interdisciplinary collaboration in biomedical engineering. The involvement of professionals from diverse backgrounds ensures a holistic approach to problem-solving and drives innovation. Furthermore, the integration of AI techniques in biomedical engineering offers exciting opportunities for enhanced diagnostics, personalized medicine, and more efficient healthcare delivery.

As biomedical engineering continues to evolve, it is crucial to foster continued research, collaboration, and knowledge exchange among researchers, professionals, and students. By investing in education and promoting interdisciplinary initiatives, we can accelerate advancements in this field and ultimately improve healthcare outcomes for individuals worldwide.

In conclusion, this chapter serves as a valuable resource for those interested in understanding the scope and impact of biomedical engineering. It provides an overview of the field's foundations, explores key areas of focus such as biomechanics and biomaterials, and emphasizes the critical role of collaboration and innovation in driving progress. By furthering our understanding of biomedical engineering, we can further advance medical technology and enhance the well-being of patients.

REFERENCES

ALL3DP. 2019. Medical 3D printing: the best healthcare applications. Accessed at https://all3dp.com/2/3d-printing-in-medicine-the-best-applications/ (on March 30, 2023).

Burdick, J.A., and Mauck, R.L. 2010. Biomaterials for tissue engineering applications: a review of the past and future trends. Vienna: Springer.

Chen, D.W. 2001. Boy, 6, dies of skull injury during M.R.I. The New York Times. B5: 1.

Dempsey, M.F. and Condon, B. 2001. Thermal injuries associated with MRI [Review]. Clinical Radiology. 56(6): 457–465.

Eboelen. 2010. 3D surface models from abdominal CT. CC0. Accessed at https://commons.wikimedia.org/w/index.php?curid=35760596 (on 15 March 2024).

Economist. 2012. Surgical robots: the kindness of strangers. Babbage Science and Technology. Accessed at https://www.economist.com/babbage/2012/01/18/the-kindness-of-strangers (on February 21, 2013).

Einhorn, T.A. 1994. Bone metabolism and metabolic bone disease. pp. 69–88. *In*: J.W. Frymoyer (ed.). Orthopaedic Knowledge Update 4 Home Study Syllabus. American Academy of Orthopaedic Surgeons.

Fatima, Sakina 2022. Da Vinci Xi surgical robot perform kidney surgery in Dubai. The Siasat Daily. Accessed at https://www.siasat.com/da-vinci-xi-surgical-robot-perform-kidney-surgery-in-dubai-2330469/#google_vignette (on May 19, 2022).

Future, C.-P.P. 2012. Intuitive Surgical. Retrieved January 14, 2015.

Gong, J.K., Arnold, J.S. and Cohn, S.H. 1964. Composition of trabecular and cortical bone. The Anatomical Record. 149(3): 325–331.

Hardy, P.T., 2nd and Weil, K.M. 2010. A review of thermal MR injuries. [Review]. Radiologic Technology. 81(6): 606–609.

Hillery, M.T. and Shuaib, I. 1999. Temperature effects in the drilling of human and bovine bone. Journal of Materials Processing Technology. 92–93: 302–308.

Hollinger, J.O. 2011. An Introduction to Biomaterials (2nd ed.). Taylor & Francis.

Independent. 2016. Rene Laennec: 5 things you need to know about the inventor of the stethoscope. Accessed at https://www.independent.co.uk/news/people/rene-laennec-google-doodle-stethoscope-today-a6878641.html (on April 16, 2023).

Iowa Orthopedic Biomechanics Laboratories. 1969. About. Accessed at https://uiobl.uiowa.edu/about (on March 18, 2023).

Irnich, W., Irnich, B., Bartsch, C., Stertmann, W.A., Gufler, H. and Weiler, G. 2005. Do we need pacemakers resistant to magnetic resonance imaging? [Review]. Europace. 7(4): 353–365.

Klucznik, R.P., Carrier, D.A., Pyka, R. and Haid, R.W. 1993. Placement of a ferromagnetic intracerebral aneurysm clip in a magnetic field with a fatal outcome. [Case Reports]. Radiology. 187(3): 855–856.

Leiden, Hart Long Centrum. 2022. Willem Einthoven. Accessed at https://hartlongcentrum.nl/over-ons/geschiedenis/ieee-milestone-award-string-galvanometer/(on April 16, 2023).

Lemelson-MIT. 2023. Rene Laennec. Accessed at https://lemelson.mit.edu/resources/rene-laennec (on April 16, 2023).

MarketWatch. 2005. Robots as surgical enablers. Accessed at https://www.marketwatch.com/story/a-fascinating-visit-to-a-high-tech-operating-room (on March 17, 2013).

Morgan, E.F., Barnes, G.L. and Einhorn, T.A. 2013. The bone organ system. Form and function. pp. 3–20. *In*: Marcus, R., Feldman, D., Dempster, D.W., Luckey, M. and Cauley, J.A. (eds). Osteoporosis (4th ed.).

Odgaard, A., Kabel, J., van Rietbergen, B., Dalstra, M. and Huiskes, R. 1997. Fabric and elastic principal directions of cancellous bone are closely related. Journal of Biomechanics. 30(5): 487–495.

OrthoInfo. (n.d.). Adult forearm fractures. Accessed at https://orthoinfo.aaos.org/en/diseases--conditions/adult-forearm-fractures/(on Retrieved April 12, 2023).

Özkaya, N., Nordin, M., Goldsheyder, D. and Leger, D. 2012. Fundamentals of biomechanics: equilibrium, motion and deformation. New York: Springer.

Ratner, B.D., Hoffman, A.S., Schoen, F.J. and Lemons, J.E. 2004. Biomaterials science: an introduction to materials in medicine. Elsevier Science.

Robertson, D.G.E. 2005. Gait laboratory. CC BY SA 3.0. Accessed at https://commons.wikimedia.org/w/index.php?curid=8469181 (on 15 March 2024).

Shellock, F.G. 2002. Magnetic resonance safety update 2002: implants and devices. Journal of Magnetic Resonance İmaging. 16(5): 485–496.

The New York Times. 2008. Prepping robots to perform surgery. Accessed at https://www.nytimes.com/2008/05/04/business/04moll.html#:~:text=Winifred%20Hayes%2C%20chief%20executive%20of,on%20their%20robots%2C%20she%20says. (on March 17, 2013).

VİKİPEDİ. 2021. Leonardo da Vinci. Accessed at https://tr.wikipedia.org/wiki/Leonardo_da_Vinci (on March 18, 2023).

Weiss, L. 1988. Cell and tissue biology. A Textbook of Histology. Urban & Fischer Verlag GmbH & Company KG.

Wikipedia 2020. da Vinci surgical system. Accessed at https://en.wikipedia.org/wiki/Da_Vinci_Surgical_System#cite_note-1 (on April 16, 2023).

Yang, G., Kabel, J., Van Rietbergen, B., Odgaard, A., Huiskes, R. and Cown, S.C. 1998. The anisotropic Hooke's law for cancellous bone and wood. Journal of Elasticity. 53(2): 125–146.

Chapter 9

Artificial Intelligence in Health Services Management

Hilal Arslan*,[1] and Fatma Kucuk[2]

[1]Department of Software Engineering,
Faculty of Engineering and Natural Science,
Ankara Yildirim Beyazit University, Ankara, Türkiye
ORCID: 0000-0002-6449-6952. Email: hilalarslan@aybu.edu.tr

[2]Department of Software Engineering,
Faculty of Engineering and Natural Science,
Ankara Yildirim Beyazit University, Ankara, Türkiye
ORCID: 0000-0002-7052-362X. Email: fatmakucuk@aybu.edu.tr

INTRODUCTION

Artificial intelligence (AI) has the potential to improve the management of healthcare services by providing efficient and effective solutions to the challenges faced by health professionals. AI-based systems are capable of analyzing large amounts of data, identifying patterns, and providing insights that can help healthcare providers make better decisions. The use of various technologies such as embedded systems, the Internet of Things (IoT), smart devices, and communication technologies alongside AI methods can significantly reduce the economic costs of healthcare systems. Recently, AI methods have been developed in various areas of healthcare service management, including patient care, diagnosis, treatment, and resource management. Next, we briefly discuss these areas.

---

*For Correspondence: Hilal Arslan (hilalarslan@aybu.edu.tr)

First, AI can improve patient care by supplying personalized care plans. AI-based technologies offer information on the best therapy options for each patient. This can assist medical professionals in providing better treatment and enhancing patient outcomes. AI may also be utilized to give real-time patient health monitoring and early warning indicators of potential health hazards. Second, AI can increase the precision of diagnosis by examining patient data and seeing trends that may not be obvious to medical specialists like physicians. Additionally, AI-based systems can assist healthcare professionals in detecting potential health risks earlier, resulting in improved health outcomes. Third, AI can assist healthcare professionals in creating patient-specific treatment plans. AI-based systems analyze each patient's medical history and current health status to determine the most effective treatment options. This may result in enhanced patient satisfaction and improved treatment outcomes. Finally, AI can help healthcare professionals to optimize resource management by analyzing data on patient demand and staff availability. AI-based systems can also help healthcare professionals to identify areas of inefficiency in healthcare operations, leading to cost savings and improved patient outcomes.

In this chapter, AI methods in health service management are reviewed in two categories: machine learning (ML) methods and deep learning (DL) methods. In the first part, traditional ML methods used in the health industry are briefly mentioned, and then the state-of-the-art ML methods with their application areas are reviewed. In the second part, after commonly used DL methods in the health industry are summarized, the state-of-the-art DL methods with application areas are also reviewed. Finally, we discuss the advantages and drawbacks of AI in health service management in the Conclusions.

ML METHODS USED FOR ANALYZING MEDICAL DATA

In the literature, several types of ML methods used in the healthcare industry have been proposed. First, we give commonly used traditional ML techniques employed for analyzing medical data. Next, we review ML methods that have been released in the literature and discuss their application areas in the health industry.

Traditional ML Methods

In this part, we briefly describe ML methods used in healthcare, which are logistic regression, support vector machine, decision tree, random forest, k-nearest neighbour, artificial neural network, and naive Bayes.

Logistic Regression

Logistic regression (LR) (DeMaris 1995) is a traditional algorithm used in various domains such as healthcare, disease prediction and treatment, and social sciences. It is easy to implement, interpretable, and can handle non-linearity. However, this method supposes that data is linearly related, and it can suffer from overfitting problems especially when the size of the data is large. LR method is used for solving classification problems and estimates the probability that a given sample data belongs to one of the classes. Thus, the output of LR is a probability score which is used as a threshold for the prediction.

Support Vector Machine

Support vector machine (SVM) (Burges 1998, Vapnik 1995) is a traditional ML method used for solving classification and regression problems. SVM aims to find an optimum hyperplane that best separates the data into different classes. The hyperplane is the decision boundary that maximises the margin between the two classes. The margin is defined as the distance between the hyperplane and the nearest data samples from each class.

The SVM can overcome both linearly separable and non-linearly separable data. In the case of non-linearly separable data, SVM performs a technique called kernel trick (Keerthi and Lin 2003, Min and Lee 2005), which converts the data into a higher-dimensional space where data is linearly separable. The most commonly used kernel functions are linear, polynomial, and radial basis function.

Decision Tree

Decision tree (DT) (Aha et al. 1991, Basu et al. 2014, Safavian and Landgrebe 1991) is a well-known ML method that is used to address classification problems. The DT method iteratively divides the data into smaller subsets based on the data and then constructs a model in the form of a tree structure. Each internal node in a DT represents a feature, and each branch is a decision rule. The projected results are represented by the tree's leaves. The most important attribute is chosen to divide the data in the DT-building process.

Random Forest

Random forest (RF) (Breiman 1996, Ho 1998) is an ML technique that combines several DTs to improve model accuracy. The final prediction is obtained by averaging the predictions of all the individual trees in the RF technique, which builds a set of DTs on various subsets of the training data. A random subset of the features and a random subset of the training data are used to build each tree in the RF. The goal of the randomization is to keep the trees different and not too associated with one another.

K-nearest Neighbour

K-nearest neighbours (KNN) (Abu Alfeilat et al. 2019, Deng et al. 2016) is a straightforward method that exploits the idea of similarity to create predictions based on nearest neighbours. In the KNN technique, the prediction for new coming data sample is based on either the average value of the K-nearest neighbours in the training set for regression issues or the majority class for classification problems. A hyperparameter called k controls how many neighbours are taken into account while making predictions. A distance metric is used to calculate the separation between the input data point and the training points. KNN does not have a training step because it uses lazy learning, which eliminates that step.

Artificial Neural Network

Artificial neural network (ANN) (Hornik et al. 1989) is a type of ML algorithm inspired by the structure and function of the human brain. ANNs are made up of layers of interconnected nodes, or neurons, and they learn patterns and relationships between inputs and outputs by being trained on a collection of input data. Backpropagation is a popular technique for training ANNs, which modifies the weights of the neurons in each layer depending on the discrepancy between the projected output and the actual output using a variant of gradient descent. The network is subjected to this procedure repeatedly over a number of iterations or epochs until the accuracy level needed is attained.

Naive Bayes

Naive Bayes (NB) is a traditional ML method used for analyzing medical data. It is based on the Bayes theorem, which estimates the likelihood that an event will occur based on knowledge of factors that may be associated with it in the past.

The State-of-the-art ML Methods in Health Service Management: Applications Areas

In this part, we discuss ML application areas and existing studies in the health industry. ML techniques have been effectively used for disease prediction, and a general overview of disease prediction is shown in Figure 9.1. Several ML methods were used effectively to fight the Covid-19 pandemic that emerged in China in 2019. These methods detected Covid-19 by analysing image data, genomic data, or laboratory information. Arslan (2021a) and Arslan and Arslan (2021) proposed Covid-19 detection methods by analyzing human genome sequences. They proposed CpG-based features that discriminate Covid-19 cases. Effectiveness of the proposed features was proven by using traditional ML methods. In another study (Arslan 2021b), a new similarity score was introduced by comparing genome sequences belonging to bat and human. Efficiency of the similarity score was shown using ML algorithms. Furthermore, various types of ML methods detecting Covid-19 cases from image data or laboratory data can be found in Alakus and Turkoglu (2020), Arslan and Aygun (2021), Arslan and Er (2022), and Jain et al. (2020). Mortality of Covid-19 patients was also predicted by using bagging and boosting methods (Arslan 2022). At the end of the Covid-19 pandemic, various types of SARS-CoV-2 variants have emerged and ML techniques have successfully detected these variants (Ali et al. 2021, Arslan 2023).

The ML techniques are also used for the diagnosis of heart disease with high accuracy. Yang et al. (2014) performed KNN, RF, and SVM methods to detect heart disease from signal data. The best accuracy of about 87.6% was achieved when RF was used. Long et al. (2015) employed ANN, NB, and SVM methods to diagnose heart disease from clinical, demographic, and image data. The NB method achieved the best accuracy with 83.3%. Jin et al. (2017) analyzed electronic health records (EHRs) and they used LR and RF. Their experimental results showed that LR and RF reach AUC scores of 0.66 and 0.62, respectively. Marikani and Shyamala (2017) used DT, KNN, RF, and SVM methods to detect heart failure from clinical and demographic data. They achieved full accuracy with SVM method.

Aneja and Lal (2014) focused on asthma disease and they performed ANN and NB methods to detect asthma from common symptoms. Their experimental results presented that ANN and NB reached accuracies of 85% and 88%, respectively. Ayer et al. (2010) used ANN and LR methods to determine breast cancer from clinical and demographic data. Their results showed that both methods achieved an accuracy of about 96%. Ahmad et al. (2013) performed ANN, DT, and SVM methods to diagnose breast cancer from clinical data. They showed that SVM achieved the best accuracy with 95%. Delen et al. (2005) performed ANN, DT, and LR methods to detect breast cancer from clinical and demographic data. They presented that DT achieved the best accuracy with 93.5%. Chen et al. (2017) detected cerebral infarction using DT, KNN, and NB. They analyzed EHRs, medical image data as well as gene data. The best result (an AUC score of 0.64) was achieved with DT.

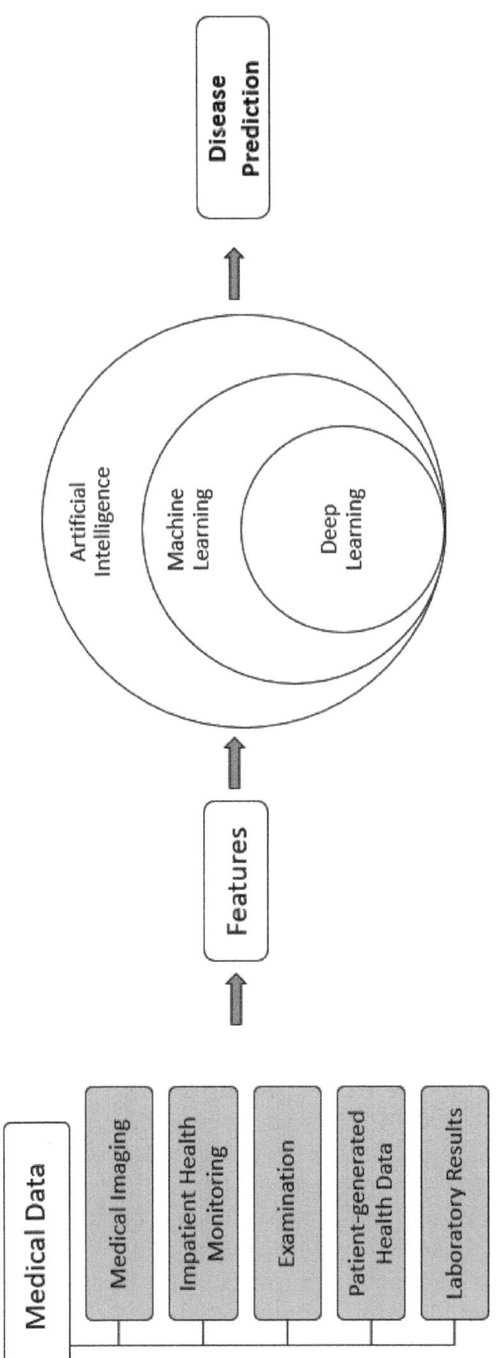

Figure 9.1 General overview of disease prediction.

The ML methods have a wide usage area for detecting diabetic disease. Sisodia and Sisodia (2018) detected diabetes from clinical test results belonging to 768 patients. They performed DT, NB, and SVM, and NB achieved satisfactory results with an accuracy of 76%. Tapak et al. (2013) diagnosed diabetes by comparing ANN, LR, RF, and SVM methods from demographic as well as clinical data. They showed that SVM had better performance with an accuracy of 98%. Cai et al. (2015) detected diabetes from gut microbiota using LR, NB, and SVM, using about 490 data points. Their experimental results showed that SVM reached an AUC score of 0.99.

The ML techniques present remarkable results for detecting haemoglobin variants, hypertension, kidney disease, lung cancer, Parkinson's disease, prostate cancer, and stroke. DT achieved the best results with an F-measure of 93%. Farran et al. (2013) detected hypertension by implementing KNN, LR, and SVM from EHRs belonging to 10,632 patients. The SVM method had a better result and reached an accuracy of 82%. Ani et al. (2016) detected kidney disease using ANN, DT, KNN, and NB from clinical and demographic data. DT reached better accuracy of 93%. Lynch et al. (2017) diagnosed lung cancer from clinical and demographic data using DT, RF, and SVM. RF had a better performance and showed significant results. Eskidere et al. (2012), Chen et al. (2013), and Behroozi and Sami (2016) detected Parkinson's disease using ML methods from voice recording as well as demographic data. ML methods presented significant results. Zupan et al. (2017a) determined prostate cancer from clinical data using DT and NB. NB achieved the best results with an accuracy of 70%. Hung et al. (2017) detected stroke from electronic medical claims and demographic data using ANN, LR, and SVM. Their results showed that ANN achieved an accuracy of 87%.

By creating patient-specific care plans, ML techniques can improve patient care. Systems based on ML techniques are able to look at patient data and figure out which treatment plans are going to work best for each patient. This can assist healthcare professionals in providing superior care and enhancing patient outcomes. Additionally, ML techniques can be used to provide early warning signs of potential health risks by monitoring a patient's health in real time. Rghioui et al. (2020) introduced a smart architecture to monitor diabetic patients to improve their life quality. They collected data from body measurements using smartphones, sensors, and smart devices. They validated simulation results using several ML algorithms and their experimental results showed that the sequential minimal optimization had a remarkable accuracy. Ahad et al. (2019) demonstrated an architecture for 5G smart healthcare and associated technologies such as software-defined network, D2D communication, and mmWaves. Furthermore, they analysed the requirements of 5G smart healthcare such as high bandwidth, high battery lifetime, ultra-high reliability, and ultra-low latency. Moreover, they demonstrated network layer solutions such as routing, scheduling, and congestion control. Lloret et al. (2017) proposed a protocol to monitor health services using 5G. They collected data from the body as well as smartphone and they required a database with an intelligence system using ML in big data that can send an alarm. They showed that using 5G network was essential to continuously monitor high number of patients since 5G networks had low delays and guarantee the availability of bandwidth for all users. Pandey and Prabha (2020) proposed a method predicting potential outcomes of cardiovascular disease. Their methods aided to mass screening systems for patients who cannot reach hospitals. Bobrie et al. (2004) predicted cardiac disease from self-measurements of blood pressure for patients who have hypertension. Logan et al. (2007) introduced a mobile phone–based remote patient monitoring system. In their study, they focused on diabetic patients with hypertension.

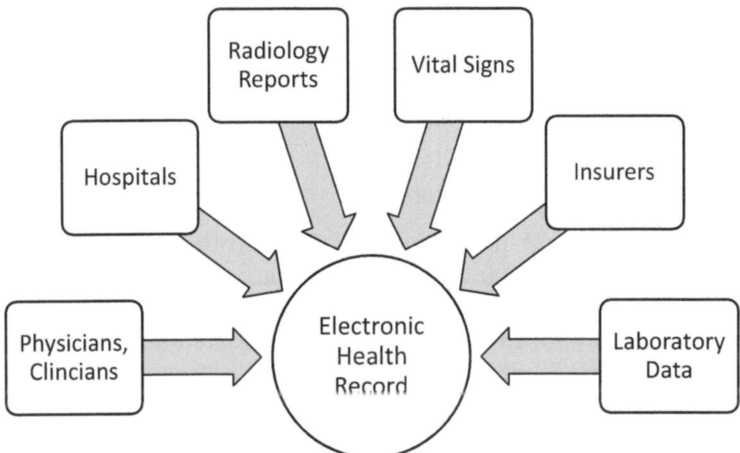

Figure 9.2   Electronic health record (EHR) that is a collection of health information belonging to each person.

Machine learning can also be used to analyze EHRs and identify patterns and trends in patient data, which helps healthcare providers to make more informed decisions about patient care. EHRs include information about the patients such as laboratory results, medical history, pathological tests, medications, and disease diagnosis, shown in Figure 9.2. Ye et al. (2020) developed an EHR-based risk evaluation tool that was constructed to alarm older adults' risk of fall. They aimed to decrease mortality in especially older people. They estimated the one-year fall model using XGBoost, which is an ML algorithm. They collected the data from the EHRs of Maine between 2016 and 2018, including about 265,000 older people. They concluded that their fall risk assessment tool may be deployed to identify personalized risk factors to provide older adults with early warnings and facilitate personalized fall interventions.

DL METHODS USED FOR ANALYZING MEDICAL DATA

Deep learning methods have received significant attention in the medical field due to their potential for analyzing large amounts of medical data. DL algorithms enable researchers and healthcare practitioners to create reliable prediction models for a variety of medical applications, including illness diagnosis and therapy planning. We begin by outlining some of the most popular DL methods for processing medical data.

Traditional DL Methods

In this section, we give a quick introduction to DL methods utilized in healthcare: convolutional neural networks, recurrent neural networks, and autoencoder.

Convolutional Neural Networks

Convolutional neural networks (CNNs) introduced by Lecun have demonstrated considerable potential in medical applications, particularly in the processing of medical images. CNNs are a kind of DL algorithm capable of automatically extracting and understanding hierarchical characteristics from incoming data. They have been applied to image segmentation, object detection, and illness classification in the context of medical imaging (Cheng et al 2018, Zhang et al. 2020). AlexNet, ResNet, VGGNet, U-Net, Graph CNN, and DeepSea can be some methods using CNNs.

Recurrent Neural Networks

Recurrent neural networks (RNNs) are another kind of DL algorithm that has shown potential in medical applications (Rumelhart et al. 1986). RNNs can analyze sequential data, such as time series data or medical records, by utilizing the previous inputs to predict the next output. They have worked in (Choi et al. 2016) the medical area on projects including developing new medications, monitoring patients, and predicting illnesses. In order to predict the likelihood of patient death using information from electronic medical records, RNNs were used. In addition, an RNN-based model for drug interaction prediction outperformed conventional ML techniques by using deep patient representation instead of raw EHRs (Miotto et al. 2016). These studies show how RNNs may be used in medical settings and imply that they could be useful tools for both researchers and medical personnel. Long short-term memory (LSTM) is the most known method that uses RNNs architecture (Hochreiter and Schmidhuber 1997).

Autoencoders

Autoencoders (AEs) are a type of DL models that can compress and reconstruct data, and they have shown considerable promise in the field of medicine. AEs have a number of important applications, including in medical imaging, where they may be used to improve and denoise images as well as detect anomalies like tumours. Genomic research has also employed AEs to find patterns in gene expression data and forecast cancer patients' medication responses (Gunavathi et al. 2021). AEs have become a potent tool in the field of medicine overall thanks to their capacity to learn intricate data representations, and they have extensive applications in a variety of fields. Stacked AE, denoised AE, and variational AE are some types of AEs in the literature.

Generative Adversarial Network

Generative adversarial networks (GANs), developed by Goodfellow, have been extremely popular in recent years for a variety of imaging-related applications. GANs have been applied to medicine to produce artificial medical pictures for study and to enlarge tiny datasets for ML algorithms. In one work that was published in the journal *Scientific Reports*, GANs were utilized to create synthetic mammograms, which may eventually lessen the necessity for mammography (Oyelade et al. 2022). In another research, GANs were employed to create artificial brain MRI images in order to enhance the precision of brain tumour segmentation (Lee et al. 2020). In general, GANs have the potential to change medical research and clinical practice by making it possible to build big, varied datasets for ML algorithms and by offering a way to produce synthetic data for use in training and simulations.

Hybrid DL Methods

All DL models used in medicine, as described in this section, fall into four broad types with the model chosen depending on the kind of data the situation at hand involves. In addition, a variety of data types must be provided as input in various applicable cases.

Hybrid architectures (HAs), which are successive assemblages of several DL models with the intention of maximizing the advantages of each model individually, provide a method for addressing issues of this nature. Three HAs—CNN+RNN, AE+CNN, and GAN+CNN—that are often used in analyzing medical issues are addressed in the part that follows. As the name implies, CNN+RNN structures are created by mixing RNNs with CNNs, which are utilized for feature extraction (Wang et al. 2017). The AE+CNN architecture combines an AE, which is employed as a pre-training model when very noisy data is present, and a CNN, which is employed as a feature extractor model (Geng et al. 2015). A GAN+CNN network is created by sequentially combining a CNN feature extractor with a GAN, which is utilized as a pre-training model to control the overfitting issue (Caballo et al. 2020).

THE STATE-OF-THE-ART DL METHODS IN HEALTH SERVICE MANAGEMENT: APPLICATION AREAS

Deep learning methods are being used in the administration of health services to enhance healthcare results, patient safety, and healthcare effectiveness. CNNs, RNNs, and GANs are among the most advanced DL techniques used in the administration of health services. RNNs are used in medical signal processing, such as electrocardiogram (ECG) analysis and prediction, whereas CNNs are utilized in medical image analysis, such as segmentation and categorization of medical pictures. In natural language processing (NLP) applications like clinical document categorization and illness prediction have also been employed as DL techniques. They were furthermore utilized in order to improve patient management, professional judgment, and healthcare policy. This section will focus on the use of DL methods in the medical industry in a variety of ways, including but not limited to applications like medical imaging analysis, predictive analytics, NLP, EHR analysis, drug discovery, and personalized medicine.

Medical imaging analysis has been transformed by DL, which allows for automated and precise image interpretation to support diagnosis and therapy planning. To find patterns and characteristics useful for certain tasks, such as picture segmentation, classification, and illness detection, DL algorithms can be trained on vast datasets of medical images. It includes X-rays, MRIs, and CT scans that may be analyzed using DL algorithms. In order to diagnose diseases including cancer, Alzheimer's disease, and cardiovascular disease, this can help discover irregularities. Various studies have shown the potential of DL in medical imaging analysis. A study revealed that DL could increase the precision of breast cancer diagnosis by applying it to mammography images (Tsochatzidis et al. 2019).

Similarly, DL algorithms may be used to precisely segment lung tumours on CT images, which could enhance treatment planning for patients with lung cancer (Duan et al. 2023). In addition, DL systems can detect lung nodules on CT scans with accuracy comparable to radiologists, according to the study in Ardila et al. (2019). DL has also demonstrated potential in the realm of cardiac imaging, where it may be used to segment and analyze the heart. Using cardiac MRI images, Bai et al.'s (2018) work showed that DL algorithms could precisely partition the left ventricle of the heart (Puyalnithi et al. 2016). With the use of this method, measures of cardiac function may be taken more accurately, and heart illness may be diagnosed more quickly. The detection and classification of brain cancers on MRI data is another use of DL in medical imaging analysis. In Vankdothu and Hameed (2022), DL algorithms were shown to perform as well as human specialists in accurately segmenting brain tumours on MRI data. This method may increase the precision and effectiveness of identifying and treating brain tumours.

Predictive analytics, a fast-growing field of healthcare management, uses statistical models, ML, and AI techniques to forecast and evaluate future events. In the subject of managing healthcare, DL has shown to be a useful tool for predictive analytics. EHRs and other health data are becoming more widely accessible, and DL algorithms may evaluate and learn from these large datasets to generate precise predictions about patient outcomes, illness diagnosis, and treatment results (Miotto et al. 2017). Predictive analytics and DL used in healthcare together can offer useful insights into patient outcomes, illness diagnosis, and treatment effectiveness. The prediction of patient readmission rates is one of the most exciting uses of predictive analytics in healthcare (Rajkomar et al. 2018). To estimate the chance of readmission, researchers have examined EHRs and other patient data using DL algorithms. By identifying high-risk patients and offering them tailored interventions to stop readmissions, this method can help healthcare professionals improve patient outcomes and save costs. Drug discovery and development is another area of DL methods employed which can benefit from predictive analytics (Segler et al. 2017). DL algorithms can forecast the efficacy of prospective new pharmaceuticals and find potential therapeutic targets by examining enormous datasets of chemical substances and their biological features (Ching et al. 2018). This strategy can quicken the drug development process and result in the identification of novel therapeutics for a range of ailments.

Natural language processing is a branch of AI that focuses on giving robots the ability to comprehend and interpret human language. In order to assist healthcare practitioners in more efficient patient data analysis, NLP is being employed in the management of health services. NLP may be used to extract data from clinical notes and EHRs, enhance clinical judgment, and improve patient outcomes (Dreisbach et al. 2019). The analysis of EHRs is one way that NLP is used in healthcare. NLP algorithms may be used to extract structured information from unstructured clinical notes, enabling medical professionals to make better judgments (Xiao et al. 2018). NLP may be used, for instance, to identify patients who are at a high risk of readmission or to find possible medication interactions. The study of examining patient feedback and satisfaction surveys is another application where NLP is used in healthcare. To find recurring themes and opportunities for development, open-ended replies may be analyzed using NLP algorithms. By using this strategy, healthcare professionals may successfully cure patients' illnesses with drug combinations.(Ding et al. 2022).

Deep learning–based EHR analysis has emerged as a potential topic of study in predicting and controlling diseases, enabling the extraction of significant knowledge from vast volumes of healthcare data (Abdel-Jaber et al. 2022). With the help of EHR analysis in DL, patient outcomes may be predicted by healthcare management, and those who are at risk of acquiring specific disorders can be identified (Liao et al. 2015). Health services management may develop individualized treatment plans that take into account an individual's particular traits and medical history by analyzing EHR data using DL algorithms. By giving physicians access to real-time data and alarms, DL EHR analysis may also be utilized to increase the precision of clinical decision-making (Suresh et al. 2017). As more EHR data becomes available, DL EHR analysis may be used to assess the impact of interventions over time and find opportunities for quality improvement in healthcare management (Donnelly et al. 2022). It is also set to play an increasingly crucial role in improving patient outcomes and optimizing healthcare delivery as the area of health services management continues to incorporate new technology and data analytics techniques (Faes et al. 2019). In summary, the application of DL techniques to EHR analysis shows considerable potential for enhancing patient outcomes and healthcare delivery in the administration of health services.

Drug discovery is a challenging and time-consuming process that involves finding prospective targets and evaluating hundreds of compounds for effectiveness and safety. DL algorithms can speed up drug development in healthcare management by foreseeing the efficacy and toxicity of drugs before they are evaluated in vitro or in vivo (Zhavoronkov et al. 2019). They can find patterns and links in massive volumes of molecular data that are hidden from human researchers, perhaps leading to the identification of new therapeutic targets. They are also becoming a crucial instrument in healthcare management for drug development as a result of the growing amount of molecular data and the demand for more effective drug discovery processes by providing accurate predictions about molecular properties (Wu et al. 2018). Finally, DL in drug discovery holds great promise for enhancing the effectiveness and efficiency of drug discovery in health services management, potentially resulting in the creation of new treatments for a variety of diseases (Chen et al. 2018).

Deep learning–based personalized medicine refers to the application of ML algorithms to examine very big and complicated datasets, such as genetic and clinical data, in order to customize medical care for specific individuals based on their particular traits and requirements (Si et al. 2021). The goal is to modify a patient's medical care based on their particular genetic, environmental, and lifestyle characteristics. It allows for the customization of medical care for individual patients based on their particular traits and requirements by applying ML algorithms to examine huge and complicated datasets, including genetic and clinical data (Chiu et al. 2022). This method may be able to spot patterns and connections that human researchers miss, which might lead to the development of more potent therapies. Recent studies have shown the promise of DL algorithms in personalized medicine, demonstrating great accuracy and reliability in patient outcome prediction (Zhang et al. 2019).

In conclusion, there are a wide range of applications for DL techniques in the administration of health services. DL has the potential to change healthcare by providing more precise diagnosis, more efficient treatments, and better patient outcomes across a variety of medical imaging analysis and customized medicine applications. The requirement for high-quality data and the possibility for bias in algorithmic decision-making are two issues that must be taken into account, as with any technology. Despite these obstacles, cutting-edge DL techniques are developing quickly and have a lot to offer in the management of health services. It will be fascinating to see how these techniques are put to use and improved upon as the field develops to meet fresh possibilities and issues in healthcare.

DISCUSSIONS

Artificial intelligence has emerged as a crucial component in the administration of healthcare particularly in the fields of ML and DL. Through real-time analysis of massive amounts of patient data, personalized diagnoses, and treatment plan recommendations, these two technologies are revolutionizing healthcare. ML algorithms are used to examine patient data, including genetics, environmental variables, and medical records, in order to detect risk factors and forecast the development of diseases. DL algorithms are utilized to effectively diagnose illnesses and identify anomalies in medical imaging like X-rays, CT scans, and MRIs. These innovations are improving patient outcomes, lowering costs, and improving the quality of care, making healthcare more effective and efficient.

Additionally, AI is crucial to the development and discovery of new drugs. By lowering the time and expense needed to bring new pharmaceuticals to market, the use of AI algorithms in drug research and development has the potential to transform the pharmaceutical business. The drug development process may be made more effective and accurate by using ML and DL algorithms to find therapeutic candidates and forecast their efficacy and toxicity. These technologies can also help medical practitioners develop patient-specific treatment plans based on each person's DNA profile, improving treatment outcomes, and reducing unfavourable side effects.

Notwithstanding its potential, AI still has certain limitations in managing healthcare. One of the major challenges is the lack of high-quality data. A vast amount of high-quality data is necessary for DL algorithms to be able to learn and produce reliable predictions. AI-based algorithms may find it challenging to provide reliable predictions in the healthcare industry due to the frequently fragmented and low-quality data. Additionally, the use of AI in healthcare management is not without difficulties. There is a chance of bias in the data and techniques utilized, and the quality and quantity of data available for training might be a limiting issue. Patients and healthcare professionals may be concerned since AI can be complicated and difficult to comprehend and explain. AI technologies continue to be an important tool for healthcare management systems despite these difficulties. This technology is projected to become more significant in enhancing patient outcomes and fostering innovation in healthcare as DL research advances.

In summary, AI is revolutionizing many aspects of healthcare administration, including medical imaging, illness diagnosis and prognosis, customized treatment regimens, and medical research. ML and DL algorithms as a subset of AI have the ability to completely change how healthcare practitioners offer care to their patients, despite the difficulties they currently confront. They will become increasingly more precise and dependable as more high-quality data becomes accessible, and their uses in managing healthcare will keep growing. In the final analysis, the application of AI to the administration of health services is altering healthcare by enabling healthcare professionals to offer individualized care and treatment plans, enhancing patient outcomes, and lowering costs.

CONCLUSIONS

The administration of health services using AI, particularly DL and ML, is changing the healthcare sector. With the use of these technologies, healthcare professionals can instantly evaluate vast volumes of patient data to provide individualized diagnoses and treatment plans. It is also transforming medicine discovery and development, speeding up the process and lowering the cost of bringing new medications to market. The technology is being used to manage health services in a way that enhances patient outcomes while also lowering costs and enhancing treatment quality. We may anticipate that it will play an ever bigger role in healthcare as technology develops, improving the efficacy and efficiency of healthcare services.

Additionally, by incorporating AI into the management of healthcare services, costs are being decreased and healthcare services are becoming more widely available. As a result of the technology, healthcare practitioners are now able to diagnose patients more quickly and accurately and develop treatment plans and drugs with more precision, which eventually results in less resource waste and reduced costs. We may anticipate even more notable changes in the healthcare sector as a result of on-going breakthroughs in AI technology, which will ultimately result in a better world for everybody.

REFERENCES

Abdel-Jaber, H., Devassy, D., Al Salam, A., Hidaytallah, L. and EL-Amir, M. 2022. A review of deep learning algorithms and their applications in healthcare. Algorithms. 15(2): 71.

Abu Alfeilat, H.A., Hassanat, A.B., Lasassmeh, O., Tarawneh, A.S., Alhasanat, M.B., Eyal Salman, H.S., et al. 2019. Effects of distance measure choice on k-nearest neighbor classifier performance: a review. Big Data. 7(4): 221–248.

Aha, D.W., Kibler, D. and Albert, M.K. 1991. Instance-based learning algorithms. Machine Learning. 6(1): 37–66.

Ahad, A., Tahir, M. and Yau, K.-L. A. 2019. 5G-based smart healthcare network: architecture, taxonomy, challenges and future research directions. IEEE Access. 7: 100747–100762.

Ahmad, L.G., Eshlaghy, A.T., Poorebrahimi, A., Ebrahimi, M. and Razavi, A.R. 2013. Using three machine learning techniques for predicting breast cancer recurrence. Journal of Health & Medical Informatics. 4(2): 124.

Alakus, T.B. and Turkoglu, I. 2020. Comparison of deep learning approaches to predict Covid-19 infection. Chaos Solitons & Fractals. 140: 110120.

Ali, S., Sahoo, B., Ullah, N., Zelikovskiy, A., Patterson, M. and Khan, I. 2021. A k-mer based approach for SARS-CoV-2 variant identification. pp. 153–164.

In: Wei, Y., Li, M., Skums, P. and Cai, Z. (eds). Bioinformatics Research and Applications (ISBRA). Springer.

Aneja, S. and Lal, S. 2014. Effective asthma disease prediction using naive Bayes amp—neural network fusion technique. 2014 International Conference on Parallel, Distributed and Grid Computing. 137–140.

Ani, R., Sasi, G., Sankar, U.R. and Deepa, O.S. 2016. Decision support system for diagnosis and prediction of chronic renal failure using random subspace classification. 2016 International Conference on Advances in Computing, Communications and Informatics (ICACCI). 1287–1292.

Ardila, D., Kiraly, A.P., Bharadwaj, S., Choi, B., Reicher, J.J., Peng, L., et al. 2019. End-to-end lung cancer screening with three-dimensional deep learning on low-dose chest computed tomography. Nature Medicine. 25(6): 954–961.

Arslan, H. and Arslan, H. 2021. A new COVID-19 detection method from human genome sequences using CpG island features and KNN classifier. Engineering Science and Technology, an International Journal. 24(4): 839–847.

Arslan, H. and Aygun, B. 2021. Performance analysis of machine learning algorithms in detection of covid-19 from common symptoms. 2021 29th Signal Processing and Communications Applications Conference (SIU). 1–4.

Arslan, H. 2021a. Machine learning methods for covid-19 prediction using human genomic data. Proceedings. 74(1): 20.

Arslan, H. 2021b. Covid-19 prediction based on genome similarity of human SARSCoV-2 and bat SARS-CoV-like coronavirus. Computers & Industrial Engineering. 161: 107666.

Arslan, H. 2022. Bagging and boosting methods for predicting mortality of patients with Covid-19. Dicle University Journal of Engineering. 13(2): 221–226.

Arslan, H. and Er, O. 2022. A comparative study on covid-19 prediction using deep learning and machine learning algorithms: a case study on performance analysis. Sakarya University Journal of Computer and Information Sciences. 5(1): 71–83.

Arslan, H. 2023. A *k*-mer based metaheuristic approach for detecting Covid-19 variants. Dicle University Journal of Engineering. 14(1): 17–26.

Ayer, T., Chhatwal, J., Alagoz, O., Kahn, C.E., Woods, R.W. and Burnside, E.S. 2010. Comparison of logistic regression and artificial neural network models in breast cancer risk estimation. RadioGraphics. 30(1): 13–22.

Bai, W., Sinclair, M., Tarroni, G., Oktay, O., Rajchl, M., Vaillant, G., et al. 2018. Automated cardiovascular magnetic resonance image analysis with fully convolutional networks. Journal of Cardiovascular Magnetic Resonance. 20(1).

Basu, M., Pan, Y. and Wang, J. (eds). 2014. Bioinformatics Research and Applications. 10th International Symposium, ISBRA 2014, Zhangjiajie, China, June 28–30. Proceedings. Springer International Publishing.

Behroozi, M. and Sami, A. 2016. A multiple-classifier framework for Parkinson's disease detection based on various vocal tests. International Journal of Telemedicine and Applications. 1–9.

Bobrie, G., Chatellier, G., Genes, N., Clerson, P., Vaur, L., Vaisse, B., et al. 2004. Cardiovascular prognosis of "masked hypertension" detected by blood pressure self-measurement in elderly treated hypertensive patients. JAMA. 291(11): 1342–1349.

Breiman, L. 1996. Bagging predictors. Machine Learning. 24(2): 123–140.

Burges, C.J. 1998. A tutorial on support vector machines for pattern recognition. Data Mining and Knowledge Discovery. 2(2): 121–167.

Caballo, M., Pangallo, D.R., Mann, R.M. and Sechopoulos, I. 2020. Deep learning-based segmentation of breast masses in dedicated breast CT imaging: radiomic feature stability between radiologists and artificial intelligence. Computers in Biology and Medicine. 118: 103629.

Cai, L., Wu, H., Li, D., Zhou, K. and Zou, F. 2015. Type 2 diabetes biomarkers of human gut microbiota selected via iterative sure independent screening method. PLOS One. 10(10): e0140827.

Chen, H.-L., Huang, C.-C., Yu, X.-G., Xu, X., Sun, X., Wang, G., et al. 2013. An efficient diagnosis system for detection of Parkinson's disease using fuzzy k-nearest neighbor approach. Expert Systems with Applications. 40(1): 263–271.

Chen, M., Hao, Y., Hwang, K., Wang, L. and Wang, L. 2017. Disease prediction by machine learning over big data from healthcare communities. IEEE Access. 5: 8869–8879.

Chen, H., Engkvist, O., Wang, Y., Olivecrona, M. and Blaschke, T. 2018. The rise of deep learning in drug discovery. Drug Discovery Today. 23(6): 1241–1250.

Cheng, G., Yang, C., Yao, X., Guo, L. and Han, J. 2018. When deep learning meets metric learning: remote sensing image scene classification via learning discriminative CNNs. IEEE Transactions on Geoscience and Remote Sensing. 56(5): 2811–2821.

Ching, T., Himmelstein, D.S., Beaulieu-Jones, B.K., Kalinin, A.A., Do, B.T., Way, G.P., et al. 2018. Opportunities and obstacles for deep learning in biology and medicine. Journal of the Royal Society Interface. 15(141): 20170387.

Chiu, I.-M., Cheng, J.-Y., Chen, T.-Y., Wang, Y.-M., Cheng, C.-Y., Kung, C.-T., et al. 2022. Using deep transfer learning to detect hyperkalemia from ambulatory electrocardiogram monitors in intensive care units: personalized medicine approach. Journal of Medical Internet Research. 24(12): e41163.

Choi, E., Bahadori, M.T., Sun, J., Kulas, J., Schuetz, A. and Stewart, W. 2016. Retain: an interpretable predictive model for healthcare using reverse time attention mechanism. Advances in Neural Information Processing Systems. 29.

Delen, D., Walker, G. and Kadam, A. 2005. Predicting breast cancer survivability: a comparison of three data mining methods. Artificial Intelligence in Medicine. 34(2): 113–127.

DeMaris, A. 1995. A tutorial in logistic regression. Journal of Marriage and the Family. 57(4): 956.

Deng, Z., Zhu, X., Cheng, D., Zong, M. and Zhang, S. 2016. Efficient KNN classification algorithm for big data. Neurocomputing. 195: 143–148.

Ding, P., Pan, Y., Wang, Q. and Xu, R. 2022. Prediction and evaluation of combination pharmacotherapy using natural language processing, machine learning and patient electronic health records. Journal of Biomedical Informatics. 133: 104164.

Donnelly, C., Janssen, A., Vinod, S., Stone, E., Harnett, P. and Shaw, T. 2022. A systematic review of electronic medical record driven quality measurement and feedback systems. International Journal of Environmental Research and Public Health. 20(1): 200.

Dreisbach, C., Koleck, T.A., Bourne, P.E. and Bakken, S. 2019. A systematic review of natural language processing and text mining of symptoms from electronic patient-authored text data. International Journal of Medical Informatics. 125: 37–46.

Duan, S., Cao, G., Hua, Y., Hu, J., Zheng, Y., Wu, F., et al. 2023. Identification of origin for spinal metastases from MR images: comparison between radiomics and deep learning methods. World Neurosurgery. 175: e823–e831.

Eskidere, O., Ertaş, F. and Hanilçi, C. 2012. A comparison of regression methods for remote tracking of Parkinson's disease progression. Expert Systems with Applications. 39(5): 5523–5528.

Faes, L., Wagner, S.K., Fu, D.J., Liu, X., Korot, E., Ledsam, J.R., et al. 2019. Automated deep learning design for medical image classification by health-care professionals with no coding experience: a feasibility study. The Lancet Digital Health. 1(5): e232–e242.

Farran, B., Channanath, A.M., Behbehani, K. and Thanaraj, T.A. 2013. Predictive models to assess risk of type 2 diabetes, hypertension and comorbidity: machine-learning algorithms and validation using national health data from Kuwait—a cohort study. BMJ Open. 3(5): e002457.

Geng, J., Fan, J., Wang, H., Ma, X., Li, B. and Chen, F. 2015. High-resolution SAR image classification via deep convolutional autoencoders. IEEE Geoscience and Remote Sensing Letters. 12(11): 2351–2355.

Gunavathi, C., Sivasubramanian, K., Keerthika, P. and Paramasivam, C. 2021. A review on convolutional neural network based deep learning methods in gene expression data for disease diagnosis. Materials Today: Proceedings. 45: 2282–2285.

Ho, T.K. 1998. The random subspace method for constructing decision forests. IEEE Transactions on Pattern Analysis and Machine Intelligence. 20(8): 832–844.

Hochreiter, S. and Schmidhuber, J. 1997. Long short-term memory. Neural Computation. 9(8): 1735–1780.

Hornik, K., Stinchcombe, M. and White, H. 1989. Multilayer feedforward networks are universal approximators. Neural Networks. 2(5): 359–366.

Hung, C.-Y., Chen, W.-C., Lai, P.-T., Lin, C.-H. and Lee, C.-C. 2017. Comparing deep neural network and other machine learning algorithms for stroke prediction in a large-scale population-based electronic medical claims database. 2017 39th Annual International Conference of the IEEE Engineering in Medicine and Biology Society (EMBC). 3110–3113.

Jain, G., Mittal, D., Thakur, D. and Mittal, M.K. 2020. A deep learning approach to detect covid-19 coronavirus with X-ray images. Biocybernetics and Biomedical Engineering. 40(4): 1391–1405.

Jin, A., Gomez, S., Luft, H., Lichtensztajn, D. and Thompson, C. 2017. External validity of electronic health record studies of cancer patients. Journal of Patient-Centered Research and Reviews. 4: 150.

Keerthi, S. S. and Lin, C.-J. 2003. Asymptotic behaviors of support vector machines with Gaussian kernel. Neural Computation. 15(7): 1667–1689.

Lee, H., Jo, J. and Lim, H. 2020. Study on optimal generative network for synthesizing brain tumor-segmented MR images. Mathematical Problems in Engineering. 1–12.

Liao, K.P., Cai, T., Savova, G.K., Murphy, S.N., Karlson, E.W., Ananthakrishnan, A.N., et al. 2015. Development of phenotype algorithms using electronic medical records and incorporating natural language processing. BMJ. 350: h1885–h1885.

Lloret, J., Parra, L., Taha, M. and Tomás, J. 2017. An architecture and protocol for smart continuous ehealth monitoring using 5G. Computer Networks. 129: 340–351.

Logan, A., McIsaac, W., Tisler, A., Irvine, M., Saunders, A., Dunai, A., et al. 2007. Mobile phone–based remote patient monitoring system for management of hypertension in diabetic patients. American Journal of Hypertension. 20(9): 942–948.

Long, N.C., Meesad, P. and Unger, H. 2015. A highly accurate firefly based algorithm for heart disease prediction. Expert Systems with Applications. 42(21): 8221–8231.

Lynch, C.M., Abdollahi, B., Fuqua, J.D., de Carlo, A.R., Bartholomai, J.A., Balgemann, R.N., et al. 2017. Prediction of lung cancer patient survival via supervised machine learning classification techniques. International Journal of Medical Informatics. 108: 1–8.

Marikani, T. and Shyamala, K. 2017. Prediction of heart disease using supervised learning algorithms. International Journal of Computer Applications. 165(5): 41–44. https://doi.org/10.5120/ijca2017913868

Min, J. and Lee, Y. 2005. Bankruptcy prediction using support vector machine with optimal choice of kernel function parameters. Expert Systems with Applications. 28(4): 603–614.

Miotto, R., Li, L., Kidd, B.A. and Dudley, J.T. 2016. Deep patient: an unsupervised representation to predict the future of patients from the electronic health records. Scientific Reports. 6(1): 1–10.

Miotto, R., Wang, F., Wang, S., Jiang, X. and Dudley, J.T. 2017. Deep learning for healthcare: review, opportunities and challenges. Briefings in Bioinformatics. 19(6): 1236–1246.

Oyelade, O.N., Ezugwu, A.E., Almutairi, M.S., Saha, A.K., Abualigah, L. and Chiroma, H. 2022. A generative adversarial network for synthetization of regions of interest based on digital mammograms. Scientific Reports. 12: 6166.

Pandey, H. and Prabha, S. 2020. Smart health monitoring system using IoT and machine learning techniques. 2020 Sixth International Conference on Bio Signals, Images and Instrumentation (ICBSII). 1–4.

Puyalnithi, T. and Madhu Viswanatham, V. 2016. Preliminary cardiac disease risk prediction based on medical and behavioural data set using supervised machine learning techniques. Indian Journal of Science and Technology. 9(31): 1–5.

Rajkomar, A., Oren, E., Chen, K., Dai, A.M., Hajaj, N., Hardt, M., et al. 2018. Scalable and accurate deep learning with electronic health records. NPJ Digital Medicine. 1(1): 18.

Rghioui, A., Lloret, J., Sendra, S. and Oumnad, A. 2020. A smart architecture for diabetic patient monitoring using machine learning algorithms. Healthcare. 8(3): 348.

Rumelhart, D.E., Hinton, G.E. and Williams, R.J. 1986. Learning representations by back-propagating errors. Nature. 323(6088): 533–536.

Safavian, S. and Landgrebe, D. 1991. A survey of decision tree classifier methodology. IEEE Transactions on Systems, Man and Cybernetics. 21(3): 660–674.

Segler, M.H.S., Kogej, T., Tyrchan, C. and Waller, M.P. 2017. Generating focused molecule libraries for drug discovery with recurrent neural networks. ACS Central Science, 4(1): 120–131.

Si, Y., Du, J., Li, Z., Jiang, X., Miller, T., Wang, F., et al. 2021. Deep representation learning of patient data from electronic health records (EHR): a systematic review. Journal of Biomedical Informatics. 115: 103671.

Sisodia, D. and Sisodia, D.S. 2018. Prediction of diabetes using classification algorithms. Procedia Computer Science. 132: 1578–1585.

Suresh, H., Hunt, N., Johnson, A., Celi, L.A., Szolovits, P. and Ghassemi, M. 2017. Clinical intervention prediction and understanding with deep neural networks. Machine Learning for Healthcare Conference. 322–337. Proceedings of Machine Learning Research (PMLR).

Tapak, L., Mahjub, H., Hamidi, O. and Poorolajal, J. 2013. Real-data comparison of data mining methods in prediction of diabetes in Iran. Healthcare Informatics Research. 19(3): 177.

Tsochatzidis, L., Costaridou, L. and Pratikakis, I. 2019. Deep learning for breast cancer diagnosis from mammograms—a comparative study. Journal of Imaging. 5(3): 37.

Vankdothu, R. and Hameed, M.A. 2022. Brain tumor MRI images identification and classification based on the recurrent convolutional neural network. Measurement: Sensors. 24: 100412.

Vapnik, V.N. 1995. The Nature of Statistical Learning Theory. New York: Springer.

Wang, C., Jiang, F. and Yang, H. 2017. A hybrid framework for text modeling with convolutional RNN. Proceedings of the 23rd ACM SIGKDD International Conference on Knowledge Discovery and Data Mining. 2061–2069.

Wu, Z., Ramsundar, B., Feinberg, E.N., Gomes, J., Geniesse, C., Pappu, A.S., et al. 2018. Moleculenet: a benchmark for molecular machine learning. Chemical Science. 9(2): 513–530.

Xiao, C., Choi, E. and Sun, J. 2018. Opportunities and challenges in developing deep learning models using electronic health records data: a systematic review. Journal of the American Medical Informatics Association. 25(10): 1419–1428.

Yang, J., Yao, D., Zhan, X. and Zhan, X. 2014. Predicting disease risks using feature selection based on random forest and support vector machine. pp. 1–11. *In*: Basu, M., Pan, Y. and Wang, J. (eds). Bioinformatics Research and Applications. Springer.

Ye, C., Li, J., Hao, S., Liu, M., Jin, H., Zheng, L., et al. 2020. Identification of elders at higher risk for fall with statewide electronic health records and a machine learning algorithm. International Journal of Medical Informatics. 137: 104105.

Zhang, S., Bamakan, S.M.H., Qu, Q. and Li, S. 2019. Learning for personalized medicine: a comprehensive review from a deep learning perspective. IEEE Reviews in Biomedical Engineering. 12: 194–208.

Zhang, S., Ma, Z., Zhang, G., Lei, T., Zhang, R. and Cui, Y. 2020. Semantic image segmentation with deep convolutional neural networks and quick shift. Symmetry. 12(3): 427.

Zhavoronkov, A., Ivanenkov, Y.A., Aliper, A., Veselov, M.S., Aladinskiy, V.A., Aladinskaya, A.V., et al. 2019. Deep learning enables rapid identification of potent DDR1 kinase inhibitors. Nature Biotechnology. 37(9): 1038–1040.

Chapter 10

Implementation of Artificial Intelligence for the Healthcare Supply Chain: Prospects and Challenges

Ourania Areta Hiziroglu

Department of Management Information Systems,
Izmir Bakircay University, Izmir Türkiye
ORCID: 0000-0001-8607-6089; Email: ourania.areta@bakircay.edu.tr

INTRODUCTION

Healthcare is one of the industries that is growing quickly and demands efficient services and goods to meet the increasing needs of patients. Moreover, healthcare providers need a reliable supply chain to ensure timely delivery of necessary medical supplies. However, the healthcare supply chain (HSC) can be complex and may not always operate effectively, as seen during the Covid-19 pandemic when hospitals worldwide confronted shortages of essential items, such as vaccines, ventilators, masks, and personal protective equipment, due to inefficient supply chain management (Gardeva 2021). Various studies have highlighted these issues (Mahmoodi et al. 2021, Khot 2020, Spieske et al. 2022).

In the meantime, artificial intelligence (AI) is becoming prevalent in the healthcare industry to address complications posed by intricate supply chains. By enhancing the stages of the supply chain process, Al has enabled medical professionals to eradicate operational inefficiencies and ensure prompt patient care (Kumar et al. 2023). Additionally, it provides critical information such as vital medical supplies requirements considering elements like patient conditions, demographics, and location that aid clinicians in better decision-making. However, various obstacles must be overcome before Al can be properly used to improve the efficiency of the HSC. These include a lack of data, high implementation costs, and a lack of experience on the side of healthcare personnel (Gardeva 2021).

The existing AI literature covers a wide range of areas, including healthcare. However, much AI research in healthcare has focused on medical diagnosis, treatments, and prescription while disregarding the HSC (Toorajipour et al. 2021). To fill the knowledge vacuum, this chapter will offer studies on the application of AI for HSC and will investigate the numerous potential and problems that this involves. Despite these obstacles, Al has the potential to transform the healthcare business by delivering a more efficient and cost-effective solution to some of the sector's core issues (Kumar et al. 2023, Toorajipour et al. 2021).

The purpose of this study is to examine the present uses of and future potential for AI in the HSC, along with related challenges and aspects that need to be considered for a successful implementation within the framework of enhancing the HSC.

The remainder of this study is arranged as follows: the next section presents the topic of healthcare supply chain and the relevant challenges that it faces. The third section examines AI and provides an overall input on its applications for healthcare in general and then for HSC in particular; this section ends with the discussion of a few case studies from the HSC environment as examples for the potential of AI in HSC. The section thereafter delves into the challenges of using AI in the HSC. The final section concludes with some observations and recommendations for further research.

THE HEALTHCARE SUPPLY CHAIN

The healthcare system's proper functioning relies heavily on the HSC, which ensures that patients have timely access to medical supplies and services (Viloria 2015). The HSC is a vast network comprising various players involved in planning, sourcing, manufacturing, distributing, and consuming health-related goods and services. This includes manufacturers, distributors, pharmacies, hospitals, clinics as well as consumers (see Figure 10.1). It encompasses all aspects of product procurement to distribution and administration of diverse medical products like medications, equipment devices, and supplies (Viloria 2015). Information systems and regulatory frameworks also constitute essential components within this network (Yadav 2007). The successful operation of such a complex supply chain contributes towards enhancing patient satisfaction while optimizing the medical outcomes with reduced costs (Viloria 2015).

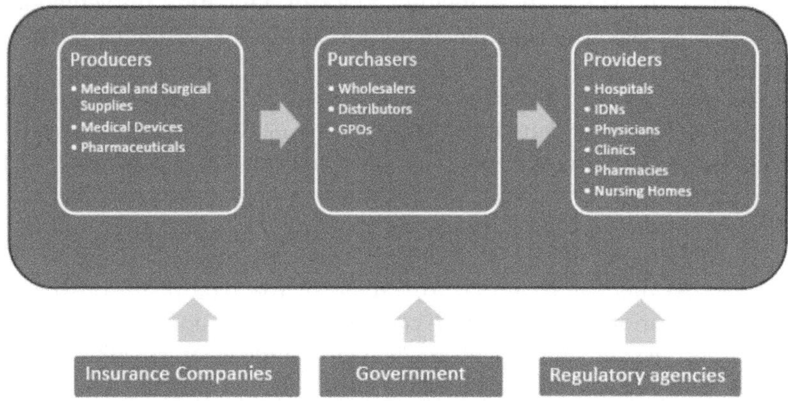

Figure 10.1   Healthcare supply chain (HSC) configuration.
Source: Mathew et al. (2013), adapted from Burns (2002).

The HSC is an essential component of the healthcare system as it ensures the availability of quality essential medicines and health supplies (Lugada et al. 2022). The primary objective of HSC is to improve access to healthcare by developing, manufacturing, and making available health commodities appropriate to the health needs of the global population (Singh 2021). A well-functioning supply chain is necessary for effective health service delivery as it not only provides appropriate health outputs but also has the potential to create and deliver cost-effective outcomes in line with the economic, social, and cultural conditions of a country (Kumar and Singh 2020).

The Covid-19 pandemic has highlighted the importance of HSC as it is vital to a well-functioning health system and advancing national and regional health security goals (Gladys Okafor et al. 2021). A well-functioning supply chain to deliver medicines, vaccines, and other health products forms the backbone of the health system (Idris and Parashar 2015).

Leadership is also important in providing direction and guidance to achieve set goals in an integrated public HSC system (Umezulike and Eronini 2022). The HSC is a complex adaptive ecosystem that facilitates the delivery of health products to the end patient in a cost-effective way (Santos and Duarte 2021).

Lean and agile can be used as process strategies to improve supply chain performance in the healthcare system (Li 2011). A scoping review has also highlighted the importance of a lean HSC (Bai et al. 2022).

In conclusion, HSC is important as it ensures the availability of quality essential medicines and health supplies, improves access to healthcare, and is vital to a well-functioning health system and advancing national and regional health security goals. Leadership, process strategies such as lean and agile, and a well-functioning supply chain are necessary for effective health service delivery.

Nevertheless, the HSC faces numerous obstacles that limit its effectiveness and influence. These challenges are listed in Table 10.1.

Table 10.1   Challenges of healthcare supply chain (HSC).

Uncertainty about demand	Demand for medical products and services is frequently unpredictable and fluctuates as a result of variables such as illness outbreaks, seasonal variations, demographic changes, and policy interventions. Uncertainty in demand can result in shortages or surpluses of medical items and services, influencing patient outcomes and healthcare expenditures (Chen et al. 2020).
Inventory management	The HSC must strike a balance between having enough inventory to fulfil demand while avoiding stock-outs and having too much inventory, which leads to waste, expiry, and obsolescence (Nahmias and Smith 2011).
Disruption in supply	The HSC is a complex and worldwide network of suppliers, manufacturers, distributors, and providers. Any disturbance in this network has the potential to impair the flow of medical products and services across the supply chain. Political instability, economic conflicts, cyberattacks, quality difficulties, or environmental dangers can all interrupt supply (Betcheva et al. 2021, Snowdon and Wright 2022).
Regulatory compliance	The HSC must adhere to a number of rules and standards designed to assure the safety, efficacy, and quality of medical products and services. Regulatory compliance can be difficult due to the complexity, variety, and expense of different markets and jurisdictions (Betcheva et al. 2021).
Integration of new technologies and innovations	The HSC must keep up with the fast development and acceptance of new technologies and innovations that can improve patient care and health system performance. In terms of compatibility, interoperability, scalability, and cost of new medical goods and services, innovation integration might present obstacles (Clauson et al. 2018).

(Contd.)

(*Contd.*)

Quality assurance	From manufacturing to consumption, the HSC must assure the quality and safety of medical products and services. Compliance with regulatory requirements, monitoring quality indicators, recognizing faults and mistakes, and performing remedial measures are all required (Karthika and Vijayakumar 2022).
Cost-cutting measures	The HSC must cut costs while maintaining or enhancing quality and service levels. This necessitates optimizing resource allocation, reducing waste and inefficiencies, negotiating pricing and contracts, and taking advantage of economies of scale (Essila 2023).
Assigning lot and serial numbers	Using lot numbers, serial numbers, or both, healthcare items must be monitored and traced along the supply chain. This necessitates the gathering and exchange of accurate and timely data across different stakeholders, as well as compliance with regulatory standards.
Counterfeit prevention	Counterfeit or inferior healthcare items endanger patient health and safety, as well as the reputation and revenue of real producers and distributors. Strong identification and verification mechanisms, as well as coordination and collaboration among regulators, law enforcement agencies, and industry participants, are required (Singh et al. 2020).
Expiration monitoring	Healthcare items have finite shelf life and must be utilized or discarded before they expire. This necessitates effective inventory management and forecasting procedures, as well as clear expiry date marking and communication (Bhakoo et al. 2012).
Gaining worldwide visibility	Healthcare items frequently transit through several nations and regions before arriving at their final destination. This necessitates the openness and traceability of product flow and status across the supply chain, as well as the alignment and integration of various systems and standards (Senna et al. 2020).

The Covid-19 epidemic has compounded these difficulties by exposing the HSC's shortcomings and deficiencies, resulting in shortages, delays, waste, and disparities. To address these challenges, stakeholders in the HSC must take a comprehensive and strategic approach that leverages data and analytics, engages clinicians and patients, fosters collaboration and partnerships, implements best practices and standards, and embraces digital transformation and innovation (Leite et al. 2020).

The deployment of AI, which is described as "the science and engineering of making intelligent machines" (Russell and Norvig 2016), can help the HSC overcome these difficulties. By offering data-driven insights, automating decision-making, and optimizing workflows across supply chain operations, AI may assist to enhance the HSC. In the HSC, AI may potentially allow new skills and chances for innovation and change. These elements will be examined in the following section.

AI AND ITS APPLICATIONS IN HEALTHCARE

Artificial intelligence is a fast-expanding area that has piqued the interest of many disciplines, and has significant implications for various domains of human activity, such as business, health, education, and entertainment. AI is broadly defined as the ability of machines or systems to perform tasks that normally require human intelligence, such as perception, reasoning, learning, decision-making, and problem solving (Russell and Norvig 2016). AI has the ability to alter many elements of research and practice, including increasing user experience, system performance, allowing new business models, and tackling social concerns. To describe and simulate intelligence, several methodologies and paradigms have been developed, including symbolic AI, connectionism, evolutionary computation, artificial neural networks, deep learning, reinforcement learning, and so on. Each strategy has advantages and disadvantages, and they are frequently combined or integrated to produce superior outcomes (Yigitcanlar and Cugurullo 2020).

With regards to AI applications, a few examples are natural language processing, computer vision, speech recognition, expert systems, robotics, and machine learning. There are numerous examples of successful and impactful AI applications in a variety of domains, including healthcare (diagnosis, treatment, prevention), education (personalized learning, assessment), security (surveillance, cyberdefence), entertainment (games, music), social good (disaster response, environmental protection), and so on. Each application has its unique set of needs and restrictions, and they frequently involve several stakeholders with disparate interests and points of view (Yigitcanlar et al. 2020).

Specifically for healthcare, AI has several applications, including improving diagnosis, increasing patient interaction, automating workflows, and expediting research:

- *Diagnostics* is a typical use of AI in healthcare. AI may help healthcare professionals by speeding up diagnosis, assessing symptoms, recommending therapies, and predicting hazards. It is also capable of recognizing anomalous outcomes. For example, by evaluating photos of skin lesions and comparing them to a database of known instances, AI can assist in the diagnosis of skin cancer (Esteva et al. 2017). AI may also help radiologists evaluate medical pictures and detect anomalies (Rajpurkar et al. 2022).

- Another use of AI in healthcare is the use of *chatbots* to improve primary care. They are computer programs that use natural language to engage with humans. Chatbots may answer questions, give health information, triage symptoms, and book appointments. They can also increase patient involvement by sending out reminders, providing comments, and providing assistance. Babylon Health, for example, is a chatbot that can analyze symptoms and offer medical recommendations depending on the user's medical history and location (Richardson et al. 2021).

- In healthcare, AI can also reduce the burden of *electronic health records* (EHRs). EHRs are computerized records that contain information about a patient's health, such as medical history, diagnosis, prescriptions, and test results. EHRs can improve the quality and efficiency of care delivery, but they also present issues for clinicians, including increased workload, documentation mistakes, and less patient engagement. By automating data input, extracting pertinent information, and creating summaries, AI can assist minimize the EHR load. Nuance, for example, is an AI-powered speech recognition and natural language processing solutions provider for EHRs (Nuance Communications Inc. 2022).

- *Robotic operations* are considered another application of AI in healthcare. Robotic operations are surgical procedures carried out by robots that are controlled by surgeons. Robotic procedures can improve surgical precision, accuracy, and flexibility while also reducing blood loss, infection risk, and recovery time (Lanfranco et al. 2004). However, robotic operations also pose challenges such as high costs, technical difficulties, and ethical dilemmas (Honda et al. 2017).

The aforementioned describe the applications of AI in healthcare overall. In the following part, we will examine the applications of AI in the HSC.

AI AND HSC

Artificial Intelligence has the potential to revolutionize the HSC by improving efficiency, reducing costs, and enhancing supply chain resilience. AI can be used to analyze data and make predictions about demand, optimize logistics and transportation routes, and identify inefficiencies in the supply chain (Roy et al. 2023). Following are some of the applications of AI in HSC.

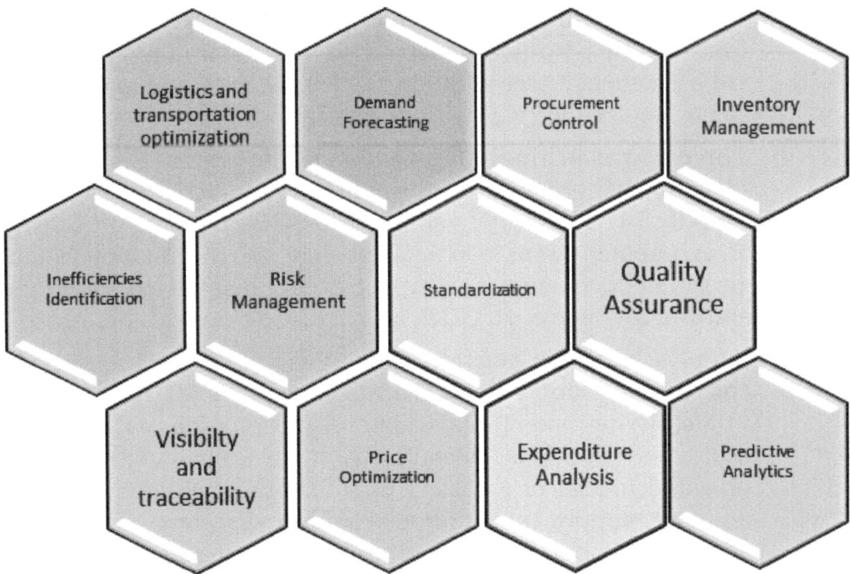

Figure 10.2　Topics for AI applications in healthcare supply chain (HSC) (own work)

(a) **Logistics and transportation optimization:** AI can optimize logistics and transportation routes (route optimization), thereby reducing costs and increasing efficiency (Pagell et al. 2020). It is also capable of predicting demand, which can be utilized to optimize transportation routes. To optimize delivery routes, reduce transportation costs, and improve delivery times, AI systems may evaluate data on transportation routes, traffic patterns, and delivery schedules based on a number of variables including cost, time, distance, capacity, dependability, and environmental impact. It can also monitor and trace shipments in real time and send alerts in the case of delays or disruptions. This can facilitate the expeditious and efficient procurement of supplies by medical personnel.

(b) **Demand forecasting:** Using historical data, current trends, seasonal fluctuations, epidemiological variables, and patient preferences, AI can help estimate the demand for pharmaceuticals and medical equipment (Santosh 2020). This can aid in the optimization of healthcare product manufacturing and distribution, inventory cost reduction, and the avoidance of stock-outs and overstocking.

(c) **Automated inventory management:** AI can help automate the difficult process of inventory management, including monitoring, replenishing, and forecasting the demand and supply of medical commodities (Stoyanov 2021). Using data from multiple sources, such as EHRs, point-of-sale systems, radio frequency identification (RFID) devices, and sensors, AI could help reduce waste, stock-outs, and human errors.

(d) **Three-way matching:** AI can automate the process of validating that purchase orders, invoices, and receipts match prior to paying suppliers. Using a combination of natural language processing and computer vision to extract and compare information from a variety of documents, AI may help reduce manual labour, errors, and fraud (Tater et al. 2022).

(e) **Supply chain risk management:** AI can be utilized to identify and mitigate supply chain risks (Shen et al. 2018). AI can assist in identifying potential disruptions and provide real-time risk mitigation solutions. Specifically, it can help determine the potential impact of a variety of situations, such as fluctuating demand, supply interruptions, natural disasters, pandemics, and cyberattacks. In addition, it can aid in the development of contingency plans and recovery techniques to minimize damage and restore normal operations (Qiu et al. 2021).

(f) **Preference card standardization:** AI can aid in the standardization of surgeons' preference cards, which identify the tools, supplies, and equipment required for each surgical procedure. Based on historical data, clinical results, and best practices, AI may assist in analyzing the preference cards and recommending ideal combinations of supplies (Rasouli et al. 2020).

(g) **Quality assurance:** AI can assist to assure the quality and safety of healthcare items across the supply chain. It can aid in the detection and prevention of counterfeit or inferior items through the use of technology such as image recognition, barcode scanning, and blockchain verification. Using sensors, smart labels, or RFID tags, it may also assist in monitoring and managing the storage conditions and handling practices of healthcare supplies (Clauson et al. 2018).

(h) **Visibility and traceability:** In addition to these uses, AI may also be used to increase supply chain visibility and traceability. Healthcare providers may receive real-time visibility into the status of their orders by utilizing AI algorithms to follow the movement of items and information across the supply chain, allowing them to immediately identify and rectify any issues (Alabaddi et al. 2023).

(i) **Price optimization:** AI may also be used to optimize healthcare product price. To ensure that healthcare items are priced competitively while simultaneously optimizing profit margins, AI algorithms may monitor market trends, demand patterns, and competition pricing. This can assist manufacturers and distributors to maintain market competitiveness while also offering high-quality products to healthcare practitioners and patients (Iliashenko et al. 2019).

(j) **Medical supply expenditure analysis:** AI can assist with analyzing the spending patterns of surgical, medical, and medication supplies, which account for approximately 15% of a health system's operational expenses. AI can help identify opportunities for cost savings, standardization, and contract and vendor optimization (Richardson et al. 2021).

(k) **Integrated predictive analytics:** AI can facilitate the integration of data from multiple sources, such as internal systems, external databases, social media, and weather forecasts, to provide predictive insights for supply chain planning and decision-making. Using machine learning and deep learning algorithms, AI can aid in predicting demand changes, supply interruptions, market trends, and customer preferences (Chang and Seol 2022).

AI solutions have transformed the HSC in a variety of ways, including boosting demand forecasting, optimizing inventory management, increasing logistical efficiency, and lowering waste and costs. The following section presents some case studies of organizations that have effectively used AI technologies in the HSC.

CASE STUDIES OF AI APPLICATIONS IN THE HSC

Here are some indicative case studies of AI implementation in the HSC:

- *McKesson:* The world's largest pharmaceutical distributor employed AI to enhance its inventory management and delivery network, saving more than $100 million each year. The firm used an AI system that examined data from its 30 distribution centres and over 40,000 pharmacies and made suggestions on ideal inventory levels, replenishment frequency, and routing tactics. McKesson was also able to adapt swiftly to shifting demand patterns and supply interruptions created by the Covid-19 epidemic (Mejia 2019).

- *Roche:* The Swiss biopharmaceutical firm in partnership with EarlySign employed AI with an initial focus on cancer diagnoses. The LungFlag software employs machine learning to analyze a variety of standard patient data, such as demographic, medical, medication, and laboratory test information. Using this analysis, the AI is able to identify individuals with an increased risk of developing lung cancer. With this information, healthcare clinicians can target their treatment efforts more precisely and order follow-up screenings only for patients who are most likely to have the disease (Park 2022).

- *OptumLabs:* OptumLabs has a history of developing AI models with regression and machine learning techniques. They have constructed models to predict the onset of Alzheimer's disease, diabetes, and patient clusters with heart failure and Chronic Obstructive Pulmonary Disease (COPD), among others. They are currently investigating the application of deep learning to the examination of EHRs, and the possibility that natural language processing, a technique for extracting content from words in physician notes, could be used to feed deep learning models (OptumLabs 2024).

- *Merck KGaA:* It is a prominent scientific and technology firm, using AI to improve its demand forecasting and supply planning operations. The organization analyzes data from several sources, including sales, marketing, production, and external variables, using sophisticated analytics and machine learning. This assists the organization in anticipating consumer demands, reducing stock-outs and overstocking, and balancing supply and demand throughout its worldwide network (McKevitt 2016).

These AI applications in the HSC may help actors in the healthcare industry to enhance patient care, operational efficiency, financial performance, and competitive advantage. However, there are certain drawbacks to using AI in HSC management. The following section presents the related challenges, and the aspects that need to be considered for its successful implementation.

AI AND HSC CHALLENGES

The HSC is intricate, involving the transfer of items, information, and funds from producers to healthcare providers and patients. In a variety of ways, the application of AI has the potential to improve the performance and efficiency of the HSC. Prior to incorporating AI in the HSC, however, a number of obstacles must be surmounted to ensure that AI is utilized successfully and ethically. Among these challenges are:

- **Data quality and accessibility:** To generate correct predictions and choices, AI systems rely substantially on data. As a result, high-quality data is critical for successful AI application in the HSC. Healthcare data, on the other hand, is frequently fragmented and non-standardized, making it challenging to access and utilize for AI applications. As a result, efforts must be taken to guarantee that healthcare data is of high quality and available to all supply chain stakeholders (Dora et al. 2021).

- **Bias and ethical concerns:** AI algorithms are only as good as the data on which they are trained, and if the data used to train AI models is prejudiced, so will be the algorithms. Bias in AI can have major ethical concerns, notably in healthcare, where AI systems' judgments might have life-changing repercussions. As a result, it is critical to guarantee that AI algorithms are created and deployed in an ethical manner, and that they do not discriminate against specific categories of people (Modgil et al. 2021).

- **Cost:** AI implementation in the HSC can be costly, especially for smaller healthcare providers that may lack the financial means to invest in AI. As a result, developing inexpensive and scalable AI solutions that can be adopted by healthcare providers of all sizes is critical (Bvuchete et al. 2020).

- **Data security and privacy:** Healthcare data is extremely sensitive and must be safeguarded to maintain patient privacy and confidentiality. As a result, AI systems must be built with strong data privacy and security safeguards to defend against data breaches and cyberattacks (Le Tan 2022).

- **Resistance to change:** Because healthcare is a highly regulated sector, many healthcare providers may be hesitant to adopt new technology such as AI owing to compliance and regulatory issues. As a result, efforts must be made to educate healthcare practitioners about the benefits of AI while also addressing their compliance and regulatory concerns (Kumar 2022).

To ensure that AI is used successfully and ethically in the HSC, it will be essential to address these concerns.

However, in order to completely exploit the potential of AI in the HSC, it is also necessary to consider four crucial success factors. These include technological elements like data quality, security, and interoperability; institutional or environmental factors like legislation, standards, and policies; human aspects like skills, trust, and acceptance; and organizational factors like culture, leadership, and strategy (Baryannis et al. 2018).

Moreover, and considering the complexity of the HSC and the many obstacles involved, such as expanding demand, rising costs, quality issues, regulatory compliance, and environmental sustainability, AI may assist in addressing these issues by delivering data-driven insights, automating processes, improving decision-making, and increasing efficiency and effectiveness (Modgil et al. 2021). However, various critical success factors (CSFs) must be considered before applying AI for the HSC. These elements are classified into four categories: technological (TEC), institutional or environmental (INT), human (HUM), and organizational (ORG).

Table 10.2 Critical success factors (CSFs) aspects for AI implementation in Healthcare supply chain (HSC).

Aspect	
Technological (TEC)	The TEC component relates to the HSC's AI technologies and infrastructure's availability, compatibility, dependability, and security. This component is the most significant element influencing AI adoption in HSC in emerging nations (Kumar et al. 2023). TEC elements include data quality and availability, system interoperability and integration, solution scalability and adaptability, and cybersecurity and privacy protection.
Institutional or Environmental (INT)	The INT dimension refers to external variables influencing AI adoption in HSC, including legal, ethical, social, and cultural considerations. Depending on the level of support or opposition from various stakeholders such as governments, regulators, consumers, suppliers, rivals, and society at large, these variables can generate possibilities or hurdles for AI adoption. Regulatory compliance and standards, ethical values and norms, customer expectations and satisfaction, supplier collaboration and coordination, and social responsibility and sustainability are some of the INT considerations.
Human (HUM)	The HUM component refers to the human resources and competencies necessary for AI implementation in HSC. This dimension includes the abilities, knowledge, attitudes, and actions of those involved in or impacted by AI adoption, including as management, workers, consumers, suppliers, and partners. Leadership and vision, training and education, change management and communication, trust and acceptance, and cooperation and teamwork are some of the HUM aspects.
Organizational (ORG)	The ORG dimension refers to the internal elements influencing AI adoption in HSC, such as organizational structure, culture, strategy, procedures, and performance. These elements can help with or impede AI adoption depending on how well they correspond with AI aims and objectives. Organizational preparedness and maturity, strategy alignment and direction, process innovation and optimization, performance measurement and assessment, and organizational learning and adaptation are some of the ORG aspects.

Finally, AI has the potential to significantly help the HSC by addressing its issues and boosting its capabilities. However, before applying AI for the HSC, various elements need to be considered. These criteria can decide whether AI use in HSC succeeds or fails in emerging economies.

FUTURE RESEARCH PROSPECTS

Artificial intelligence and HSC are two growing domains with considerable promise to improve the quality, efficiency, and accessibility of health care services. However, there are other hurdles and hazards associated with integrating AI with the HSC, including ethical, legal, social, and technological concerns. To overcome these difficulties and to optimize the benefits of emerging technologies for health care, it is critical to conduct thorough and multidisciplinary research on AI and HSC.

The following are some potential implications of and areas for future study on AI in the HSC:

- Creating frameworks and standards for assessing, validating, and regulating AI and HSC applications such AI-based diagnosis, treatment, monitoring, and logistics.

- Investigating the influence of AI and the HSC on the health care workforce, including the skills, duties, and responsibilities of health care professionals and management in the AI and HSC era.

- Investigating the ethical, legal, and societal implications of AI and HSC systems and data, such as privacy, security, accountability, and trustworthiness.

- Creating human-centred, inclusive AI and HSC solutions that take into account the requirements, preferences, and values of many stakeholders, including patients, providers, payers, and policymakers.

- Promoting collaboration and coordination among the various players and sectors participating in the AI and HSC, including academia, industry, government, and civil society.

- **Integration with EHR systems:** One potential future research topic is to investigate the integration of AI with EHR systems. Integrating AI with EHR systems might help healthcare providers improve demand forecasting and inventory management, as well as increase patient safety and quality of treatment.

- **Development of AI-powered decision support tools:** Another prospective research path is the development of AI-powered decision support systems for HSC management. These solutions might provide supply chain teams with real-time insights and suggestions, allowing them to make more educated and data-driven choices.

- **Implementation in low- and middle-income nations:** The HSCs in many low- and middle-income countries (LMICs) confront considerable obstacles due to insufficient resources and infrastructure. Future studies might look into the feasibility and efficacy of deploying AI-powered solutions in low-income countries, with an emphasis on increasing access to crucial medicines and supplies.

- **Ethical and social implications:** The application of AI in HSC management presents ethical and social concerns, as with any developing technology. Future studies might investigate these implications and assess the possible hazards and advantages of AI-powered solutions, such as privacy, prejudice, and equality concerns.

Finally, future research on AI and the HSC might investigate a variety of avenues and ramifications, such as integration with EHR systems, the creation of decision support tools, adoption in LMICs, and the assessment of ethical and social implications.

REFERENCES

Alabaddi, Z., Obidat, A. and Alziyadat, Z. 2023. Exploring the effect of blockchain technology on supply chain resilience and transparency: evidence from the healthcare industry. Uncertain Supply Chain Management. 11(2): 787–798.

Bai, C., Tang, O. and Lau, H. 2022. Lean and resilience in the healthcare supply chain—a scoping review. International Journal of Lean Six Sigma. 13(5): 1058–1078.

Baryannis, G., Validi, S., Dani, S. and Antoniou, G. 2018. Supply chain risk management and artificial intelligence: state of the art and future research directions. International Journal of Production Research. 57(7): 2179–2202.

Betcheva, L., Erhun, F. and Jiang, H. 2021. OM Forum—supply chain thinking in healthcare: lessons and outlooks. Manufacturing and Service Operations Management. 23(6): 1333–1353.

Bhakoo, V., Singh, P. and Sohal, A. 2012. Collaborative management of inventory in Australian hospital supply chains: practices and issues. Supply Chain Management: An International Journal. 17(2): 217–230.

Burns, L. 2002. The Health Care Value Chain: Producers, Purchasers, and Providers. John Wiley & Sons.

Bvuchete, M., Saartjie Grobbelaar, S. and Van Eeden, J. 2020. Best practices for demand-driven supply chain management in public healthcare sector: a systematic literature review. South African Journal of Industrial Engineering, 31(2): 11–27.

Chang, S.E. and Seol, H. 2022. Artificial intelligence, firm resilience to supply chain disruptions and firm performance. 2022 55th Hawaii International Conference on System Sciences (HICSS). 5679–5688.

Chen, Y., Li, X. and Zhang, X. 2020. Effective demand forecasting in health supply chains: emerging trend and future directions. Healthcare (Basel, Switzerland). 8(1): 12.

Clauson, K.A., Breeden, E.A., Davidson, C. and Mackey, T.K. 2018. Leveraging blockchain technology to enhance supply chain management in healthcare. Blockchain in Healthcare Today. 1. Accessed at https://blockchainhealthcaretoday.com/index.php/journal/article/view/20   (on March 5, 2024)

Dora, M., Kumar, A., Mangla, S.K., Pant, A. and Kamal, M.M. 2021. Critical success factors influencing artificial intelligence adoption in food supply chains. International Journal of Production Research. 60(14): 4621–4640.

Essila, J.C. 2023. Strategies for reducing healthcare supply chain inventory costs. Benchmarking: An International Journal. 30(8): 2655–2669. https://doi.org/10.1108/BIJ-11-2021-0680.

Esteva, A., Kuprel, B., Novoa, R.A., Ko, J., Swetter, S.M., Blau, H.M., et al. 2017. Dermatologist-level classification of skin cancer with deep neural networks. Nature. 542: 115–118.

Gardeva, A. 2021. 4 challenges impacting the healthcare supply chain (IBM blog). Accessed at https://www.ibm.com/blog/4-challenges-affecting-the-healthcare-supply-chain/ (on May 11, 2023).

Gladys Okafor, U., Aderonke Olaleye, M., Chukwuemeka Asobara, H. and Fidelis Umeodinka, E. 2021. Global Impact of COVID-19 Pandemic on Public Health Supply Chains. IntechOpen. doi: 10.5772/intechopen.97454.

Honda, M., Morizane, S., Hikita, K. and Takenaka, A. 2017. Current status of robotic surgery in urology. Asian Journal of Endoscopic Surgery. 10(4): 372–381. https://doi.org/10.1111/ases.12381

Idris, J. and Parashar, S. 2015. Health product supply chains in developing countries: diagnosis of the root causes of underperformance and an agenda for reform. Health Systems and Reform. 1(2): 142–154.

Iliashenko, O., Bikkulova, Z. and Dubgorn, A. 2019. Opportunities and challenges of artificial intelligence in healthcare. E3S Web of Conferences. 110: 02028.

Karthika, B. and Vijayakumar, A.R. 2022. ISO 13485: Medical devices—quality management systems, requirements for regulatory purposes. pp. 19–29. *In*: Timiri Shanmugam, P.S., Thangaraju, P., Palani, N. and Sampath, T. (eds). Medical Device Guidelines and Regulations Handbook. Springer, Cham.

Khot, U.N. 2020. A cardiologist's perspective on navigating healthcare supply shortages during the Covid-19 pandemic. Circulation: Cardiovascular Quality and Outcomes. 13(6): 280–283.

Kumar, S. and Singh, A. 2020. Enabling health supply chains for improved well-being. Supply Chain Forum: An International Journal. 21(4): 229–236.

Kumar, A. 2022. Keynote speech: application of artificial intelligence (AI) in supply chains. 2022 International Conference on Computational Modelling, Simulation and Optimization (ICCMSO). xxv–xxvi.

Kumar, A., Mani, V., Jain, V., Gupta, H. and Venkatesh, V. 2023. A study of crucial success elements in healthcare supply chain management using artificial intelligence (AI). Computers and Industrial Engineering. 175: 108815.

Lanfranco, A.R., Castellanos, A.E., Desai, J.P. and Meyers, W.C. 2004. Robotic surgery: a current perspective. Annals of Surgery. 239(1): 14–21. https://doi.org/10.1097/01.sla.0000103020.19595.7d.

Le Tan, T. 2022. Critical factors affecting artificial intelligence in supply chain management (case study in Danang SMEs). Journal of Interdisciplinary Socio-Economic and Community Study. 2(1): 27–33.

Leite, H., Lindsay, C. and Kumar, M. 2020. Covid-19 outbreak: implications on healthcare operations. The TQM Journal. 33(1): 247–256.

Li, S. 2011. Developing lean and agile health care supply chains. Supply Chain Management: An International Journal. 16(3): 176–183.

Lugada, E., Ochola, I., Kirunda, A., Sembatya, M., Mwebaze, S., Olowo, M., et al. 2022. Health supply chain system in Uganda: assessment of status and of performance of health facilities. Journal of Pharmaceutical Policy and Practice. 15(1): 58. https://doi.org/10.1186/s40545-022-00452-w

Mahmoodi, F., Blutinger, E., Echazu, L. and Nocetti, D. 2021. Covid-19 and the health care supply chain: impacts and lessons learned. Supply Chain Quarterly. Accessed at https://www.supplychainquarterly.com/articles/4417-covid-19-and-the-health-care-supply-chain-impacts-and-lessons-learned/ (on May 11, 2023).

Mathew, J., John, J. and Kumar, S. 2013. New Trends in Healthcare Supply Chain. Paper presented at the International Annual Conference, Production and Operations Management Society, Denver, Colorado.

McKevitt, J. 2016. Merck KGaA: AI will run demand planning in 2017. Supply Chain Dive. Accessed at https://www.supplychaindive.com/news/Merck-KGaA-AI-machine-learning-demand-planning/432885/ (on March 5, 2024).

Mejia, N. 2019. Artificial Intelligence at McKesson – AI Initiatives and Investments. Emerj Artificial Intelligence Research. https://emerj.com/ai-sector-overviews/artificial-intelligence-at-mckesson/

Modgil, S., Singh, R.K. and Hannibal, C. 2021. Artificial intelligence for supply chain resilience: learning from Covid-19. The International Journal of Logistics Management. 33(4): 1246–1268.

Nahmias, S. and Smith, J. 2011. Operations and supply Chain Management (3rd ed.). John Wiley & Sons.

Nuance Communications Inc. 2022. Nuance healthcare solutions overview. Accessed at https://www.nuance.com/healthcare.html (on January 25, 2022).

OptumLabs. 2024. Harnessing artificial intelligence (AI) in health care. Accessed at https://www.optumlabs.com/work/artificial-intelligence.html (on March 5, 2024).

Pagell, M., Wu, Z., Yildiz, H. and Vachon, S. 2020. AI in operations management: applications, challenges and opportunities. Journal of Data, Information and Management. 2(2): 67–74.

Park, A. 2022. Roche, EarlySign expand partnership to include AI-powered lung cancer diagnosis. Accessed at https://www.fiercebiotech.com/medtech/roche-earlysign-expand-partnership-include-ai-powered-lung-cancer-diagnosis (on May 10, 2023).

Qiu, Y., Zhu, K., Leung, S. and Sun, L. 2021. Is artificial intelligence an enabler of supply chain resiliency post Covid-19? An exploratory state-of-the-art review for future research. Operations Management Research. 1–2(15): 378–398.

Rajpurkar, P., Chen, E., Banerjee, O. and Topol, E.J. 2022. AI in health and medicine. Nature Medicine. 28: 31–38. https://doi.org/10.1038/s41591-021-01614-0.

Rasouli, J.J., Shao, J., Neifert, S., Gibbs, W.N., Habboub, G., Steinmetz, M.P., et al. 2020. Artificial intelligence and robotics in spine surgery. Global Spine Journal. 11(4): 556–564.

Richardson, J.P., Smith, C., Curtis, S., Watson, S., Zhu, X., Barry, B. and Sharp, R.R. 2021. Patient apprehensions about the use of artificial intelligence in healthcare. npj Digital Medicine. 4(1): 140.

Roy, D., Chatterjee, D. and Naskar, M. 2023. Impact of artificial intelligence on supply chain management performance. Journal of Service Science and Management. 16(1): 44–58.

Russell, S.J. and Norvig, P. 2016. Artificial Intelligence: A Modern Approach. Pearson Education Limited, Malaysia.

Santos, A. and Duarte, S. 2021. A network maturity mapping tool for demand-driven supply chain management: a case for the public healthcare sector. Sustainability. 13(21): 11988.

Santosh, K.C. 2020. AI-driven tools for coronavirus outbreak: need of active learning and cross-population train/test models on multitudinal/multimodal data. Journal of Medical Systems. 44(5): 93.

Senna, P., Reis, A., Santos, I.L., Dias, A.C. and Coelho, O. 2020. A systematic literature review on supply chain risk management: is healthcare management a forsaken research field? Benchmarking: An International Journal. 28(3): 926–956.

Shen, Y., Gunasekaran, A., Papadopoulos, T. and Childe, S.J. 2018. Supply chain risk management and artificial intelligence: state of the art and future research directions. International Journal of Production Research. 57(7): 2179–2202.

Singh, R., Dwivedi, A.D. and Srivastava, G. 2020. Internet of things based blockchain for temperature monitoring and counterfeit pharmaceutical prevention. Sensors. 20(14): 3951.

Singh, S.K. 2021. Effective demand forecasting in health supply chains: emerging trend, enablers and blockers. Logistics. 5(1): 12.

Snowdon, A. and Wright, A. 2022. Digitally enabled supply chain as a strategic asset for the Covid-19 response in Alberta. Healthcare Management Forum. 35(2): 90–98.

Spieske, A., Gebhardt, M., Kopyto, M. and Birkel, H. 2022. Improving healthcare supply chain resilience in a pandemic: evidence from Europe during the Covid-19 outbreak. Journal of Purchasing and Supply Management. 28(5): 100748.

Stoyanov, S. 2021. Integration of artificial intelligence in the supply chain management. Journal Scientific and Applied Research. 20(1): 53–58.

Tater, T., Gantayat, N., Dechu, S., Jagirdar, H., Rawat, H., Guptha, M., et al. 2022. AI driven accounts payable transformation. Proceedings of the AAAI Conference on Artificial Intelligence. 36(11): 12405–12413.

Toorajipour, R., Sohrabpour, V., Nazarpour, A., Oghazi, P. and Fischl, M. 2021. A thorough survey of the literature on artificial intelligence in supply chain management. Journal of Business Research. 502–517.

Umezulike, A.C. and Eronini, O.I. 2022. Framework for integration of vertical public health supply chain systems: a case study of Nigeria. International Journal of Supply Chain Management. 7(1): 1–27.

Viloria, J. 2015. Health product supply chains in developing countries: diagnosis of the root causes of underperformance and an agenda for reform. Health Systems and Reform. 2(1): 142–154.

Yadav, P. 2007. Promise and problems with supply chain management approaches to health care purchasing. Health Care Management Review. 32(3): 192–202.

Yigitcanlar, T. and Cugurullo, F. 2020. The sustainability of artificial intelligence: an urbanistic viewpoint from the lens of smart and sustainable cities. Sustainability. 12(20): 8548.

Yigitcanlar, T., Kankanamge, N., Regona, M., Ruiz Maldonado, A., Rowan, B., Ryu, A., et al. 2020. Artificial intelligence technologies and related urban planning and development concepts: how are they perceived and utilized in Australia? Journal of Open Innovation: Technology, Market and Complexity. 6(4): 187.

Chapter 11

Artificial Intelligence in Public Health and Health Policies

Emine Cetin

Department of Healthcare Management,
Faculty of Health Science, University of Bakircay,
Izmir Bakircay University, Izmir Türkiye
ORCID: 0000-0003-4326-2070
Email: emine.aslan@bakircay.edu.tr; cetinemine@gmail.com

INTRODUCTION

The widespread use of artificial intelligence (AI) has created significant changes in the field of health in general and public health in particular. While AI in health is prominent in fields such as radiology, pathology (Schwalbe and Wahl 2020), and dermatology, public health applications are not visible enough. The reason why public health applications are less prominent is that the results of public health practices occur over a longer term than curative health services (Küçükali 2021). However, public health interventions have the advantages of affecting large segments of society and enabling intervention before health problems are identified and become devastating. Therefore, the spread of AI applications in the field of public health is important in terms of improving public health.

Although not as prominent as other areas of health, AI technologies have application areas that contribute positively to public health (Küçükali 2021). Areas of contribution include surveillance systems, epidemic management, early diagnosis of diseases, monitoring of disease risk factors, and vaccine studies (Alıcılar and Çöl 2021). Apart from these direct intervention areas, there are also areas of indirect contribution such as facilitating the collection and processing of health records, enabling non-medical records to identify health risks and diseases in the community, accurate and rapid diagnosis of diseases, and increasing academic studies (Thiébaut and Cossin 2019).

As a result of the increasing use of AI in public health, new concepts have emerged in public health areas. These concepts include digital epidemiology, precision public health, infodemiology, and infoveillance or syndromic surveillance. Precision public health is about making the proper intervention for the right population at the right time (Thiébaut and Thiessard 2018). At this point, AI plays an essential role in precision public health as it facilitates "better determining the health status of different segments of society, diagnos[ing] health problems multidimensionally, and plan[ning] and timely implement[ing] problem-specific preventive interventions" (Küçükali 2021).

Another frequently seen concept in the public health literature is digital epidemiology. Epidemiology (non-digital epidemiology), one of the main scientific fields of public health, is the science that studies the distribution and determinants of diseases in society. It is defined by the World Health Organization as "the study of the distribution and determinants of health-related conditions or events in particular populations and the application of this study to the prevention and control of health problems" (Bonita et al. 2006). Epidemiology provides public health professionals and policymakers with tools and data to guide public health and policy decisions (Eysenbach 2009). Digital epidemiology is defined as the use of data produced for non-health purposes in epidemiology. The data used constitutes an important part of big data (Hayran 2021). Data used in digital epidemiology can be obtained from a wide range of sources such as Internet search engines, social media platforms, mobile phone data, and electronic health records from mobile devices.

Infodemiology (information epidemiology) is a combination of the words information and epidemiology (Eysenbach 2009) and it means epidemiology using digital data (Hayran 2021). As a clearer description, infodemiology can be defined as the "science of distribution and determinants of information in an electronic medium, specifically the Internet, or in a population, with the ultimate aim to inform public health and public policy" (Eysenbach 2009, Mavragani 2020). One of the important goals of infodemiology research is the collection and monitoring of data that is epidemiologically important or that could otherwise affect public health (Eysenbach 2009). The syndromic surveillance concept, which is used synonymously with infoveillance, is infodemiological studies in which the main purpose is surveillance.

In these studies, before the symptoms of the disease appear, health-related data are monitored in order to take timely measures against problems that may threaten public health. For example, health line calls, emergency service visits, Internet queries, and monitoring of social media posts (Hayran 2021). In infodemiology and infoveillance studies, unstructured, free text data available on the Internet is constantly analyzed. The data collected from the Internet can be search queries (demand side), as well as publications such as web pages and blogs (supply side) (Eysenbach 2009).

As can be understood from the new concepts added to the public health literature, the development of technology and AI has significantly changed the data sources used by public health and the way this data is processed. Today, with technological developments, health data can be collected much faster, as well as daily life data can be used to monitor events that affect public health. In addition, the data collection and analysis process, which previously took years, even decades, has been shortened considerably, and it has become much faster, almost in real time. Thus, it is possible to easily detect the factors that threaten public health and to bring more proactive and more accurate solutions to the problems.

In this study, the effects of AI on public health data acquisition and analysis, the advantages it provides to developing countries, and areas that need improvement have been reviewed.

USING AI FOR DATA ACQUISITION AND ANALYSIS

Access to accurate and up-to-date data is very important in the implementation of evidence-based public health initiatives. AI has an important role in increasing knowledge in the field of public health. AI can make significant contributions to public health by enabling the use of non-health data, summarizing the results of scientific publications, and analysing the collected data in real time, as well as keeping health records more accurate and complete.

PROVIDING INFORMATION THROUGH THE COMPILATION OF PUBLISHED STUDIES

It is important to compile the information obtained from published scientific studies and to obtain a conclusion. In this sense, literature reviews and meta-analyses are used as academic methods. These methods are seen as providing reliable results because they make an important contribution to evaluating the differences between and results of studies conducted in different settings and in different case groups. However, doing these studies may require significant effort and a long time. In addition, it is possible that the subject is out of date when the study is completed. In terms of public health, it is also possible that the health problem causes irreversible harm to society. With AI, these studies can be carried out much faster. For example, Michelson et al. (2020) have done a meta-analysis with a method they call "rapid meta-analysis" performed by AI to determine the side effects of an active substance used in the treatment of Covid-19 disease. They used AI to scan published articles and select relevant ones, determine their results, and analyse the data with statistical methods. The meta-analysis was completed in less than 30 minutes and a significant clinical result was achieved (Michelson et al. 2020).

It is seen that AI has an important role in the creation of new studies as well as in compiling existing scientific studies. It has been determined that most of the articles published in 2018, reviewed in the Public Health and Epidemiological Informatics section of the *International Medical Informatics Association Yearbook*, are about epidemiological surveillance based on digital data obtained through the analysis of big data from social media and electronic health records (Thiébaut and Cossin 2019).

ELECTRONIC HEALTH RECORDS

Perhaps the most important contribution of AI to public health is that it provides large and detailed data that could not be imagined until recently. Complete and timely data is essential to inform decision-making on public health issues and improve healthcare delivery (Haskew et al. 2015). Health records are health-related data and have an important place in monitoring the services provided in the health sector, determining the resources used, and determining the course and outcome of diseases.

Health records, medical records, and medical charts are different terms used to describe the documentation of a patient's medical history and care (Evans 2016). The health records are the electronic health records, patient demographic information and images, prescriptions, discharge summaries, insurance information, and data from sensory devices (Hussain et al. 2019). In recent years, health records have gained importance based on the fact that a patient's medical information should include health and lifestyle information beyond the health problems at admission (Evans 2016).

Traditionally, health records have been kept on a paper basis. There was generally only one copy of the records kept in paper form (Evans 2016). This situation caused the storage, sharing, and analysis of health records to become quite problematic. It could be seen that some health records were kept only by the patient, and the health institution did not keep these records (Haskew et al. 2015). Also, the opportunity for data validation was very low. Especially in developing countries, there may be problems in collecting data and there may be situations where data collection should be determined as a goal rather than a tool. For example, a survey of routine primary care data in South Africa showed that only 26% of the data in the mother-to-child AIDS/HIV transmission prevention registry was complete and only 12.8% of this recorded data was accurate (Haskew et al. 2015, Mate et al. 2009).

The new computer technology developed in the 1960s and 1970s led to the transfer of health records to electronic media. Thus, electronic health records were born. Electronic health records are defined as digital versions of patient and community health information (Wahl et al. 2018).

The emergence of electronic health records has not only changed the environment in which health records are kept but also expanded the features and uses of health records. Identity information required to be included in the health records can be easily verified, the health history is available for a longer period of time, and comparisons can be made with retrospective records. It is possible to integrate the data related to the health service that the patient receives from different institutions.

Health records, which can be kept longer and in more detail in the electronic environment, reach enormous dimensions. For example, it is reported that a normal patient produces 80 MB of electronic health data annually; 1.2 billion clinical documents are produced each year in the United States. Because of this huge body of data, electronic health records account for approximately 30% of all stored data (Hussain et al. 2019). Therefore, health records are typical examples of big data. Storing patient records, which used to be large in physical archives, has now become a serious managerial problem in electronic media. As a result of the fact that it is not possible to store the huge information clusters on CDs or hard disks, cloud technology has become a solution for healthcare institutions. Cloud technology can be defined as the storage of data on a network of remote servers rather than a single computer or data storage unit (Wahl et al. 2018). With this technology, health institutions have the opportunity to store electronic patient records without using any physical space and with high security.

MHEALTH (MOBILE HEALTH) DATA

Today, besides the data held by health institutions, health data produced by mobile devices also contributes significantly to the health records. Mhealth can be briefly defined as health-related services offered through mobile communication devices (Bhavnani et al. 2016, Whittaker 2012). A mobile device is used to monitor and collect biological or health data of the patient or person. Mobile devices can be items that are used in daily life and carried by the person, such as smart watches, glasses, bracelets, or clothes. In addition, the use of small probes developed to measure blood sugar or heartbeat, attached to the patient's body, has become widespread (Dinh-Le et al. 2019). With mobile devices, the desired features of the person can be monitored (remotely and) continuously while the person is out of the health institution. Most of the smart devices can send alerts to the person, the health institution, or both when vital signs go out of normal limits (Greiwe and Nyenhuis 2020).

While the Mhealth application makes a significant contribution to health data accumulation, it has a special place in the field of public health as it can collect information about people's health that may not be realized in health institutions, provide continuous monitoring, and provide data about the environment. Conditions such as pollen, temperature, and humidity level, which are risk factors for diseases, can be monitored in the person's environment. Monitoring the person's daily exercise and calorie intake can help provide an early warning for people in the risk-prone group. This contributes to the improvement of health status through closer monitoring of diseases and patient behaviours.

NATURALLY OCCURRING DATA AND SOCIAL MEDIA DATA

Having diverse, fast, and accurate data is the main determinant in the effectiveness of interventions to improve the health of the population. In this sense, obtaining data from different sources is valuable. With the increase in the use of AI, one of the data types that have entered our lives is "naturally occurring data". Naturally occurring data is formed as a result of daily activities without a research purpose and turns into data with the involvement of a researcher in the process. The events in which this data is collected will continue even if there is no research (Kiyimba et al. 2019). Examples of the events in which naturally occurring data are collected are health line calls, emergency service applications, Internet queries, and monitoring social media posts (Hayran 2021).

Prior to the development of AI, health records were traditionally used. However, it may take a long time to reflect the events affecting society on the health records, to analyse these records, and to determine the precautions. In fact, in periods when technology could not be utilized sufficiently, this process could take years or even decades. Due to the difficulty in monitoring the data continuously, reports can only be published annually or biennially (Dai and Wang 2019). In addition, although health records are very valuable, they reflect the health problems of only those individuals who approach health institutions. This shows that traditional health records alone are not sufficient to provide rapid response to many public health problems.

Social media is a very important source of naturally occurring data. Today, social media is frequently used by community members to create and share general messages about their health (Dai and Wang 2019). People use the Internet for health-related issues as well as other purposes or to share their health-related status (Dai and Wang 2019). According to a survey conducted in the United States, 3.63% of respondents use online health chat rooms to find solutions to health problems and 43.55% search the Internet for health-related information (Amante et al. 2015).

The data obtained from social media, the advantages of AI, and the data produced for non-health purposes are used to monitor public health. As stated in the introduction, digital epidemiology is considered a new field of public health that emerged with the use of these data. In digital epidemiology, data produced by people in their daily lives such as Google searches, social media shares, and text analyses from published articles can be used for status determination before health records. Thus, the data obtained from these searches and sharing creates a unique data source to determine the health problems seen in society, their prevalence, and even the anxiety they cause in society. The use of this data makes it possible to monitor the health of a wider population; it is also faster and involves lower costs than traditional methods (Choi et al. 2017).

The best-known example of disease prediction and surveillance using social media data is Google Trends (Choi et al. 2017). It is an AI application developed to detect trends, the rate of spread of the flu disease, and the regional situation at a real-time and realistic level using Google searches. The fact that the data obtained from the application showed a significant correlation with the actual data showed the usability of such tools in public health monitoring. In the United States, it models outpatient flu-like illness (ILI) using publicly available ILI surveillance data provided by the Centers for Disease Control and Prevention (CDC) (Cook et al. 2011).

Social media data has been used to monitor the disease and its spread, as well as to monitor the public's response to the disease. The relationship between mass media and public sentiment was analysed during the Middle East Respiratory Syndrome (MERS) epidemic that occurred in Korea in 2015 (Thiébaut and Thiessard 2018). By analysing the content of Twitter messages, Kang et al. (2018) revealed that vaccine sensitivity in the United States can be tracked using social media data.

In a study conducted in Turkey during the Covid-19 pandemic, the response of the public to the disease was successfully analysed using Google Trends (Avcı 2021). White et al. (2013) demonstrated that the negative effects of drug interactions can be determined using Internet searches and that this method is a much cheaper follow-up tool than health records.

The differences between naturally occurring data and data collected for research purposes are summarized in Table 1.1. Both data types have features that are superior to each other. It is possible that the combined use of data obtained for research purposes, health records, and naturally occurring data will provide higher benefits in terms of public health.

Table 11.1 The difference between naturally occurring data and data produced by researchers.

Produced by Researchers	Naturally Occurring Data
The researcher selects some participants (universe, sample) and collects data by asking questions and/or observing.	The researcher uses the outputs of some spontaneous and already existing activities, all kinds of written, visual, and verbal records as data.
The environment and conditions in which the data will be collected are determined by the researcher.	The researcher determines which sources such as audio, video, or written records will be used as data.
The researcher assumes that consistent views can be obtained from the participants if appropriate questions are asked.	The researcher is aware that the records examined may have been created by different communities and with different content.

Source: Hayran (2021).

ANALYSIS OF DATA

Electronic health records, records on human mobility, and environmental conditions created with the help of AI-assisted technologies create quite large data groups. Although the collection and storage of health records are very important, it is necessary to correctly classify and process these data in order to be used in the planning and evaluation of health services. The most important social effects of big data, which is obtained from different sources and is expected to be used for health purposes, are likely to occur when used with AI (Benke and Benke 2018). Methods such as machine learning, automated planning and scheduling, expert systems, and natural language processing (NLP), which are considered sub-applications of AI technology, enable large data to be processed easily and accurately (Wahl et al. 2018).

Data flow combined with the increase in data processing and analysis power of AI creates an opportunity to identify health threats and take precautions against threats (Lu et al. 2019). The analysis methods offered by AI provide important benefits in "detecting the patterns in the data and the elements that disrupt the patterns and ensuring the continuous follow-up of the diseases in the society", which is called surveillance. AI is a very effective method in detecting public health problems early and before the problem grows, as it can perform surveillance continuously, fairly quickly, and accurately. The incidence of diseases can be determined instantly by using health records kept in an electronic environment with AI (Küçükali 2021).

The fact that fuzzy logic, which is a set of mathematical methods for representing information based on probability and uncertainty, can also be used in cases where data is incomplete and uncertain (Wahl et al. 2018) makes it possible to use larger data masses. For example, Lu et al. (2019) were able to predict the course of the flu epidemic by modelling using Google searches, Google trends, and health records. Using data from the 1918 influenza epidemic in California and the 2013–2015 Ebola outbreak in West Africa, Smirnova et al. were able to model the course of infectious diseases. It is possible to predict future infectious diseases with modelling (Smirnova et al. 2019).

Artificial intelligence is also used to predict public health problems other than infectious diseases. AI and deep learning offer clinical predictions and diseases can be predicted before they occur. By monitoring patients for a short time with AI, diseases that may develop in the future, especially diabetes and cancer types, can be predicted (Alıcılar and Çöl 2021). Studies have aimed to estimate the risk of anaemia in children using standard household survey data, to identify children at highest risk of missing vaccination sessions, and to identify high-risk births using cardiotocography data. A study conducted in Brazil succeeded in correctly classifying the behavioural risk of sexually active youth in the range of 65–99% (Schwalbe and Wahl 2020).

One of the important problems with electronic health records used in many studies is hiding the identity information in these records. Before the use of health records, there is a need for anonymization of data, which can be defined as the elimination of information that will indicate the person. Electronic health records are not allowed until they are anonymized. Therefore, anonymization is the primary step in making clinical data accessible to more people and is of great interest (Liu et al. 2017). Coding for anonymization was first made by humans. However, anonymizing data can be a long, complex, and difficult process. Again, at this point, the help of AI is taken. It has been found that AI encodes in a shorter time, at a lower cost, and more accurately than human coders (Ahmed et al. 2020).

AI FOR DEVELOPING COUNTRIES

Tackling major public health problems is characteristic of developing countries. Developing countries have the bulk of the world's communicable disease burden. About 90% of AIDS/HIV infection cases are in developing countries, and prevalence rates of other communicable diseases are also high in developing countries. Millions of people die every year due to diseases such as malaria and tuberculosis, which can be treated with modern medical practices (Japan International Cooperation Agency 2005). In addition to the prevalence of communicable diseases, non-communicable diseases seriously threaten public health in these countries. Child and maternal deaths are common (World Health Organization 2017). Despite the intensity of communicable and non-communicable diseases, health workers, health institutions, and drugs are not enough (Japan International Cooperation Agency 2005). Existing healthcare workers tend to have low education and skills.

Because of the advantage of preventing diseases before they start, public health interventions are ideal healthcare services both to improve public health and to avoid large health expenditures. Given the lack of resources and the large disease burden in developing countries, it is possible that these countries will benefit from appropriate public health initiatives. AI can be used in these countries to identify risk factors, monitor diseases, and support healthcare workers. It is hoped that the proliferation of information technology, mobile computing power, and the Internet will offer opportunities to address the problems of developing countries (Schwalbe and Wahl 2020).

In developing countries, the lack of adequate training of health workers and the compensation of shortage of doctors by intermediate health workers may lead to failures in diagnosis and treatment. Decision support systems can be critical for improving public health for healthcare professionals who have to provide healthcare services with a lack of information in countries where there is a lack of resources (Knoble et al. 2010, Knoble and Bhusal 2015). In resource-poor settings, expert systems can be used to support health programs in a variety of ways. As in high-income countries, AI can support healthcare professionals in diagnosis and treatment planning (Wahl et al. 2018). For example, in Nepal, an electronic algorithm that can work on smartphones and tablets has been developed to assist rural healthcare workers in making a diagnosis. In this algorithm, more than 260 different diseases can be diagnosed with the answers given to the questions about the health problems of the patients (Knoble and Bhusal 2015).

Artificial intelligence can be used in planning to alleviate the workload of a small number of healthcare workers in developing countries and to enable them to work more efficiently. An AI application is being developed that aims to optimize home visits and drug delivery by community health workers in Africa. Again, mobile health applications were used to convey health information to those living in remote areas (Wahl et al. 2018).

With the opportunity brought by the widespread use of smartphones, AI applications for patients can be used to improve public health. With these applications, healthcare professionals can guide lifestyle changes and nutrition, and the patient can self-evaluate symptoms during pregnancy and recovery (Hosny and Aerts 2019). As it is practised in developed countries, AI in developing countries may offer the opportunity to detect infectious disease outbreaks earlier and to intervene in a timely manner (Schwalbe and Wahl 2020). Thus, contributions can be made to improve public health and reduce the burden on the health system.

PROBLEMS AND IMPROVEMENT AREAS FOR THE APPLICATION OF AI TO PUBLIC HEALTH

It is clear that AI has the potential to make significant contributions to health in general and public health in particular. However, more research, infrastructure, and research are still needed in order to see the expected effects in all environments. While the success of AI has been proven in academic research and its practice in some fields, more evidence is needed about the basic functions of public health, namely protecting and supporting the health of populations (Panch et al. 2019). A significant portion of these doings are small-scale practices. Therefore, there are still concerns about the extent to which the expected effects will be realized in widespread use.

Although projections and models provide certain predictions, factors that have not been calculated can negatively affect the reliability of the results. For example, the consistency of survival estimates in breast cancer has been found to differ according to the stage at which the cancer is diagnosed and varies according to the method used (Kleinlein and Riaño 2019). Similarly, tools aimed at predicting and surveillance of outbreaks need to be supported and complemented by strong surveillance systems to guide an adequate public health emergency response if an outbreak is accurately predicted (Schwalbe and Wahl 2020).

Although the existing technological infrastructure can be used for AI practices, investment will be required to strengthen the health system to be able to rely on AI-powered applications (Schwalbe and Wahl 2020). Rural and resource-limited environments in low-income countries are expected to be even more difficult to leverage these technologies due to various socio-organizational and technical factors affecting the practice and adoption of technologies. In these countries, which are most in need of AI-supported public health, there is a greater lack of infrastructure and trained manpower, and there is also a problem in providing the necessary resources for investment (Sukums et al. 2014). Consequently, although great opportunities are to be expected from this new resource, a lot of work needs to be done to exploit and validate them (Thiébaut and Cossin 2019).

REFERENCES

Ahmed, T., Aziz, M.M.Al and Mohammed, N. 2020. De-identification of electronic health record using neural network. Scientific Reports. 10(1): 1–11.

Alıcılar, H.E. and Çöl, M. 2021. Halk sağlığında yapay zekanın kullanımı. Uludağ Üniversitesi Tıp Fakültesi Dergisi (Usage of artificial intelligence in public health. Journal of Uludağ University Medical Faculty). 47(1): 151–158.

Amante, D.J., Hogan, T.P., Pagoto, S.L., English, T.M. and Lapane, K.L. 2015. Access to care and use of the Internet to search for health information: results from the US National Health Interview Survey. Journal of Medical Internet Research. 17(4): e106.

Avcı, K. 2021. Investigation of Covid-19 related web search behaviors in Turkey: a digital epidemiology study using Google Trends. Turk Hijyen ve Deneysel Biyoloji Dergisi (Turkish Bulletin of Hygiene and Experimental Biology). 78(2): 133–146.

Benke, K. and Benke, G. 2018. Artificial intelligence and big data in public health. International Journal of Environmental Research and Public Health. 15(12): 1–9.

Bhavnani, S.P., Narula, J. and Sengupta, P.P. 2016. Mobile technology and the digitization of healthcare. European Heart Journal. 37(18): 1428–1438.

Bonita, R., Beaglehole, R. and Kjellström, T. 2006. Temel Epidemiyoloji (2nd Ed.) (Basic epidemiology (2nd Ed.) World Health Organization). Başak Matbaacılık ve Tanıtım Hiz. Ltd. Şti. Accessed at https://ekutuphane.saglik.gov.tr/ Ekutuphane/kitaplar/epidemiyoloji.pdf (on 10 March 2024).

Choi, S., Lee, J., Kang, M.G., Min, H., Chang, Y.S. and Yoon, S. 2017. Large-scale machine learning of media outlets for understanding public reactions to nation-wide viral infection outbreaks. Methods. 129: 50–59.

Cook, S., Conrad, C., Fowlkes, A.L. and Mohebbi, M.H. 2011. Assessing Google Flu trends performance in the United States during the 2009 influenza virus A (H1N1) pandemic. PLoS ONE. 1–8.

Dai, H.J. and Wang, C.K. 2019. Classifying adverse drug reactions from imbalanced twitter data. International Journal of Medical Informatics. 129: 122–132.

Dinh-Le, C., Chuang, R., Chokshi, S. and Mann, D. 2019. Wearable health technology and electronic health record integration: scoping review and future directions. JMIR mHealth and uHealth. 7(9): 1–13.

Evans, R.S. 2016. Electronic health records: then, now, and in the future. Yearbook of Medical Informatics. 1: S48–S61.

Eysenbach, G. 2009. Infodemiology and infoveillance: framework for an emerging set of public health informatics methods to analyze search, communication and publication behavior on the internet. Journal of Medical Internet Research. 11(1): 1–10.

Greiwe, J. and Nyenhuis, S.M. 2020. Wearable technology and how this can be implemented into clinical practice. Current Allergy and Asthma Reports. 20(8): 1–10.

Haskew, J., Rø, G., Saito, K., Turner, K., Odhiambo, G., Wamae, A., et al. 2015. Implementation of a cloud-based electronic medical record for maternal and child health in rural Kenya. International Journal of Medical Informatics. 84(5): 349–354.

Hayran, O. 2021. İnfodemiyoloji, dijital epidemiyoloji ve metabilim: İnsanın insanı, bilimin insanı aldatması nasıl önlenir? ESTÜDAM Halk Sağlığı Dergisi (Infodemiology, digital epidemiology and metascience: How to manage human-based and science-based misinformation? ESTUDAM Public Health Journal). 6(3): 322–330.

Hosny, A. and Aerts, H.J.W.L. 2019. Artificial intelligence for global health: socially responsible technologies promise to help address health care inequalities. Science. 366(6468): 955–956.

Hussain, S., Hussain, M., Afzal, M., Hussain, J., Bang, J., Seung, H., et al. 2019. Semantic preservation of standardized healthcare documents in big data. International Journal of Medical Informatics. 129(July): 133–145.

Japan International Cooperation Agency. 2005. Japan's experience in public health and medical systems: towards improving public health and medical systems in developing countries. Accessed at https://openjicareport.jica. go.jp/pdf/11868221.pdf (on 10 March 2024).

Kang, J.G., Ewing-Nelson, S., Mackey, L., Schlitt, J., Marathe, A., Abbas, K., et al. 2018. Semantic network analysis of vaccine sentiment in online social media. Physiology & Behavior. 176(1): 139–148.

Kiyimba, N., Lester, J.N. and O'Reilly, M. 2019. Using Naturally Occurring Data İn Qualitative Health Research (1st ed.). Springer.

Kleinlein, R. and Riaño, D. 2019. Persistence of data-driven knowledge to predict breast cancer survival. International Journal of Medical Informatics. 129(January): 303–311.

Knoble, S.J. and Bhusal, M.R. 2015. Electronic diagnostic algorithms to assist mid-level health care workers in Nepal: a mixed-method exploratory study. International Journal of Medical Informatics. 84(5): 334–340.

Knoble, S., Pandit, A., Koirala, B. and Ghimire, L. 2010. Measuring the quality of rural-based, government health care workers in Nepal. Internet Journal of Allied Health Sciences and Practice. 8(1): 1–9.

Küçükali, H. 2021. Halk sağlığında yapay zekâ. Sağlık Düşüncesi ve Tıp Kültürü (Artificial intelligence in public health. Journal of Health Thought and Medical Culture). 58: 92–95.

Liu, Z., Tang, B., Wang, X. and Chen, Q. 2017. De-identification of clinical notes via recurrent neural network and conditional random field. Journal of Biomedical Informatics. 75, S34–S42.

Lu, F.S., Hattab, M.W., Clemente, C.L., Biggerstaff, M. and Santillana, M. 2019. Improved state-level influenza nowcasting in the United States leveraging internet-based data and network approaches. Nature Communications. 10(1): 1–10.

Mate, K.S., Bennett, B., Mphatswe, W., Barker, P. and Rollins, N. 2009. Challenges for routine health system data management in a large public programme to prevent mother-to-child HIV transmission in South Africa. PLoS One. 4(5): 1–6.

Mavragani, A. 2020. Infodemiology and infoveillance: scoping review. Journal of Medical Internet Research. 22(4): 1–15.

Michelson, M., Chow, T., Martin, N.A., Ross, M., Ying, A.T.Q. and Minton, S. 2020. Artificial intelligence for rapid meta-analysis: case study on ocular toxicity of hydroxychloroquine. Journal of Medical Internet Research. 22(8): e20007.

Panch, T., Pearson-Stuttard, J., Greaves, F. and Atun, R. 2019. Artificial intelligence: opportunities and risks for public health. The Lancet Digital Health. 1(1): e13–e14.

Schwalbe, N. and Wahl, B. 2020. Artificial intelligence and the future of global health. Lancet. 395(10236): 1579–1586.

Smirnova, A., deCamp, L. and Chowell, G. 2019. Forecasting epidemics through nonparametric estimation of time-dependent transmission rates using the SEIR model. Bulletin of Mathematical Biology. 81(11): 4343–4365.

Sukums, F., Mensah, N., Mpembeni, R., Massawe, S., Duysburgh, E., Williams, A., et al. 2014. Promising adoption of an electronic clinical decision support system for antenatal and intrapartum care in rural primary healthcare facilities in sub-Saharan Africa: The QUALMAT experience. International Journal of Medical Informatics. 84(9): 647–657.

Thiébaut, R. and Cossin, S. 2019. Artificial intelligence for surveillance in public health. Yearbook of Medical Informatics. 28(1): 232–234.

Thiébaut, R. and Thiessard, F. 2018. Artificial intelligence in public health and epidemiology. Yearbook of Medical Informatics. 27(1): 207–210.

Wahl, B., Cossy-Gantner, A., Germann, S. and Schwalbe, N.R. 2018. Artificial intelligence (AI) and global health: How can AI contribute to health in resource-poor settings? BMJ Global Health. 3(4): 1–7.

White, R.W., Tatonetti, N.P., Shah, N.H., Altman, R.B. and Horvitz, E. 2013. Web-scale pharmacovigilance: listening to signals from the crowd. Journal of the American Medical Informatics Association. 20(3): 404–408.

Whittaker, R. 2012. Issues in mhealth: findings from key informant interviews. Journal of Medical Internet Research. 14(5): e129.

World Health Organization. 2017. Least developed countries—health and WHO: country presence rofile. Accessed at https://apps.who.int/iris/bitstream/handle/10665/255802/WHO-CCU-17.07-eng.pdf?sequence=1 (on 10 March 2024).

Chapter 12

The New Era: Effect of Increasing Use of Artificial Intelligence in Healthcare on Quality and Accreditation

Ibrahim Halil Kayral[1], Figen Cizmeci Senel[2], Gulsen Koralay[3] and Didem Incegil[*,4]

[1]Department of Health Management, Izmir Bakircay University, Izmir Türkiye
and
Health Institutes of Türkiye, Ankara, Türkiye
ORCID: 0000-0003-1734-6844
Email: ikayral@gmail.com

[2]Faculty of Dentistry of Karadeniz Technical University, Trabzon, Turkıye
and
Health Institutes of Türkiye, Ankara, Türkiye
ORCID: 0000-0002-1859-2003
Email: fcsenel@hotmail.com

[3]Health Institutes of Türkiye, Ankara, Türkiye
ORCID: 0000-0001-5109-528X
Email: koralayg@gmail.com

[4]Health Institutes of Türkiye, Ankara, Türkiye
ORCID: 0000-0002-8778-7066
Email: didemincegil@gmail.com

---

*For Correspondence: Didem Incegil (didemincegil@gmail.com)

DIGITAL TRANSFORMATION IN HEALTHCARE DELIVERY

There is a great need for digital change in delivery and management of health services due to many problems such as rapid changes in health science, developing technology with industrialization, follow-up process of diseases related to increasing chronic disease burden, increase in life expectancy at birth, increase in population in need of home healthcare, possible epidemic threats such as Covid-19 pandemic, change in society's expectations from health services, and insufficient number of health professionals (Akalın and Veranyurt 2021).

Today, one of essential changes in the field of health services is digital transformation. Digital transformation refers to a process that aims to produce effective and efficient services in digital environment by triggering significant changes in characteristics of information, information processing, communication, and connection technologies combinations (Kraus et al. 2021). Internet of things, machine-to-machine communication, cloud computing, big data, and wearable and portable technologies are the building blocks of digital transformation, and they directly and deeply affect health system and cause quality standards of healthcare services to increase gradually (Aslan and Güzel 2019).

Digital transformation in health services includes concepts such as industrialization, which started with the Industrial Revolution in the eighteenth century, and the use of autonomous systems and unmanned workflows that entered our lives with industry 4.0 today (Akalın and Veranyurt 2021). In general, the factors that make digital transformation compulsory in health services all over the world are:

- to increase access to care, improve the quality and safety of care, and reduce costs; pressures from service recipients, payment institutions, and health system regulatory authorities;
- increased patient comfort with telehealth and other digital technologies implemented during the Covid-19 pandemic;
- emergence of new technologies, such as artificial intelligence (AI), that provide the ability to overcome problems and take advantage of previously unattainable opportunities;
- sharp increase in private equity investments promoting digital health applications such as telehealth and remote monitoring;
- the aggressive launch of digital health products and services by technology giants such as Google, Microsoft, Apple, Oracle, and Amazon, and tech-savvy retailers, pharmacies, and new healthcare providers (Glaser and Shaw 2022).

In health services delivery processes, management, and application areas, the existence of a technology-integrated health system is considered a strategic resource for both healthcare providers and health managers in order to make the right decisions and decide on the most effective treatment method among existing treatment methods (Long et al. 2018).

Artificial intelligence, which is one of main dynamics of digital transformation phenomenon in health, is developing as a separate field on its own. AI is based on human brain functions, it is the transfer of human-specific abilities such as learning, thinking, interpreting, communicating, analyzing, and decision-making to systems such as computers, robots, and programs that have ability to perform complex tasks generally associated with intelligent beings, and that use different learning methods and algorithms (Akalın and Veranyurt 2021, Hui Jin et al. 2020).

It can be said that AI applications are used in almost all of the services offered in the field of digital health. All modern health-related fields such as medical health services, digital health, and mobile health that make up health services intersect with AI (Figure 12.1). AI-based solutions appear with applications such as voice response systems in mobile health and diagnosis and treatment in medicine (Shin 2019).

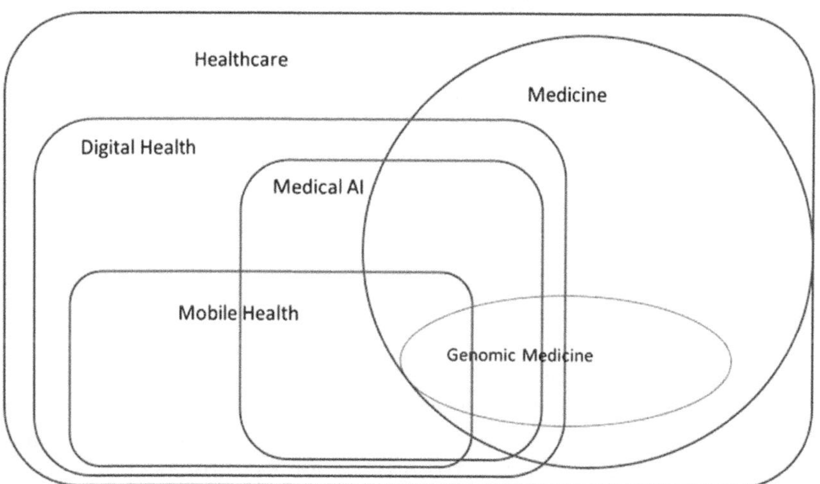

Figure 12.1. Relationship between digital health and other terms.
Source: Adapted with permission from Shin (2019).

AI APPLICATIONS IN HEALTHCARE

Today, AI applications are used in diagnosis, treatment, and rehabilitation of diseases, in improvement and development of public health, and in management of health services to reduce costs, increase quality, reduce human-induced errors, and increase performance (Akalın and Veranyurt 2021).

With the use of AI in health services, many analytical predictions such as clinical decision-making, course of diseases, protection from disease risks, and predictive disease risk scoring can be created. At the same time, AI systems can reduce human-related diagnosis and treatment errors, which are inevitable in clinical applications (Akgerman et al. 2022, Robert 2019).

The usage areas of AI in health services can be grouped under four main categories (Figure 12.2).

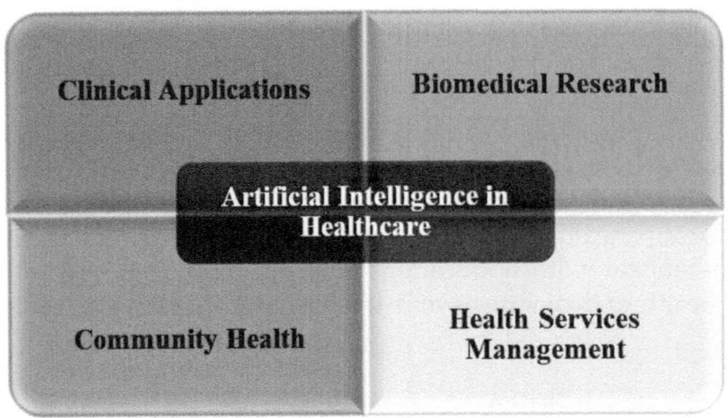

Figure 12.2   Artificial intelligence usage areas in health services.
Source: STOA (2022).

CLINICAL APPLICATIONS AND AI

Use of AI in clinical research processes in decision-making and diagnosis phase of clinical applications is quite common. Besides clinical records required for diagnosis and treatment in healthcare institutions, data comes from many other sources such as laboratory tests, pharmacy data, medical imaging, and genomic information. Although AI has an important role in tasks such as image analysis (radiology, ophthalmology, etc.) and signal processing (electrocardiography, electroencephalography, etc.), it can also be used to integrate and rank results with other clinical data to facilitate clinical workflows (STOA 2022).

Various machine learning algorithms are used to diagnose diseases in advance. Especially in cancers, early diagnosis is extremely important for success of treatment. Detection of disease before visible signs of disease appear is often life-saving. The most well-known AI application used in diagnosis of diseases is IBM Watson for Health application. It is an application that uses machine learning and natural language processing capabilities. It is designed to help physicians review patients' electronic health records and analyze search-related medical research publications and guidelines. This application has a multi-model structure and provides support to doctors in diseases that are difficult to diagnose (Büyükgöze and Dereli 2020, Akalın and Veranyurt 2021).

The AI tools used in radiology can prioritize and monitor findings that require attention and enable radiologists to concentrate on images that are most likely to be abnormal (STOA 2022). On the other hand, examination and reporting of radiology images and evaluation of reports by patient's physician requesting imaging is a process that takes a long time. Sending images with AI applications can save both time and workload (Akalın and Veranyurt 2021).

It is possible to minimize the likelihood of error in surgical procedures performed with AI-supported robots (Şimşir and Mete 2021). Biomedical research and AI.

Within the field of biomedical research, AI applications are widely used in areas such as drug research, clinical research, and personalized treatment. Drug development involves expensive, time-consuming, and labor-intensive processes. AI technologies can contribute to drug development studies at the molecular level. Many drugs or nutritional supplements can cause oxidative damage to cell components in the human body. Hydrogen atom transfer is used to predict the damages that such substances can cause, and quantum computers are required to evaluate the results. A model is proposed using machine learning to simulate and predict this effect. Thus, hardware and time costs have been significantly optimized for this calculation (Şimşir and Mete 2021, Akalın and Veranyurt 2021, STOA 2022). Community health and AI.

Artificial intelligence applications can be used in areas such as raising awareness of individuals about diseases, and conducting and evaluating screening tests by reaching out to a large number of target audiences. With AI applications, individuals can be encouraged to develop positive health behaviors and proactive management of healthy lifestyles can be supported (Büyükgöze and Dereli 2020, Akalın and Veranyurt 2021).

Internet of medical objects technology is used in many areas related to health services such as health protection, and development and support for a healthy life. With the sensors in wearable technologies, medical values such as heart rate, blood pressure, calories burned and step counts can be monitored; these values can be shared with health professionals remotely (Bozbuğa et al. 2021).

HEALTHCARE MANAGEMENT AND AI

In recent years, the concept of a digital hospital, wherein papers, films, files, and manual operations are absent, and where all tasks are carried out, controlled, and managed with a fully automated system, has been frequently mentioned. In integrated digital hospitals, diagnostic and treatment applications such as hospital information management system, electronic health records, laboratory and radiology information systems Picture Archiving and Communication Systems (PACS), digital medical archive, e-prescription, e-referral, e-appointment systems, radio frequency identification (RFID), and barcode systems are used. They also employ corporate applications such as e-finance, quality assurance policies, device tracking, smart building, e-purchasing, internet, as well as external connection applications such as banks, insurance companies, social security institution, suppliers, smart health cards, MEDULLA and home care. Technological applications such as smart hospital buildings, network, call centers, storage, and Internet Protocol (IP) communication are also frequently used (Aslan and Güzel 2019, Uysal and Ulusinan 2020, Akalın and Veranyurt 2021, STOA 2022).

FUTURE OF AI IN HEALTHCARE

Increasing use of AI in healthcare services accelerates the digitalization process day by day. With digitalization of health services, patient information is entered into the system, and necessary medical information (radiological images, laboratory results, daily medical follow-ups, etc.) can be easily accessed from within or outside an institution. It is anticipated that this situation will reduce medical errors arising from lack of access to information. Similarly, absence of temporal or spatial restrictions in accessing information will minimize waiting and hospitalization times of patients. The working processes of health professionals will be shortened, costs will reduce as use of paper, x-ray, and other stationery materials will be done away with, and information security will increase by digitally storing records. With barcode, QR code, and RFID systems used in digital hospitals, drugs and medical supplies will be easily monitored and medical errors related to them will decrease, leading to the emergence of a decision support system. Hospitals can also improve the monitoring of statistical data, thereby enabling better measurement of their performance (T.C. Sağlık Bakanlığı 2014), Şimşir and Mete 2021, Zeybek and Zeybek 2022).

ACCREDITATION IN HEALTH SERVICES

Accreditation, which is a formal process by which performance level of a healthcare provider is evaluated and approved by a recognized independent legal entity in line with predetermined and published standards, is a management model and method that provides hospitals with a competitive advantage and the ability to adapt to sustainable environmental changes (Pasinringi et al. 2021).

Accreditation practices, which primarily focus on benefits such as reducing differences in medical practices, reducing inappropriate healthcare outcomes, and decreasing costs, are mainly interventions for patient and employee safety. For institutions that provide health services and for those who receive these services, accreditation has several benefits such as improving health service production process, improving clinical results, enhancing the quality of healthcare, increasing trust of care recipients in the institution, and reducing risks of harm and infection for both service recipients and service providers (Demir 2020).

FUTURE OF ACCREDITATION IN HEALTHCARE

Technological changes that gain speed day by day in the field of health services with effects that resonate in the whole world necessitate reorganization of accreditation programs to adapt to these changes. The literature states that in the coming years, the field of healthcare will be shaped on the basis of five main trends: sustainable health systems, genomic revolution, technological developments, global demographic dynamics, and new care models. Considering the effects of these trends on accreditation, standards, and policies, it can be said that digitalization, AI, and tele-medicine applications will gain importance in setting up new standards and methodologies. It will require that accreditation methodology be arranged in a way that focuses on individuality such as healthy behavior and making sound decisions, and is oriented towards evaluation of the whole system, rather than being specific to the institution. Similarly, in terms of sustainability, it will tend to transform accreditation standards into a more flexible structure that will facilitate adaptation to changes (Nicklin et al. 2020, Braithwaite et al. 2018).

EFFECT OF USING AI IN HEALTHCARE ON ACCREDITATION

For global health systems to be sustainable in the years to come, they will need to adapt to constant challenges and pressures created by rapid and unprecedented changes. Inadequacy of financial and human resources that put pressure on health systems can be summarized as expectations of the society from health services and establishing healthy relationships with multiple stakeholders in order to maintain service processes (Braithwaite et al. 2018). It is possible to say that rapidly increasing digitalization process with AI applications, which have a serious effect on minimizing these negative impacts that put pressure on health systems, is life-saving. However, one of the most important issues is to consider the disadvantages and risks of using AI in health services and management. Misuse and interpretation errors may cause serious consequences due to fact that the engineers involved in the development of algorithms do not have sufficient knowledge and experience, and the health professionals who will be responsible for the use of workflows do not have a good grasp of the subject. It takes a certain amount of time to form correct and sufficient number of datasets that will be required for AI applications to be used in clinical diagnosis and treatment processes, and the processes of checking accuracy of datasets is also very laborious. If this situation is not brought under control, it may lead to unreliable results and erroneous applications. The fact that images obtained with AI give satisfactory empirical results in diagnosis processes is also related to correct evaluation of images by the specialist. Therefore, multidisciplinary teamwork can be considered as a necessity. On the other hand, it should not be forgotten that uncertainties about moral and ethical dimensions of increasing use of AI may cause human rights problems (Ellahham et al. 2020, Akalın and Veranyurt 2021, Semiz 2022).

Accreditation programs designed to achieve objectives such as patient and employee safety, efficiency, effectiveness, sustainability, timeliness, and equity can be beneficial in overcoming difficulties that may be experienced in the field of health services. In addition, use of AI in the field of health services requires the changes taking place due to increasing digitalization to reshape accreditation programs (Braithwaite et al. 2018, Nicklin et al. 2020.)

REFERENCES

Akalın, B. and Veranyurt, Ü. 2021. Sağlık hizmetleri ve yönetiminde yapay zeka (Artificial Intelligence in Health Services and Management). Acta Infologica. 5(1): 231–240.

Akgerman, A., Özdemir Yavuz, E.D., Kavaslar, İ. and Güngör, S. 2022. Yapay zekâ ve hemşirelik (Artificial Intelligence and Nursing). JAIHS. 2(1): 21–27.

Aslan, Ş. and Güzel, Ş. 2019. Development process of the industry 4.0 and digital transformation. *In*: Health. 2nd International Congress On New Horizons In Education And Social Sciences (ICES-2019) Proceedings. Accessed at https:// www.researchgate.net/profile/Serife-Guezel/publication/335225721_ ENDUSTRI_40_GELISIM_SURECI_VE_SAGLIKTA_DIJITAL_DONUSUM/ links/600170b845851553a0456ecd/ENDUeSTRI-40-GELISIM-SUeRECI- VE-SAGLIKTA-DIJITAL-DOeNUeSUeM.pdf?_sg%5B0%5D=started_ experiment_milestone&origin=journalDetail (on May 14, 2024).

Braithwaite, J., Mannion, R., Matsuyama, Y., Shekelle, P., Whittaker, S., Al-Adawi, S., et al. 2018. The future of health systems to 2030: a roadmap for global progress and sustainability. International Journal for Quality in Health Care. 30(10): 823–831.

Bozbuğa, N., Tekbaş, M. and Gülseçen, S. 2021. Tıbbi nesnelerin İnterneti (Internet of Medical Things). Accessed at https://cdn.istanbul.edu.tr/file/JTA6CLJ8T5/E859DD9F6A5749E7A54059214B051FA9 (on November 21, 2022).

Büyükgöze, S. and Dereli, E. 2020. Dijital sağlık uygulamalarında yapay zeka (Artificial Intelligence in Digital Health Applications). Accessed at https://www.researchgate.net/publication/339091309 (on November 19, 2022).

Demir, B. 2020. Sağlığın kavramsallaştırılması ve İnsan odaklı sağlık hizmetlerinde kalite ve akreditasyon perspektifi (Conceptualization of health and perspective of quality and accreditation in human-centered health services). İnsan&İnsan. 7(24): 62–83.

Ellahham, S., Ellahham, N. and Şimşekler, M.C.E. 2020. Application of artificial intelligence in the health care safety context: opportunities and challenges. American Journal of Medical Quality. 35(4): 341–348.

Hui Jin, M.L., Vogel, S., Kitikiti, N. and Mauthalagu, A.P. 2020. Artificial intelligence in healthcare: landscape, policies and regulations in Asia-Pacific. Accessed at https://www.duke-nus.edu.sg/docs/librariesprovider5/default-document-library/niha_white-paper_ai-in-healthcare_vfinal-23102020.pdf?sfvrsn=1c5e2636_0 (on November 19, 2022).

Glaser, J. and Shaw, S. 2022. Digital transformation success: what can health care providers learn from other industries? *NEJM Catalyst*. Accessed at https://catalyst.nejm.org/doi/full/10.1056/CAT.21.0434 (on November 18, 2022).

Kraus, S., Schiavone, F., Pluzhnikova, A. and Invernizzi, A.C. 2021. Digital transformation in healthcare: analyzing the current state of research. Journal of Business Research. 123: 557–567.

Long, L.A., Pariyo, G. and Kallander, K. 2018. Digital technologies for health workforce development in low- and middle-income countries: a scoping review. Global Health, Science and Practice. 6(1): 41–48.

Nicklin, W., Engel, C. and Stewart, J. 2020. Accreditation in 2030. International Journal for Quality in Health Care. 33(1): 1–5.

Pasinringi, S.A., Rivai, F., Arifah, N. and Rezeki, S.F. 2021. The relationship between service quality perceptions and the level of hospital accreditation. Gaceta Sanitaria. 35(S2): 116–119.

Robert, N. 2019. How artificial intelligence is changing nursing. Nursing Management. 50(9): 30–39.

Semiz, T. 2022. Sağlıkta yapay zeka (Artificial intelligence in health). pp. 195–211. *In*: Uysal, B. and Semiz, T. (eds). Sağlık Hizmetlerinde Dijitalleşme ve Geleceği (Digitalization and Its Future in Healthcare). Ankara: İksad Yayınevi.

Shin, S.Y. 2019. Current status and future direction of digital health in Korea. Korean Journal of Physiology and Pharmacology. 23(5): 311–315.

STOA. 2022. Panel for the future of science and technology. Accessed at https://www.europarl.europa.eu/RegData/etudes/STUD/2022/729512/EPRS_STU(2022)729512_EN.pdf (on November 21, 2022).

Şimşir, İ. and Mete, B. 2021. Sağlık hizmetlerinin geleceği: dijital sağlık teknolojileri (The Future of Healthcare Services: Digital Health Technologies). Journal of Innovative Healthcare Practices. 2(1): 33–39.

T.C. Sağlık Bakanlığı. 2014. Neden dijital hastane (Why Digital Hospital)? Accessed at https://dijitalhastane.saglik.gov.tr/TR,5009/neden-dijital-hastane.html (on November 23, 2022).

Uysal, B. and Ulusinan, E. 2020. Güncel dijital sağlık uygulamalarının İncelenmesi (Examining Current Digital Health Applications). Selçuk Sağlık Dergisi. 1: 46–60.

Zeybek, M. and Zeybek, D.Ö. 2022. Dijital hastanelerin değerlendirilmesi ve geleceği (Evaluation and future of digital hospitals). pp. 213–227. *In*: Uysal, B. and Semiz, T. (eds). Sağlık Hizmetlerinde Dijitalleşme ve Geleceği (Digitalization and Its Future in Healthcare). Ankara: İksad Yayınevi.

Index